Acknowledgements

KU-077-217

This book is the result of a research project carried out in four countries by an international team of researchers from 2000 to 2002. The research was supported by the European Commission DG Research, as part of the European TSE Project, grant PL987028, and led by the World Health Organization.

The team consisted of the following contributors:

i.   Daniela Balata, Dipartimento di Economia Istituzioni Società, Università di Sassari, Sassari, Italy;

ii.   Martin W. Bauer, Department of Social Psychology, London School of Economics, London, United Kingdom;

iii.   Elizabeth Dowler, Department of Sociology, University of Warwick, Coventry, United Kingdom;

iv.   Alizon Draper, School of Integrated Health, University of Westminster, London, United Kingdom;

v.   Kerstin Dressel, Süddeutsches Institut für empirische Sozialforschung, Munich, Germany;

vi.   Giolo Fele, Dipartimento Discipline della Comunicazione, Università di Bologna, Bologna, Italy;

vii.   Giancarlo Gasperoni, Dipartimento Discipline della Comunicazione, Università di Bologna, Bologna, Italy;

viii.   Maria Grazia Gianichedda, Dipartimento di Economia Istituzioni Società, Università di Sassari, Sassari, Italy;

ix.   Pier Paolo Giglioli, Dipartimento Discipline della Comunicazione, Università di Bologna, Bologna, Italy;

x.   Judith Green, Health Services Research Unit, London School of Hygiene and Tropical Medicine, London, United Kingdom;

xi.   Vera Hagenhoff, Institut für Agraroekonomie, Kiel, Germany;

xii.   Susan Howard, London School of Economics, London, United Kingdom;

xiii.   Meri Koivusalo, Globalism and Social Policy Programme, National Research and Development Centre for Welfare and Health (STAKES), Helsinki, Finland;

xiv.   Erik Millstone, Science Policy Research Unit, Sussex University, Brighton, United Kingdom;

xv.   Eeva Ollila, Globalism and Social Policy Programme, National Research and Development Centre for Welfare and Health (STAKES), Helsinki, Finland;

xvi.   Maria Rusanen, Department of Environmental Health, National Public Health Institute, Helsinki, Finland;

xvii.   Timo Rusanen, Environmental Policy Research Programme, Finnish Environment Institute, Helsinki, Finland;

xviii.   Patrick van Zwanenberg, Science Policy Research Unit, Sussex University, Brighton, United Kingdom;

xix.   Reimar von Alvensleben, Institut für Agraroekonomie, Kiel, Germany.

Overall direction of the project was by Carlos Dora, World Health Organization.

The contributions of the following persons to the research are also gratefully acknowledged by the authors: Simona Barbatano, Eugenia Cannata, Cristina Demaria, Lisa Donath, Francesca Gleria, Minna Ilva, Pina Lalli, Elisabetta Trippa, Isacco Turina.

We thank Andrew Wilson for his able editorial assistance and coordination during the writing of this book, and Maria Teresa Marchetti for administration of the research project and support during the publication process.

Foreword

Communicating about health hazards is an integral part of the daily work of any health department or agency, from the local to the international level. It is a central function of the World Health Organization (WHO) which, as part of its mandate and mission, interacts with Member States to inform them about a wide range of health risks. Risk communication is thus a key public health tool, and an understanding of communication processes is essential to good public health work. So far, the majority of analysis and scholarship has addressed two aspects of communication: what influences people's perceptions of risk and how to convey a message adequately for the potential users. Indeed, there is today good understanding of those issues, and much guidance has been produced for health systems about how to consider public perceptions of risk in the effective communication of public health messages.

The bovine spongiform encephalopathy (BSE) saga has made painfully evident the limitations of risk communication as a one-way avenue, where information to the public about the risks they face comes after critical policy decisions have already been made. In fact, communication has even been identified as one of the key elements of what went wrong and generated the loss of trust in government discourse and in beef in Europe. Clearly, there was a need to learn from that experience and share those lessons. This challenge was taken up by WHO and a group of European scholars, with the support of the European Commission DG Research.

This book takes the debate about risk communication a step further, dealing with it as an evolving and interactive process between decision-makers and their publics. The book underlines the critical importance of creating mechanisms for interaction between policy-makers and stakeholders early on, and at all stages of policy-making, in order for risk communication to be effective. The book sets the stage for the development of practical recommendations that health information actors may adopt in order to engage with the public over perceptions of health risks and hazards.

The analyses presented in this book will come to food and public health audiences as a welcome surprise. The book reports on research into the strategies used by different actors to communicate about BSE and Creutzfeldt-Jakob disease (CJD) in four European countries between 1985 and 2000. These actors include the mass media, health information systems, and political actors. The research also assessed the way people construct their perceptions about risk, who they listen to and how they make decisions on risk avoidance.

A range of qualitative and quantitative methods was used to describe what was said as well as the perspectives and framework assumptions espoused by those different actors. These are reported in the book, which also includes a detailed analysis of the mass-media reporting of the issue over the period that is quite unique.

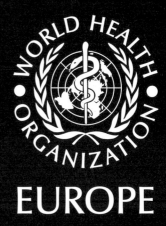

EUROPE

Health, Hazards and Public Debate

Lessons for risk communication from the BSE/CJD saga

Keywords

ENCEPHALOPATHY, BOVINE SPONGIFORM
CREUTZFELDT-JAKOB SYNDROME
RISK ASSESSMENT
COMMUNICATION
HEALTH EDUCATION
MASS MEDIA
POLICY-MAKING
EPIDEMIOLOGIC SURVEILLANCE
EUROPEAN UNION
UNITED KINGDOM
GERMANY
ITALY
FINLAND

ISBN 92-890-1070-3

Address requests about publications of the WHO Regional Office to:

· by e-mail   **publicationrequests@euro.who.int** (for copies of publications)
                permissions@euro.who.int (for permission to reproduce them)
                pubrights@euro.who.int (for permission to translate them)

· by post   **Publications**
                WHO Regional Office for Europe
                Scherfigsvej 8
                DK-2100 Copenhagen Ø, Denmark

Contents

One of the basic problems identified in the BSE case was the lack of connection between those communicating about risk and people's perspectives and concerns about the potential health hazards presented by BSE. In particular, the known prescriptions for good communication did not work in the BSE case. This research examined this issue in detail and from different angles. The historical case studies provide good insights into how some communication strategies succeeded, while others adopted in a different part of the same country and in the same time period failed. It is also remarkable to realize how the same communication pitfalls were repeated later, elsewhere, and how the lessons had not been disseminated. The potential use of mass-media sampling as a way to inform about public perceptions of risk was explored, and the findings give a rich account of the existing complexities. Perhaps the best insights presented in the book come from the analyses of the empirical findings and how they relate to existing communication theory and analytical frameworks.

The end result is rewarding. First, the book presents clear accounts of good practice; second, it gives in-depth understanding of how and why some of the communications managed to relate to people's concerns while others did not; third, it examines the roles of the different actors in the communications process, identifying where they could improve; and finally it proposes a robust framework for understanding how communication inputs contribute to different stages of policy-making.

The framework is derived from case-study findings and from theory, and can serve as a key tool for developing communication strategies that take account of public opinion effectively. The framework explores the rationale for engaging the public at different stages of policy-making and identifies opportunities for engaging with public opinion. Ultimately this has the potential to help increase the public's faith in the policy-making process.

Roberto Bertollini
Director, Special Programme on Health and Environment
WHO Regional Office for Europe

1

Introduction: seeking lessons from BSE/CJD
for communication strategies on health and risk

Introduction: seeking lessons from BSE/CJD for communication strategies on health and risk

Carlos Dora

▾ Background

Public perceptions and risk communication are high-profile topics in today's public and policy arenas. Governments, agencies and policy-makers need to know how people will perceive and react to contemporary uncertainties. They want to find ways of engaging with public concerns in such a way as to avoid scares and prevent the situation evolving into a political crisis. The history of BSE and variant CJD (vCJD) in Europe since the mid-1980s — in which communication issues were at the origin of a political crisis — provides a clear illustration of the importance of rethinking how science-based policy issues are communicated.

Since the first cases were identified in 1986, BSE has been a recurrent and important item of public concern, in particular regarding the possibility of cross-species transfer and the risks posed to humans by beef consumption. For many years, however, official communications tended to downplay the risks, characterizing public concerns as irrational "overreactions". Scientific evidence that BSE was unlikely to be transmitted to humans was interpreted as indicating that there was no threat to public health, and official communications emphasized the safety of national food production systems.

However, the March 1996 announcement, in the British House of Commons, that exposure to BSE was the most likely explanation for 10 cases of a new variant of CJD, led to a massive crisis in public confidence in information sources and in government. A dramatic drop in beef consumption and a serious health scare regarding the risks of contracting CJD ensued. Similar events occurred in other European countries in the years that followed.

• New risk communication needed

The BSE/CJD situation is one of a number of recent controversies involving a health risk, scientific uncertainty and economic interests. These have provoked intense debate among various interest groups and distrust of official pronouncements. Other diseases have also been associated with growing public distrust in scientific "experts" and in the ability of governments to manage the social, physical, natural and technological environment. Issues such as nuclear power generation and genetically modified foods have made visible a wide divergence between scientific and lay perceptions of risk.

The response of many policy-makers and scientists has been to stress the need for better "communication of risk", with a focus on how to express the conclusions once the scientific and policy deliberations have been completed. This is relevant, but is only one part of the communication process. Limiting communication to a tertiary activity (after the scientific and policy stages) assumes that public reactions should be anticipated and if possible "managed". Yet there is considerable doubt that this is possible — or even desirable — without the engagement of the public in a dialogue about the assessment of risks and risk management options. In fact, the BSE case dramatically demonstrates the limitations of focusing solely on risk communication. It illustrates the cost to public authorities of not adopting a more open and transparent dialogue with the public.

• Seeking lessons

This book is based on empirical research in the United Kingdom, Germany, Italy and Finland.[1] Undertaken by an international team of researchers, using a range of quantitative and qualitative methodologies. The broad objectives of this research were:

1. to identify determinants of consumer perceptions, attitudes, knowledge and behaviour;

2. to describe the communication process regarding BSE/CJD in different countries since the mid-1980s, including the role of the media and of different stakeholders;

3. to describe relevant policy measures and institutional communication, including the surveillance systems in place and framework assumptions prevalent among public policy officials;

4. to investigate whether monitoring of media coverage, government discourse, public perceptions and behaviour could inform health, environment and food policy, and be part of an existing surveillance system; and

5. to correlate and draw conclusions from the results of the above-mentioned objectives that can improve information policy with regard to areas of real or perceived risk to public health.

---

[1] This ordering of the countries reflects the chronological order in which the crisis developed, and is maintained throughout.

The research was sparked by a need to provide practical advice to policy-makers on how to incorporate consumer perceptions of risk into their regular communication activities. A particular emphasis was to facilitate timely and adequate risk communication, both to prevent and to respond to food and environmental health scares. This need grew out of a number of uncertainties engendered by the BSE/CJD crisis.

By the end of the 1990s it was widely accepted that communication issues had been intrinsically involved in the origin and amplification of the crisis. However, there was great uncertainty about what had generated the miscommunication. There was agreement on only a limited number of communication-related issues, such as the need for a broader range of expertise in scientific advisory committees on BSE, and the need to separate sources of food safety information from those concerned with food production advice. The need for better communication of scientific uncertainty was also widely accepted. On the other hand, dealing with such process-oriented issues did not address the obvious problem that public concern about BSE and trust in information sources were situated in broader political and cultural contexts. These contexts, which had been the subject of a considerable amount of research, included the valued role of meat in many traditional European diets (Wilson, 1976) and its symbolic significance (Twigg, 1983; Fiddes, 1991); the decline in red meat consumption in most of western Europe (Burnett, 1989); reduced faith in "experts" more generally in the late twentieth century (Giddens, 1991; Beck, 1992); and the role of food as a

Introduction: seeking lessons from BSE/CJD for

marker of cultural identity and of national boundaries (Douglas & Wildavsky, 1982). It was also clear that, in the context of economic changes in the European Union (EU), debates about national agricultural and food policies had symbolic significance for individual national identities.

Little information had been gathered on people's perceptions of BSE/CJD risk specifically, and the role of the media had not been examined in detail. Not much was known about the influence of a variety of stakeholders in different parts of Europe, and what role they played in policy-making. It was not clear how or if policy-makers took into account the beliefs, concerns and attitudes of citizens, and no detailed analysis had been made of the role that health and food information systems played in the crisis.

In summary, there was both a need and an opportunity to draw lessons by examining the types of communication strategies adopted in different countries, to gain a greater understanding of the interplay between public perceptions, the media, communication strategies and policy initiatives, and to investigate how public authorities could earn trust and legitimacy when communicating about uncertainty and risks to health.

All of these needs informed the research for this book, and have contributed to its content and structure. The intended audience for this study is broad, taking in all those interested in understanding the wide spectrum of risk communication issues and practices, and the links

with policy-making. In particular, the study is intended to provide useful information to policy-makers, as well as to communications professionals and persons working with health and food risks, or engaged in information and intelligence systems.

▾ A historical perspective

The BSE/CJD story is complex, and spans almost two decades and many countries. In order to provide an overview of the events, issues and actors, Chapter 2 ("A chronology of BSE policy in four countries and the European Community") provides a brief historical description of the different ways in which public policy has evolved in response to the BSE/CJD crisis in the United Kingdom, Germany, Italy and Finland. Because of the importance of the European Community (EC) in shaping policy development in individual Member States, Chapter 2 also includes a discussion of the EC's BSE/CJD-related activities. It outlines the different institutional and procedural arrangements for food safety and animal health issues, and the ways in which those arrangements and institutions have evolved. In addition, it summarizes the key reasons why the emergence of the new disease posed such acute challenges for public policy.

▾ Understanding public perceptions

Since the mid-1980s, public perception of the relationship between food, risk and health has been a critical element in the BSE/CJD affair. The misjudgement of the public's expectations about information arguably led to a crisis of faith, not only in British food production but in

communication strategies on health and risk

the very processes of democratic decision-making (Eldridge et al, 1998). What "people seem generally to think or believe" influences their behaviour — and plays a vital role in shaping events. Policy-makers, especially those responsible for information policy, face significant challenges in assessing public perceptions and in shaping policy that takes information needs into account and responds adequately to people's key concerns.

• Issues and methods

Chapter 3 ("Assessing public perception: issues and methods") reviews key issues in understanding public perceptions and behaviours, how they are constructed and influenced by beliefs and social interaction, and how they are affected by social frameworks, including trust in information sources. It discusses issues such as the need for indicators of perception and trust, along with methods for capturing and interpreting what these mean and how they can be used in policy-making. It covers current issues such as the relevance of describing the public as "consumers" or as "citizens", the potential contribution of lay epidemiology, and the value of monitoring the symbolic environment (made up of perceptions and beliefs) in which various actors operate. It also discusses issues of representation in policy-making, particularly representation by direct participation of certain individuals as against representation through researching the opinions of a wider group.

In particular, it discusses three different methods for accessing existing views: focus group discussions, surveys or opinion polls, and content analysis of mass media coverage. The strengths and weaknesses of each method are examined briefly, along with practical considerations such as their cost and the ease with which they can be "contracted out" to private service providers. Examples drawn from the United Kingdom are provided to illustrate how and why each method has been used in the "real world". A summary of the characteristics of each is provided in Table 3.1 at the end of the chapter.

Chapters 4–6 stem directly from the empirical research carried out for this project, and demonstrate the potential for using the three methodologies discussed above as input to policies that address health and food risks.

• Focus groups

Chapter 4 ("Risk and trust: determinants of public perception") is based on the results of focus group discussions, mostly with natural groups (i.e. those who either socialize or have some prior social relationship with each other outside the research setting, such as work, school or church). Across the four countries, 36 focus groups explored how risk is communicated and constructed in everyday contexts. The chapter investigates consumer perceptions of food risks and safety, including BSE- and CJD-related risk. Grounded analysis was used to develop models that reflect the ways in which people conceptualize and manage risk in everyday life. This provided insights into how perceptions are socially constructed, how the social setting influences perceptions of risk and trust in information sources, and the impact of these perceptions on consumer behaviour.

Introduction: seeking lessons from BSE/CJD for

The analysis reveals the complexity and sophistication of public constructions of food safety and risk, as well as the strategies and shortcuts used to assess those in routine food choices. These are important parameters against which to measure communication strategies, which need to take into account that level of sophistication and understanding.

• Survey methods

The research reported in Chapter 5 ("Sample surveys of public perceptions and opinion") begins by exploring the availability of survey data regarding perceptions of risk and trust in information sources relevant to BSE/CJD in the four countries. It reports on what part of the existing information is available, and on the findings of the few accessible results. It goes on to present results of secondary analysis, in which data from 11 Eurobarometer surveys in each of the four countries were acquired and re-analysed, along with an EU survey that included data on meat-purchasing behaviour by consumers. The chapter provides a useful discussion of issues such as public knowledge and awareness of food safety issues, public trust in various sources of information (including food producers and distributors, scientists, health officials, etc.) and of food consumption, especially of meat. The chapter also discusses in detail the strengths and weaknesses of survey methods as tools in public policy-making on food and related issues. Finally, it illuminates the important issue of what use is made by policy-makers of existing and easily accessible information on risk perceptions and trust in information sources.

• Content analysis of mass media coverage

Chapter 6 ("The BSE and CJD crisis in the press") tackles an important question raised by BSE/CJD: to what extent can the mass media be used as an index of public perception by policy-makers? The chapter presents results of empirical analysis of mass media coverage of the BSE/CJD issue in the four study countries since the early days of BSE. The analysis included the assessment of content, intensity and timing of media coverage, and the trajectory of the issues and frames used by the media. On a practical level, the chapter provides a methodology for the analysis of mass media reporting on risks, and tests the feasibility of implementing it in the four countries. On a conceptual level, the chapter looks beyond the case of BSE/CJD and surveillance systems in general to explore the idea of a "parallel epidemiology". It is conceived as "parallel" because, in addition to surveillance of BSE in the animal population and CJD in humans, there appears to be value in monitoring social representations of the problem. This is not an indicator of public perception but a measure of the waves of change in discourse by the media that have an impact on the public sphere and that both affect and draw from public perceptions. The chapter discusses the dual role of the media as a mirror of public opinion and as a contributor to the formation of public perceptions (including setting the public agenda).

▾ Problems in risk communication strategies

The BSE/CJD crisis has demonstrated that current approaches to risk communication and to conducting science-based policy-making are no longer sustainable.

communication strategies on health and risk

The dominant assumption until now has held risk communication to be strictly a downstream or "tertiary" activity, to be carried out once scientific and policy deliberations have been completed (WHO, 2002). This assumption — and the communication strategies and practices that flow from it — has lost much of its plausibility across the entire spectrum of policy-making, for reasons explored in the next three chapters.

• **Approaches and strategies in risk communication**

Chapter 7 ("Risk communication strategies in public policy-making") provides an analytical context for the following chapters' description and analysis of BSE risk communication strategies in the study countries. After a brief historical and theoretical account of major developments in thinking about risk communication, it discusses three analytically distinct ways in which risk communication has been conceptualized and practised, and how these are, in turn, connected to more general ideas about the relationship between science and policy-making. This description is a particularly appealing analytical tool, as the different models still coexist in practice.

At one extreme, in what is called the "technocratic" approach, the purpose of risk communication is understood to be correction of the public "deficit" of information. In other words, what is needed is to provide science-based representations of risk that are sufficiently simplified to be readily transferable to the minds of the public, in order to diminish their ignorance. The chapter describes how psychological research on risk perceptions helped to adjust the messages, and how sociologi-

cal research indicated the importance of trust in information sources. On the basis of these advances, a second approach, called "decisionist" in this chapter, goes a step further to accept that public views are (a) legitimate, and (b) necessary for deciding on policy options and the acceptability of costs and benefits. However, such an investigation of public perceptions still comes after a strictly scientific assessment of risks, in which the public has no role to play. The last approach, called "deliberative", acknowledges the range of judgements and values that could usefully be incorporated into all stages of the risk assessment and decision-making process. It also identifies the need for input from different publics, and the role of dialogue in defining a number of crucial steps in risk policy-making.

The chapter concludes with an outline of the dimensions of risk communication strategies that were applied in the analyses carried out in the study countries.

• **The role of health surveillance and information systems**

Human and veterinary health surveillance systems have a prominent role in health-risk communication. Much of the raw material of the BSE/CJD story was provided by those systems. Chapter 8 ("Surveillance systems: their information and communication practices") provides a comparative analysis of BSE and CJD surveillance systems in the four countries and of their role in communicating about BSE/CJD. These findings are based both on reviews of documentation and on in-depth interviews with staff from the relevant institutions. To provide a

Introduction: seeking lessons from BSE/CJD for

wider perspective on the role these systems have played in risk communication, interviews were conducted with staff operating at both national and regional levels of surveillance, and with journalists and medical and veterinary scientists who were not specifically concerned with surveillance.

In particular, the chapter describes the types of information that surveillance systems gather and communicate, and examines if there were communication strategies on the issue, or if no strategy seemed to frame the communication. In the first instance it explores how and why those communication strategies have emerged, the effects of those choices on policy-making, and how successful the different strategies were. The chapter also explores the possibility that such systems could serve as a means for gathering information on perceptions. It provides valuable insights into the possibilities of risk communication when opened to such authorities, even at regional or local level.

Overall, the chapter examines the role in the BSE crisis played by surveillance institutions responsible for providing information about risks, and explores the potential of health information institutions to take up a wider role in risk communication.

• Risk communication strategies
Communication strategies take on an enhanced significance following the conclusion of the BSE Inquiry in the United Kingdom by Phillips et al. that most of what went wrong in BSE policy-making was due to failures in com-

munication (Phillips et al., 2000). Chapter 9 ("Evolution and implications of public risk communication strategies on BSE") describes the evolution of official BSE risk communication strategies in the study countries. These strategies were directed towards each country's citizens, but embedded in administrative and scientific structures and affected by stakeholder interests.

The chapter is based on a great deal of information collected in key informant interviews with policy-makers, reporters, scientific advisers, regulatory officers, and consumer and producer groups. This information was triangulated against official risk communications and against the results of the other research tasks in this project, allowing an understanding of the interplay of those actors. The chapter's broad analysis adds value to the understanding of the role that specific actors played in the adoption of public risk communication strategies related to BSE and CJD. The different phases in risk communication strategies adopted over time in each country are analysed in the light of the approaches to risk communication modelled in Chapter 7.

▾ Towards better risk communication
Drawbacks in risk communication strategies in the United Kingdom, Germany and Italy (and less so in Finland) ultimately undermined public confidence in BSE policies and risk governance more generally. Today, new and reformed institutions are attempting new approaches to risk communication, both to mitigate the loss of public trust in food regulation and to engage more fully with consumer/citizen concerns.

communication strategies on health and risk

Chapter 10 ("Improving communication strategies and engaging with public concerns") discusses how public policy-making institutions can improve their strategies for communicating with the public and with key stakeholder and public interest groups in risk policy-making. Drawing on the "co-evolutionary" approach to policy-making discussed in Chapter 7, the chapter suggests a fairly straightforward but useful distinction between three sequential stages of the policy-making process (termed "upstream", "midstream" and "downstream"). Risk considerations at each of those stages are identified, together with the rationale for engaging public views and those of scientists. This provides a robust framework for understanding risk communication strategies and for identifying how and when they can be improved. The risk communication strategies that do engage with the public from the outset (notably those employed by the Food Standards Agency (FSA) in the United Kingdom and by the government of North Rhine-Westphalia in Germany) are living examples of how communication practices do evolve, and of the need to evaluate such experiments as the learning goes on.

▾ How much progress has been made? The contribution of this research

One of the main contributions of this research is its identification of important gaps in the practice of risk communication in European countries. These practices ranged from having no communication strategy or having communication with no strategy, to having strategies that misconstrued the scientific evidence and underestimated the public. The research demonstrates how risk communication errors (notably those in the United Kingdom) were repeated elsewhere at later dates. This highlights the importance of learning lessons and proposing solutions.

The research also contributes to finding solutions to these gaps and errors. In particular, Chapter 9 proposes a robust theoretical framework for understanding how communication inputs contribute to different stages of policy-making. The framework explores rationales for engaging the public at those stages and identifies opportunities for engaging with public opinion and incorporating it into policy-making. This framework is vital for developing communication strategies that address public opinions effectively. Ultimately, it has the potential to increase the public's faith in the policy-making process and to ensure that information about risk resonates with public concerns.

On the basis of existing knowledge and of the empirical work carried out in the study countries, the researchers examined in detail the potential for using specific techniques for engaging public opinion in policy-making. This includes the use of focus group discussions, surveys of public opinion and media analysis. In addition, the study examines the use of deliberative techniques for the same purpose. The study team's experience in trying out these techniques provides insight into their utility and limitations.

The research findings can be applied in three different ways. The first stems from the team's analysis of the communication practices and framework assumptions of different stakeholders in the four countries, particularly those with a responsibility for communicating about risks. This analysis provides insights into the institutional constraints against adopting communication that engages public perceptions, and indicates which areas to focus on in order to address those constraints. The second relates to the examples of good practice the study team identified (notably by the FSA in the United Kingdom, North Rhine-Westphalia in Germany, some local government efforts in Italy, and possibly the Ministry of Agriculture and Forestry in Finland). These, although few, could potentially have a major influence on future communication strategies if the lessons learnt are applied. Third, the team's findings suggest a number of opportunities for operational research into some of the remaining questions, especially about testing and evaluating specific methods for engaging public opinion in policy-making.

Overall, it is hoped that this research moves the debate on risk communication a step further, and has immediate relevance to its day-to-day practice. The issues raised generated lively and heated debates within the research group, both face-to-face in project working meetings and in e-mail exchanges. It is hoped that the exploration of these issues here will excite interest in the wider arena of risk research and communication and stimulate a similar shift in focus.

References

Beck U (1992) *Risk society: towards a new modernity*. London, Sage.

Burnett J (1989) *Plenty and want: a social history of diet in England from 1815 to the present day*, 3rd ed. London, Routledge.

Douglas M, Wildavsky A (1982) *Risk and culture: an essay on the selection of technological and environmental dangers*. Berkeley, CA, University of California Press.

Eldridge J, Kitzinger J, Philo G, Reilly J (1998) The re-emergence of BSE: the impact on public beliefs and behaviour. *Risk and Human Behaviour Newsletter*, 3:6–10.

Fiddes N (1991) *Meat: a natural symbol*. London, Routledge.

Giddens A (1991) *Modernity and self identity: self and society in the late modern age*. London, Polity Press.

Phillips N, Bridgeman J, Ferguson-Smith M (2000) *The BSE Inquiry: Report: evidence and supporting papers of the inquiry into the emergence and identification of Bovine Spongiform Encephalopathy (BSE) and variant Creutzfeldt-Jakob Disease (vCJD) and the action taken in response to it up to 20 March 1996*. London, The Stationery Office. (http://www.bseinquiry.gov.uk/report/index.htm)

Twigg J (1983) Vegetarianism and the meanings of meat. In: Murcott A, ed. *The sociology of food and eating*. Aldershot, Gower:18–30.

Wilson CE (1976) *Food and drink in Britain*. Harmondsworth, Penguin.

WHO (2002) *The world health report 2002: Reducing risks to health, promoting healthy life*. Geneva, World Health Organization:27–43.

Chapter 2

A chronology of BSE policy in four countries
and the European Community

A chronology of BSE policy in four countries and the European Community

Patrick van Zwanenberg, Kerstin Dressel, Pier Paolo Giglioli, Meri Koivusalo, Eeva Ollila

Since BSE was first identified in the south of England in November 1986, almost 180 000 British cattle, from over 35 000 farms, have been officially diagnosed with the disease (DEFRA, 2002). The mean incubation time for BSE is about five years, and most infected cattle therefore did not manifest symptoms of the disease because they were slaughtered between two and three years of age. As a consequence, an additional 750 000 undetected animals are estimated to have contracted BSE, most of which would have entered the human food-chain (Anderson et al., 1996; Donnelly et al., 2002). In the United Kingdom, the epidemic reached its peak in 1993, when over 34 000 cases were reported. Since then, levels have been declining, but it is widely expected that there will be a long tail to the epidemic and it is possible that the United Kingdom may never completely eliminate BSE.

In the late 1980s it was not obvious that BSE would cause more difficulties than any of a large number of other food safety scares that had arisen in the United Kingdom and elsewhere since the early 1980s. That changed with the British Government's 20 March 1996 announcement (Hansard, 20 March 1996) that a novel fatal disease in humans (now called vCJD) had emerged and was almost certainly caused by consuming BSE-contaminated food.

At the time of writing (mid-2002), 127 cases of vCJD had been reported in the United Kingdom. There had also been six cases in France, one case in China (Hong Kong Special Administrative Region) in a former resi-dent of the United Kingdom, one case in Ireland, one case in the United States of America in a former resi-dent of the United Kingdom, one case in Canada and one case in Italy.

The incidence of vCJD in the United Kingdom has, thus far, been rising at an annual rate of around 20–30% (Spongiform Encephalopathy Advisory Committee, 2001), but the total number of people who will eventually contract vCJD remains uncertain.

Although BSE has been primarily a British problem, it has caused difficulties for many other jurisdictions too. As a consequence of trade in contaminated British ani-mal feedstuffs and infected cattle, BSE is now present in the domestic herds of virtually all European coun-tries.[1] Several Member States have rising numbers of reported BSE cases, whilst a number of countries that previously thought they might be free of the disease have recently discovered cases amongst their domestic cattle populations (see, for example, Office International des Epizooties, 2002). In 2001, the Food and Agriculture Organization of the United Nations (FAO) warned that more than 100 countries that had imported meat and bone meal or live cattle from west-ern Europe during the 1980s were at risk from BSE (FAO, 2001). Many countries are likely to face consider-able animal and public health problems for some time.

---

[1] At the time of writing, every EU Member State except Sweden had reported cases of BSE.

For many years Germany, Italy and Finland appeared to be free of BSE in their domestic herds. During the 1990s, a handful of cases had been reported in animals that had been imported into Germany and Italy, but until the introduction of a Europe-wide rapid postmortem monitoring regime in late 2000, no cases had been noticed in Italy's domestic cattle populations and few in Germany. In late 2000 and 2001 the situation changed dramatically. Germany discovered 132 BSE cases (7 in 2000 and 125 in 2001) in its domestic herd. Within 12 months, 48 domestic cases of BSE had been detected in Italy. Finland initially appeared to be an exception, but in December 2001 it too reported a case of BSE in an animal born and raised in Finland.

Just as the reported incidence of BSE has varied considerably between countries, so too have policy responses. BSE has been a serious policy challenge in the United Kingdom since the mid-1980s. Several other European countries such as France, Ireland and Portugal had sufficiently high rates of incidence that their governments recognized the need to place controls on their domestic production systems during the early 1990s. Other countries with lower incidences of BSE registered some concern and undertook regulatory activities, but primarily in relation to traded animals and feedstuffs, and in response to European Community legislation. Germany, Italy and Finland fall generally into this latter category, although there have been differences in policy responses across the three jurisdictions.

This chapter provides a brief chronological description of the different ways in which public policy in five jurisdictions — the European Commission, the United Kingdom, Germany, Italy and Finland — has evolved in response to the emergence of possible threats from BSE. Although the European Commission is not one of the jurisdictions examined elsewhere in this book, a discussion of its activities with regard to BSE is included in this chapter because of its importance in shaping policy development in individual Member States. In discussing BSE policy development, this chapter also outlines the different institutional and procedural arrangements in place to deal with food safety and animal health issues, and the ways in which those arrangements and institutions have evolved. This chapter begins by summarizing some of the key reasons why the emergence of the new disease posed, and continues to pose, such acute challenges for public policy.

▾ Challenges to policy-making

• Early dilemmas
BSE-related policy-making has always been exceptionally difficult because scientific knowledge about transmissible spongiform encephalopathies (TSEs) has been, and remains, incomplete and uncertain.

When a novel, fatal neurological disease in cattle was first recognized in the United Kingdom in late 1986, the symptoms of diseased animals and postmortem pathology closely resembled scrapie, a TSE that has been endemic in British sheep flocks for several hundred

A chronology of BSE policy

years. TSEs are a group of untreatable brain diseases that afflict both animals and humans. They are very poorly understood and invariably fatal.

The agent responsible for TSEs has not been identified, although many believe that it is an abnormal and virtually indestructible type of protein known as a prion. TSEs have long incubation periods and an animal can be infectious well before its clinical symptoms appear. Until advances in testing were made in the mid-1990s, the presence of the disease could not be detected before the onset of symptoms. The mechanisms by which transmission of the disease occurs are not fully understood, but include the oral route. Transmission occurs most readily between members of the same species but, in some cases, can also occur between species.

In the late 1980s, government scientists in the United Kingdom suspected that BSE had been caught from sheep infected with scrapie and was being transmitted through contaminated feed. The rendered remains of sheep, cattle and other animals, known as meat and bone meal, were routinely incorporated into animal feedstuffs in order to provide a protein-rich nutritional supplement. Contaminated cattle feed was quickly confirmed as the principal vector of the disease, but whether BSE had in fact derived from scrapie or from a spontaneous TSE in cattle, or from another source, remains unclear.

Although sheep scrapie was not thought to be patho-

genic to humans, policy-makers could not be sure that the agent causing BSE had in fact derived from scrapie. Each TSE was thought to possess a distinct host range. Moreover, even if the scrapie agent had jumped species into cattle, policy-makers could not be sure that BSE would subsequently have the same transmission characteristics as scrapie. It was not possible to predict what the host range of a given strain of scrapie would be once it had jumped to another species. Experimental precedents for such altered host ranges, following passage to other species, were well known (Kimberlin, Cole & Walker, 1987).

For all these reasons, the key policy and public health question — whether the new disease presented a risk to human health — could not be answered. Even if policy-makers in the late 1980s and early 1990s assumed that BSE might be pathogenic to humans, they faced acute difficulties in estimating the magnitude of that possible risk. For example, no one knew how many cattle had been exposed to contaminated feed, or indeed whether there were additional vectors of transmission, aside from the recycling of contaminated meat and bone meal. No one knew how many cattle were already infected with the disease. There was no test that could reliably detect the pathogen in live animals before clinical symptoms appeared, and asymptomatic infected cattle could not be differentiated from uninfected cattle.

Analogies with scrapie and other TSEs indicated that the pathogen that causes BSE is found in its most concentrated form in the brain, central nervous system and

in four countries and the European Community

lymphatic tissues of cattle. However, it is not necessarily confined to those tissues. Various other tissues might contain infectivity, as they did in scrapie-affected sheep, albeit at lower levels. No one knew which cattle tissues, if any, would be free of the infectious agent. These topics — on which veterinary science in most respects remains profoundly ignorant — were, and remain, enormously important for public health, for public policy, and for the meat trade. In summary, regulatory regimes in the late 1980s and early 1990s had the unenviable task of responding to the emergence of a novel disease whose nature and implications were entirely unknown.

A wide choice of possible policy responses was available, with a similarly wide range of costs. The total eradication of the disease and its pathogen from agriculture and food would have required, amongst other things, the slaughter and exclusion from the food-chain of all the animals that had received feed known or suspected to have been contaminated with the pathogen. As there was no way of knowing which batches of feed were contaminated, that scenario would have entailed slaughtering and restocking almost the entire national herd.

There were other measures available, that did not involve slaughtering the entire herd and that would have contributed to diminishing human exposure to the pathogenic agent. The extent to which risks were diminished would depend on which tissues were removed from the food-chain and from which animals (e.g. from animals exhibiting conspicuous clinical symptoms of

BSE, or from animals that had received feed known or believed to have been contaminated with the BSE pathogen, or from animals above a certain age, or from all animals).

The scientific considerations were never, by themselves, sufficient to indicate what an appropriate policy response would be. Judgements had to be made about how significant the risks might be. Those judgements then had to balance the risks against the costs and difficulties of removing bovine material from the human food-chain and animal feed-chains, or the cost of taking action to reduce or eradicate the disease in the cattle herd. Policy-makers had to make political judgements about which level of protection was worth paying for, and how the costs should be distributed between public and private sources.

One of the many difficulties of BSE policy-making was that much of the relevant scientific research was only indirectly relevant to human risk. Nevertheless, throughout the 1990s, evidence was produced or gathered that might have had a bearing on policy developments. From the late 1980s onwards, for example, evidence repeatedly emerged suggesting that BSE behaved differently from the scrapie agent; thus the fact that scrapie was not pathogenic to humans provided less and less reassurance that BSE was not pathogenic to humans.[2]

Since it was not possible to carry out research that deliberately infected humans, the question of whether

A chronology of BSE policy

BSE was pathogenic to humans could only be resolved by monitoring for a new CJD-like disease amongst the human population. As the head of pathology at the British Ministry of Agriculture's Central Veterinary Laboratory told his Director in 1988, "[we] cannot answer the question 'is BSE transmissible to humans?'. That natural experiment is underway in the human population and it remains for epidemiologists to collect data and produce a hypothesis based on it" (Bradley, 1988).

Several commentators expected that it would take decades for any such evidence to emerge. As it turned out, atypical cases of CJD began appearing in young British people aged 19–41 years in the mid-1990s. By the spring of 1996,[3] British scientists had concluded that those atypical cases were most likely to have been caused by BSE. This hypothesis is now very strongly supported by scientific evidence.

---

[2] From 1988 onwards it became increasingly clear that BSE and scrapie had a different host range, different transmission properties and a different pathogenesis (Phillips et al., 2000, Vol. 2, paras. 3.48–3.61). For example, experiments conducted in 1988 failed to show transmission of BSE to hamsters, a species that is susceptible to scrapie, and they also demonstrated positive transmission to a strain of sheep that is resistant to scrapie. In early 1990 it emerged that a number of domestic cats had succumbed to a TSE. Since cats were not vulnerable experimentally to scrapie, that evidence further suggested that the scrapie model could not be relied upon.
[3] All references to seasons (spring etc.) relate to the northern hemisphere.

• Contemporary dilemmas

After the spring of 1996, the difficulties for BSE policy-making were marginally less acute, but they were still there and they will continue to present considerable challenges in the foreseeable future. Current patterns of exposure to the BSE agent, and the magnitude of the risks that those exposures entail, are still unknown. It is not known how levels of infectivity vary over the period of incubation in different tissues, or if there might be a threshold of human exposure below which the risk will be negligible. It is still not certain which cattle tissues are free of the BSE agent in infected animals.

Although infectivity has been demonstrated experimentally in relatively few bovine tissues — all of which should, under current regulations, be removed from the carcass — the existing tests are not always sufficiently sensitive to detect low levels of the BSE agent (European Commission, 1999). The most sensitive available tests (inoculating cattle with cattle tissues from infected animals) have been carried out on small numbers of animals and a narrow range of tissues, or have not been carried out at all (FSA, 2000, para. 36). For example, infectivity has not been found thus far in cows' milk or muscle tissue, but the experiments to date have all been conducted by inoculating those materials into mice. If the experiments were to be repeated using calves rather than mice the experiments would be approximately 1000 times more sensitive. Without these more sensitive experiments, there is no certainty that milk, muscle and other cattle tissues from infected animals do not have the potential to

in four countries and the European Community

transmit prion diseases. Despite this lack of certainty, however, policy-makers and their advisers have been making decisions based on assumptions that can be described as optimistic rather than cautious.

Although rapid postmortem tests for BSE now exist, they can only detect infectivity in animals shortly before their clinical symptoms appear. It is not possible, therefore, to estimate empirically the numbers of subclinically infected cattle that are more than a few months away from clinical onset. And, in the absence of a total ban on the consumption of cattle, it is impossible to remove such animals from the human food-chain.

Uncertainties about the transmission of BSE within the animal population also continue to complicate policy-making. Although the main vector of transmission of BSE is known to be contaminated feed, it is now known that maternal transmission (from cow to calf) is likely to occur. There may well be other routes of transmission that are currently unidentified. BSE-contaminated feed has also been fed to other species of farm animals, such as sheep and pigs. BSE has been transmitted orally to sheep under experimental conditions and there is consequently a theoretical possibility that BSE is being maintained in sheep flocks by sheep-to-sheep transmission. There has, however, been insufficient testing of sheep to settle that issue. Nonetheless, it is known that if the BSE pathogen is present in sheep, it is probably distributed far more widely within sheep than within cattle tissues, and

that it would be virtually impossible to separate all potentially infected tissues without destroying the saleable carcass (Food Standards Agency, 2000, paras. 21–30).

Many of the policy dilemmas faced by officials and ministers prior to March 1996 therefore still persist. Which cattle (and other farm animals that might have been exposed to the BSE agent) should be allowed into the food-chain? Which tissues should be removed from those animals? How important is complete compliance with any such controls and how can the chosen level of compliance be ensured? Should there be an attempt to eradicate BSE from national herds as fast as possible, and if so, which steps should be taken? What level of protection is worth paying for, and can stability in the beef market be interpreted as evidence of the social acceptability of risks and policies?

▾ The United Kingdom
The United Kingdom is a unitary state and constitutional monarchy. Its national government directs most government activity, although there are some administrative differences between its four constituent countries. The institution with primary responsibility for BSE policy-making has been the Ministry of Agriculture, Fisheries and Food (MAFF). Until April 2000, MAFF was expected simultaneously to promote the economic interests of farmers and the food industry whilst also protecting public health. That had been the case since MAFF was first created in the immediate aftermath of the Second World War.

A chronology of BSE policy

Public health policy is the responsibility of the Department of Health in the United Kingdom. However, on food safety policy, it usually shared responsibilities with MAFF, and on most of those issues usually took a subordinate role to MAFF. That was the case with BSE; indeed, MAFF was primarily responsible for the development, implementation and enforcement of most of the relevant policies.

Many other institutions and actors have been important players in BSE policy-making. These include the Treasury, which was responsible for authorizing public expenditure by departments such as MAFF, as well as a number of expert committees that were established to advise on the animal and human health implications of BSE. The principal committees were the Southwood Working Party (1988–1989), the Tyrrell Research Committee (1989–1990) and the Spongiform Encephalopathy Advisory Committee (SEAC). SEAC began its work in 1990 and is still in existence.

BSE policy-making in the United Kingdom has been a highly complex and politically fraught issue. As described below in more detail, in the period following the discovery of BSE in the British cattle herd in November 1986, the Government introduced a series of regulatory measures to control the epidemic amongst cattle and to limit human exposure to the BSE agent. The key controls were introduced belatedly, however, and the policy was never one of eradicating TSE pathogens from the herds or from the food supply. Controls fell substantially short of removing all potentially infect-ed material from the animal feed-chains and human food-chains. Nor were the controls properly enforced. As new evidence emerged and as political developments unfolded, the controls were gradually tightened but only in a reactive, not a proactive, fashion.

In March 1996, the Government banned the consumption of all cattle aged over 30 months and further tightened the existing controls in the United Kingdom after its scientific advisers concluded that BSE had probably infected humans. Exports of British beef were banned by the European Commission, which also demanded that the United Kingdom embark on a plan to eradicate BSE as a precondition to lifting the ban. The ban was eventually lifted in 1999, after the Commission had concluded that British beef presented no greater risk than beef produced in other European countries which, by then, were also affected by BSE.

The political fallout of the BSE saga has been considerable in the United Kingdom. One of the consequences was the creation of the Food Standards Agency in April 2000. The new agency took responsibility for "post-farm gate" regulation of BSE as well as for general oversight of BSE policy. MAFF was abolished in 2001, and its functions were transferred to a new Department for Environment, Food and Rural Affairs (DEFRA).

• United Kingdom policy responses prior to March 1996
BSE was first recognized as a novel cattle disease in November 1986 by scientists at MAFF's Central Veterinary Laboratory. In the months that followed, reported cases of

in four countries and the European Community

BSE steadily increased in herds throughout the country. Senior MAFF officials and scientists immediately realized that BSE posed a possible risk to human health. Over the following 12 months, however, the secretaries of state for agriculture, fisheries and food, other ministers in MAFF, and senior civil servants in both administrative and scientific grades, decided to take no regulatory action. Even though MAFF scientists suspected that BSE was being transmitted through food, cattle continued to receive contaminated feed and animals clinically affected with BSE simply went into the human food-chain.

By early 1988, however, senior MAFF officials began to be concerned that, unless clinically diseased animals were removed from the food-chain, the Government would be held responsible if it later transpired that BSE was transmissible to humans (Phillips et al., 2000, Vol. 3, para. 5.41). Recommendations to that effect were nevertheless rejected by the Minister for Agriculture. By the spring of that year, events internal to the politics of MAFF and the Department of Health led to the establishment of an ad hoc expert committee, known as the Southwood Working Party, to advise on the implications of BSE. Once that committee began meeting in June 1988, two key sets of controls were quickly introduced by the British Government.

• A ruminant feed ban, introduced by MAFF, made it unlawful to feed ruminants with ruminant protein.[4] BSE was also made a notifiable disease.

• A slaughter policy, introduced at the behest of the committee, removed clinically affected cattle from the human food-chain.

The ruminant feed ban applied to cattle and sheep only. Non-ruminants, such as pigs and poultry, could still be fed with the contaminated protein even though no one knew whether they might also be susceptible to BSE.[5] No controls were placed on exports of ruminant protein either, even though government officials expected the domestic ban to divert ruminant-derived feedstuffs overseas (Lawrence, 1998).[6]

The slaughter policy was applied only to clinically diseased cows. Moreover, the level of financial compensation was set for the first 18 months at only 50% of the animals' value, thus providing a disincentive for farmers to report cases. No controls were placed on animals that were infected but asymptomatic, although these were far greater in number and potentially almost as infectious as clinically affected animals.

Although the Southwood Working Party did not recommend that controls should be imposed on potentially asymptomatic animals, regulations to that effect were

---

[4] Ruminants are hoofed animals that chew the cud, and include cattle, sheep and goats.
[5] MAFF officials had in fact considered, and then rejected, a ban on feeding ruminant-protein meal to all animals. As the bulk of animal protein was being fed to pigs and poultry, such a ban would have deprived the rendering industry of its principal market (BSE Inquiry Transcript, 29 June 1998, p. 35).
[6] Officials' expectations of a diversion of meat-based meal overseas was correct: in 1988, 12 553 tonnes of meat-based meal were exported from the United Kingdom to Europe and in 1989 that figure had risen to 25 005 tonnes (European Parliament, 1997, p. 8, para. 3).

A chronology of BSE policy

announced by MAFF in June 1989, less than four months after the Working Party's report had been published. The ban on specified bovine offal, introduced in November 1989, was the third and final key control. It banned certain central nervous system and lymphatic tissues from all cattle from being used in human food-chains.

The tissues selected for inclusion in the ban (brain, spinal cord, tonsils, spleen, thymus and intestines) were not all those that might have harboured the infectious agent. Analogies with other species indicated that other tissues might also have carried the agent, but those were either commercially valuable or could not easily or cheaply be removed and they were excluded from the offal ban.[7] Animals under six months old were also excluded from the ban on the grounds that they should not have been given contaminated feed; however, policy-makers also assumed, in the absence of any evidence, that maternal transmission would not occur, even though scrapie was thought to be transmitted by that route.

The principal controls described above were tightened on several occasions between 1989 and 1996, in the wake of new scientific data and evidence that the existing controls had not been properly implemented and enforced, as well as in response to political pressures of various kinds. Controls to protect the animal feed-chain were amended at least six times. In September 1990, for example, MAFF banned the use of bovine offal from all mammals in the feed-chain after evi-

dence emerged showing that BSE had been transmitted to pigs under experimental conditions. MAFF was aware that the bovine offal regulations were not being observed, because it collected and analysed figures revealing substantial divergences between the quantities of offal recorded as destroyed at incinerators and the amounts supposedly removed from animals in abattoirs (Fleetwood, 1998). It also became clear that there was cross-contamination between feed destined for non-ruminants and feed destined for ruminants, thus prolonging the epidemic in cattle. In 1996, when the acute BSE crisis erupted, all mammalian meat and bone meal was banned from use in the feed of all farm animals.

Controls on the human food-chain were altered at least 11 times. For example, in March 1992, regulations were brought in to prohibit the use of the head after the skull had been opened (minimizing the risk of head meat being contaminated by the process of brain removal).[8] In June 1994 the specified bovine offal ban was extended to include the thymus and intestines of calves under six months old. In December 1995, MAFF suspended the use of bovine vertebral column (a potentially rich source of nervous tissue) in the manufacture of mechanically recovered meat.[9]

From 1994, a few cases of CJD in young people slowly began to emerge. By March 1996, the CJD Surveillance Unit[10] informed the Government's Spongiform Encephalopathy Advisory Committee of 10 cases that appeared to be a new variant of CJD. On 20 March 1996

in four countries and the European Community

the Government announced in Parliament that the most probable explanation of such cases was exposure to the BSE agent, albeit in the period before 1989. The British Government had no contingency plan for responding to the emergence of evidence in March 1996 that BSE had infected humans.

• Policy after March 1996

The announcement precipitated a major crisis for the United Kingdom and for the European Union as a whole. The European Commission immediately prohibited British exports of live cattle, meat and mammalian-derived meat and bone meal to anywhere in the world (European Commission Decision 96/239/EC). Within the United Kingdom, the Government, acting on SEAC advice, announced that it would require carcasses from cattle aged over 30 months to be deboned, with the trimmings (comprising the nervous and lymphatic tissue including 14 specified nodes) to be kept out of the

human food-chain. A few days later, however, the Government announced that, instead of cattle over 30 months being deboned, all cattle over that age would be slaughtered and destroyed. Several leading retailers had indicated that they were no longer prepared to accept beef from animals over 30 months of age. The Over-Thirty-Month Scheme (OTMS) was introduced in May 1996 to organize the slaughter of animals that could no longer enter the food-chain or feed-chain, and to provide compensation to farmers.

The European Commission insisted that its ban on all exports of British cattle products would be maintained at least until the Government provided a comprehensive plan for eradicating BSE. An action framework was agreed with Brussels that included a selective cull of cohorts of older animals, the introduction of a computerized cattle tracking system, and rigorous implementation of regulations. Once those conditions had been met, a step-by-step removal of the export ban could occur, beginning with animals and meat from herds with no history of BSE and no exposure to meat and bone meal. Exports of British beef produced in accordance with the controls outlined at the EU's Summit Meeting in Florence in June 1996 have been permitted by the EC, and by most EU Member States, since November 1999.

Regulations have been tightened on several occasions, since 20 March 1996. Prohibited bovine tissues now include: the entire head excluding the tongue but including the brains, eyes, trigeminal ganglia and

---

[7] For example, lymph nodes and peripheral nerves would almost certainly be highly infectious but could not practicably be removed. Organs such as the liver might, by analogy with other TSEs, also contain the infectious agent but were commercially valuable.

[8] The Bovine Offal (Prohibition) (Amendment) Regulations 1992 (SI 1992 No 306). (http://www.legislation.hmso.gov.uk/si/si1992/Uksi_19920306_en_1.htm).

[9] The Specified Bovine Offal (Amendment) Order 1995 (S.I. 1995/3246). (http://www.legislation.hmso.gov.uk/si/si1995/Uksi_19953246_en_1.htm).

[10] The unit was set up in 1990 by the Department of Health to monitor for atypical cases of CJD.

A chronology of BSE policy

tonsils; the thymus; the spleen and spinal cord of animals aged over six months; the vertebral column, including dorsal root ganglia, of animals aged over 30 months; and the intestines from the duodenum to the rectum of bovine animals of all ages. The heads and spinal cords from sheep and goats aged over 12 months are also prohibited for use in food.

Since 1993 the incidence of BSE has been falling, from a peak in that year of over 34 000 cases per annum to approximately 1000 reported cases in 2001. It is likely, however, that many BSE-affected animals would have been slaughtered before showing symptoms, under various culling schemes.[11] The ruminant feed ban is believed to have been thoroughly enforced only since August 1996, and animals born after that date should not have contracted BSE from contaminated feed. There have, however, been over a dozen cases of BSE in animals born after August 1996, perhaps as a result of maternal or other routes of transmission. For the time being they constitute an anomaly that remains inexplicable (European Commission, 2001). It is therefore likely that some animals under 30 months will be subclinically infected with BSE and will be entering the human food-chain, although numbers will be very small relative to historical levels of exposure.[12]

• New institutional and procedural arrangements
Following the General Election in May 1997 in the United Kingdom, proposals to separate regulation from sponsorship in the food safety arena were drawn up in

the form of a proposed Food Standards Agency (FSA). A Public Inquiry into BSE was also announced in December 1997.

The original intention was that the FSA would be responsible for the entire food-chain, "from the plough to the plate". In practice it did not quite work out like that. When the FSA was established in April 2000, the Government decided that MAFF would retain primary responsibility for veterinary and agricultural aspects of food policy, so that the FSA's responsibility runs only from the "farm gate to the plate". MAFF retained its industrial sponsorship remit and primary responsibility for three key areas of food safety policy — BSE, pesticides and veterinary medicine — while the FSA had indirect oversight of those policy domains.

---

[11] These include: the Selective Culling scheme, which has removed over 77 000 British cattle at greatest risk of developing BSE, based on their herd and feeding histories; the OTMS which has removed nearly 5.6 million older cattle from the national herd; the BSE Offspring Cull, which has found over 25 000 offspring of BSE cases that have been, or will be, slaughtered; and an unspecified number of older cattle culled under the foot and mouth disease culling regime. (Figures from DEFRA at http://www.defra.gov.uk/animalh/bse/bse-statistics.)

[12] Current models based on assumptions about the rate of maternal transmission predict very low numbers of animals entering the food-chain. See, for example: SEAC (2001) Minutes of the 71st meeting held 21 November 2001 at DEFRA. (http://www.seac.gov.uk/papers/mins21-11-01.pdf). Estimates (i.e. numbers of cows likely to contract BSE and that subsequently enter the human food-chain) are based on models that assume a 10% maternal transmission risk within six months of clinical onset in the dam, zero feed risk, and no other route of transmission.

in four countries and the European Community

Another significant change, prompted by the epidemic of foot and mouth disease in 2000, was the abolition of MAFF in May 2001. MAFF's remaining functions, as well as its responsibility for environmental policy (formerly located in the Department of the Environment, Transport and the Regions), were transferred to the new DEFRA.

Nevertheless, the FSA is now the primary source of policy in relation to food safety. When the FSA was established, it outlined three core values that would guide its work: to put the consumer first, to be open and accessible, and to be an independent voice. Those guidelines represented an abrupt change and reflected an analysis of some of the principal shortcomings in MAFF's approach to policy-making. In relation to BSE, for example, the FSA has been far more explicit than MAFF about the uncertainties, the available policy options and the reasons for particular decisions (FSA, 2000).

▾ The European Commission

The role of the European Commission in establishing EU-wide controls on BSE has obviously been an important influence on BSE policy in the Member States. Before March 1996, the Commission paid scant attention to emerging public health signals about the possible risks posed by BSE. Political and policy activity on the part of the Commission only appeared to take place either when trade was threatened or when other Member States insisted that the issue be discussed at Community level. After 1996, and criticism by a

European Parliament Inquiry of the Commission's activities on BSE, a process of institutional and procedural reform began. The Commission also became more proactively involved in the development of common EU policy on BSE.

• EU controls prior to March 1996

Prior to 1997, European BSE policy fell within the remit of two Directorates: DG III, which was responsible for the EU's internal market, and DG VI, which was responsible for agriculture and fisheries. Regulations and legislation were developed by those Directorates in collaboration with two committees: the Scientific Veterinary Committee, which comprised experts appointed by the Commission, and the Standing Veterinary Committee, which comprised official representatives of Member States' veterinary services.

Following the emergence of BSE within the United Kingdom, the Commission could reasonably have been expected to consider adopting regulatory measures in two key areas: in relation to a known animal disease and in relation to a potential risk to human health.

With regard to control of the animal epidemic, the Commission could have established (a) rules that governed trade in potentially contaminated ruminant protein and live cattle, and (b) controls that governed the practices within individual countries as regards, for example, use of recycled ruminant protein in feed for ruminants and other farm animals.

A chronology of BSE policy

In July 1989 the Commission made its first intervention in BSE policy by banning the export from the United Kingdom of live cattle that had been born before July 1988 (the date that the ruminant feed ban was introduced in the United Kingdom). However, despite the concerns expressed by several Member States about the fact that potentially contaminated ruminant meat and bone meal from the United Kingdom could be exported and fed to ruminants in other Member States, no measures were taken at that time to control trade in ruminant feed. Nor did the Commission insist that Member States other than the United Kingdom should halt the widely adopted practice of recycling ruminant protein to other ruminants.

The Commission had asked the United Kingdom to ban exports of ruminant-derived meat and bone meal, but this was refused (European Parliament, 1996). Exports to the EU of British meat and bone meal had jumped from 12 553 tonnes in 1988 (the year of the domestic controls in the United Kingdom) to 25 005 tonnes in 1989. It was only in 1996, however, that the Commission banned British exports of meat and bone meal.

In 1989, the Commission had also wanted to introduce a European-wide measure banning the feeding of ruminant meal to ruminants (European Parliament, 1997). There was, however, only limited support for that proposal. Instead, the Commission's Scientific Veterinary Committee advised, in January 1990, that all Member States should take whatever action was deemed appropriate in their own countries (European Parliament,

1996). The European Commission did not ban the practice of feeding ruminants with mammalian meat and bone meal until 1994.

With the benefit of hindsight, it is clear that exports of contaminated feed from the United Kingdom spread the BSE agent to almost all European countries, and that the agent was again recycled within national herds, thus allowing the disease to become established.

The second key area in which the Commission could reasonably have been expected to consider adopting regulatory measures was in relation to the human food-chain. Here the key issues were the control of trade in potentially contaminated carcass meat and meat products, and controls on the products entering the food-chain within individual jurisdictions.

Outside the EU, many countries banned or restricted imports of British cattle products in the period between 1988 and 1990.[13] Nonetheless, exports of meat from the

---

[13] Sweden banned the import of all British cattle in October 1988; Australia and New Zealand followed suit in December 1988 and this was followed by similar decisions from Finland in January 1989, the United States of America in June 1989, Canada and Tunisia in February 1990, and the Russian Federation in March 1990. Bans were also placed on British cattle by Israel and Saudi Arabia. Other countries required certification that cattle came from herds without BSE. These included Brazil, Japan, Morocco and South Africa (Ministry of Agriculture, Fisheries and Food, 1990).

in four countries and the European Community

United Kingdom to the rest of the EU went unregulated until April 1990, when the Commission banned the import of specified bovine offal from the United Kingdom — some five months after the same legislation had been introduced in the United Kingdom. Those controls were marginally tightened in June 1990 in an effort to prevent unilateral action on the part of France and Germany.

After that, in the period 1990–1994, there was no further Community legislation on exports of British beef and virtually no consideration of BSE by the EU's Agricultural Council, despite the fact that the BSE epidemic reached its peak during that period. Following further threats of unilateral action by Germany, controls on exports of British beef were again marginally tightened by requiring exports of bone-in beef to have come only from herds with no cases of BSE in the previous six years rather than the two years stipulated in the 1990 regulations. No further action was taken by the European Commission until the immediate aftermath of 20 March 1996, when British exports of live cattle, cattle meat and mammalian-derived meat and bone meal were prohibited to anywhere in the world (European Commission Decision 96/239/EC).

• EU controls after March 1996

The European Commission has struggled to deal with the consequences of a serious loss of public confidence in the safety of foods and in food safety policy-making institutions since March 1996. It has responded in a number of ways.

Institutionally there have been substantial changes. For example, in 1997, the Commission relocated its scientific advisory committees to the Directorate General for Health and Consumer Protection (DG SANCO). In 2000, industrial sponsorship, regulation and inspection duties were separated. Regulation was relocated to DG SANCO, while a Food and Veterinary Office based in Dublin, Ireland, became responsible for inspecting Member States' implementation of food safety-related European Commission legislation. A European Food Safety Authority was established in 2002 to advise DG SANCO.

In terms of legislation, the European Commission has introduced a complex array of controls on BSE. These fall under at least three broad headings: surveillance, controls on animal feed-chains, and protection of the human food-chain.

   • **Surveillance**. Although BSE was made notifiable across the European Community in March 1990, a common surveillance strategy has only been in place since April 1998. From that date, all Member States were required to implement a monitoring system and to test, by histopathological examination of the brain, all animals older than 20 months displaying behavioural or neurological symptoms. Since January 2001 the Commission has also required Member States to monitor for BSE using the new rapid postmortem tests. Such testing must be carried out on all healthy animals over 30 months that are destined for human consumption, as well as on several samples of healthy and ill animals.

A chronology of BSE policy

• **Animal feed-chain**. Beyond the 1994 ban on using mammalian meat and bone meal in ruminant feed, no major additional restrictions were introduced until 2000. Mammalian meat and bone meal continued to be allowed for use in feed for non-ruminant farm animals, despite the fact that experience in the United Kingdom had demonstrated that a ruminant feed ban on its own was problematic.[14] Indeed the EU's Food and Veterinary Office repeatedly found that there was a significant risk of contamination of ruminant feed by mammalian meat and bone meal. In December 2000, the European Council temporarily banned the use of animal proteins in feed for all farmed animals and that ban was made permanent as of January 2001.

• **Human food-chain**. The European Commission proposed in 1996 that EU-wide restrictions be placed on the use in food of "specified risk materials" (SRMs), which are analogous to the specified bovine materials that had been prohibited in British cattle since 1989. Those proposals were, however, rejected by the European Council in December 1996. Proposed again in July 1997, the controls were to have been implemented from January 1998 but were postponed four times until October 2000. Thus, acceptance of the Commission's proposals to remove SRMs took almost four years after first being proposed. In the interim, three Member States introduced their own bans to protect their consumers.[15]

---

[14] There was a risk of cross-contamination in feed mills between ruminant and non-ruminant feed, and also a risk that farmers might have fed non-ruminant feed to cattle.
[15] France in 1996, the Netherlands in 1997 and Belgium in 1998.

▼ Germany

Germany is a federal republic consisting of 16 states (*Länder*), each of which possesses its own constitution and its own government and parliament. The states have, however, ceded a substantial part of their legislative competence to the Federal Government. The Federal Government is responsible for legislation in certain areas, the state governments in others, and there is a system of mixed competence in a third set of areas that includes food legislation. Most food legislation in Germany is federal law, with the state governments responsible for its implementation.

Until 2001, BSE policy-making in Germany was shared between two departments, the Ministry of Food, Agriculture and Forestry (*Bundesministerium für Ernährung, Landwirtschaft und Forsten*) and the Ministry of Health (*Bundesgesundheitsministerium*). The tensions between taking care of long-term public health on the one hand and sponsoring the economic interests of farmers and the food industry on the other were therefore played out between two distinct government departments rather than within one single department, as occurred in the United Kingdom. The arrangement dates from the 1960s and was designed to diminish some of the conflicts between economic and public health interests. The two ministries were often characterized, and saw themselves, as so-called "mirror-departments" (*Spiegelreferat*). Each of those two ministries had its own Chief Veterinary Officer. Since 2001, the Ministry of Consumer Protection, Food and Agriculture has had primary responsibility for BSE

in four countries and the European Community

policy-making, and there is now only one Chief Veterinary Officer in the Federal Government.

Each state possesses its own administrative arrangements for dealing with health and agricultural policies, and they are similarly structured to the federal ministries. Each state also has its own Chief Veterinary Officer located — depending on the state — inside the State Ministry of Agriculture, State Ministry of the Environment or State Ministry for Social Affairs.

German policy on BSE was, for many years, concerned primarily with protecting its borders from imports of contaminated animal feed, live animals and meat. Unlike in many jurisdictions, German regulators did not always assume, prior to March 1996, that BSE was only a veterinary problem and would pose a zero or negligible risk to human health. The Federal Government attempted to impose unilateral trade controls on British products on several occasions and played an important role in pushing the European Commission towards taking a more proactive policy role over BSE control. Germany was also the first EU Member State that responded to BSE as a public health issue. What emerged as EU-wide controls were often a compromise between German and other more recalcitrant interests.

Yet, despite recognizing that BSE might pose a risk to human health, Germany did not put in place precautionary controls on its own domestic beef supply. Although countries such as Austria, Denmark, the Netherlands and Sweden banned the use of ruminant-derived meat and bone meal for use as cattle feed in 1989–1990, Germany — together with Belgium, Greece, Italy, Luxembourg and Spain — had no feed ban in place until the EU-wide ban on mammalian proteins for ruminants was introduced in 1994 (Court of Auditors, 2001).

Officials have claimed, however, that it had not been usual agricultural practice in Germany to feed meat and bone meal to ruminants, but only to pigs and poultry (Speakers of the highest regional authorities responsible for veterinary issues and food surveillance, 1996). The German BSE crisis of the last half of 2000 undermined that claim, however, because traces of mammalian protein were detected in ruminant feed.

In late 2000, scores of domestic cases of BSE began to be reported in Germany, following the introduction of rapid postmortem tests. The political fallout from that discovery saw domestic beef consumption plummet and led to the Ministry of Food, Agriculture and Forestry being reconstituted as the Federal Ministry for Consumer Protection, Food and Agriculture.

• German policy prior to March 1996

The Federal Government, in common with those of other Member States, implemented European Commission legislation relating to BSE as and when it was introduced. On a number of occasions, however, it took unilateral action to restrict trade with the United Kingdom. The first such occasion was in May 1989 when Germany prohibited imports of British meat and bone

A chronology of BSE policy

meal. The Commission did not introduce an EU-wide prohibition of British meat and bone meal until March 1996. In 1989, several German states also temporarily banned imports of British beef.

In August 1989, Germany announced that, as of November of that year, it would only allow imports of British beef that had been certified as originating from BSE-free herds and only if brain, spinal cord and internal organs had been removed prior to export. The United Kingdom had by that time announced but not yet introduced a specified bovine offal ban. Germany stated that it was entitled to take unilateral measures until such time as Community-wide measures had been introduced that protected the entire European public (Anon, 1989). An EU-wide ban on bovine offal from British cattle was not introduced until April 1990.

The following month, however, Germany banned imports of all British beef, as did France and Italy. Several British domestic cats had been diagnosed with a novel spongiform encephalopathy; this indicated not only that BSE might be transmissible by food to non-ruminant species but also that BSE was unlike scrapie, since the latter cannot be transmitted to cats. This was significant because reassurances about the safety of BSE for humans had been based on the premiss that BSE would behave in the same way as scrapie. Germany lifted its ban the following month, although this was after the Council of Agricultural Ministers had reached a compromise on trade in beef and calves from the United Kingdom. The decision required the United

Kingdom to certify that all boneless beef for export to Member States had "obvious nervous and lymphatic tissue" removed. It also required certification that bone-in beef for export came from farm holdings where BSE had not been confirmed in the previous two years.

The last major unilateral German policy initiative on BSE did not take place until four years later, following an international symposium on TSEs held at the Federal Health Office (*Bundesgesundheitsamt*) in December 1993. The effect of those discussions was to reinforce the view of German health officials that eating British beef might be hazardous to public health. In March 1994, following the publication of a risk assessment by the Federal Health Office (Federal Health Office, 1993), the German Government attempted to secure a complete EU-wide ban on the sale of British beef (Carvel, 1994). That attempt failed and a compromise was reached whereby the Commission marginally tightened the rules covering exports of British beef. In the period from mid-1994 until the BSE crisis of March 1996, the German Government continued to be in the vanguard of countries calling within the EU for tighter and more precautionary restrictions on bovine exports from the United Kingdom, to prevent the spread of the disease.

All the major policy initiatives, aside from implementing Commission legislation, were concerned with protecting German borders from imports of diseased animals and feedstuffs. As mentioned previously, Germany did not take seriously, at this time, the possibility that BSE

in four countries and the European Community

might be already present in the domestic herd. Thus the Federal Government did not end the use of mammalian meat and bone meal from rendered animal remains in ruminant feed or other agricultural feedstuffs until 1994, shortly before it was required to do so by EU-wide controls. Nor did it ban the consumption of what the United Kingdom termed "specified bovine offal". The Federal Government also continued to permit the use of what is known in English as "mechanically recovered meat" and in German as *Separatorenfleisch*.

Surveillance for possible cases of BSE had been undertaken in Germany since 1990 and in particular since 1992 when the first case of BSE in an imported British cow was detected. Three further cases of BSE were reported in 1994, but they too were in cows imported from the United Kingdom. According to a German scientist who was interviewed, only about 1500 brains of neurologically suspect cattle were examined between 1991 and 1999.[16] Surveillance was passive rather than active; it received and checked diagnoses, but it did not actively search for evidence of infectivity. Furthermore, pathologists working at the regional State Veterinary Laboratories were not required to undertake specialist training in the diagnosis of BSE, although some did so voluntarily. Thus domestic surveillance was relatively weak. In practice, official BSE surveillance

implied the monitoring and control of international trade in meat, meat products and live cattle — therefore not surveillance in the classical sense but rather control by the customs.

• German policy after March 1996

After the crisis of 20 March 1996, the German health and agricultural ministers prohibited all imports of British beef or live cattle, but not milk. The Federal Health Office had recommended such a ban in December 1993. Similar restrictions were imposed by the European Commission soon after the German announcement.

German BSE policy after March 1996 continued to focus on the threat from abroad. For example, following the fifth case of BSE in an animal imported from the United Kingdom in January 1997, a decision was taken to cull all 5200 cattle that had been imported from Switzerland (which also had a relatively high incidence of BSE) and the United Kingdom. The 14 000 descendants of the slaughtered cattle were to be kept under official surveillance.

In general, German regulators continued to act as if their country was free of BSE. As discussed in the previous section, the European Commission had proposed an EU-wide bovine offal ban in 1996, but that proposal was not actually introduced until June 2000. A few Member States introduced their own bans to protect their consumers, in the interim, but Germany was not one of those countries.

---

[16] It is possible that more tests were carried out, but numbers were not officially provided by the state governments.

A chronology of BSE policy

In April 1996, at a meeting on TSEs hosted by WHO in Genoa, Italy, the German Robert Koch Institute recommended that a surveillance system for BSE should be set up in all Member States; in the absence of such a system, no country's situation should be classified as BSE-free but as "unknown". The Federal Government did not accept that advice. A fully active surveillance system was introduced only as a consequence of a decision by the Council of Ministers (98/272/EC) in 1998, which obliged all Member States to establish a systematic monitoring programme. Even then the regime was not implemented in Germany until May 1999, and the Federal Government failed to implement all the requirements, such as those regarding training (European Commission Food and Health Office, 2001). According to a German scientist who was interviewed, the states were only asked by the Federal Government to test as many cattle as possible in order to fulfil the European Commission's requirements.

In May 2000, the European Commission's Scientific Steering Committee completed a geographical risk assessment of BSE in Germany, which concluded that "it is likely that domestic [German] cattle are (clinically or pre-clinically) infected with the BSE-agent but it is not confirmed" (European Commission, 2000a). The Food and Veterinary Office's assessment was based on the assumption that the current surveillance system was passive and therefore unable to detect all clinical BSE cases. It argued that there was a "significant" probability that BSE would be confirmed in Germany in the next few years, in particular if active

surveillance was adopted.

In November 2000, only a few months after the publication of the Scientific Steering Committee's Geographical Risk Assessment, the first domestic case of BSE was detected in the north of Germany. The case was identified using one of the new rapid diagnostic tests that were being used in anticipation of the European Commission legislation that would require active surveillance from January 2001 (European Commission, 2000b).

• New institutional and procedural arrangements
The disclosure of the first genuine German BSE cases triggered a crisis of credibility in the risk assessment and risk management abilities of official German institutions, and led to substantial reorganization and restructuring of various political institutions. By mid-January 2001, as domestic demand for beef slumped, both the Agriculture Minister and the Health Minister resigned from the Federal Government. In January 2001, under Green minister Renate Künast, the Agriculture Ministry was abolished and replaced by the Ministry for Consumer Protection, Food and Agriculture (*Bundesministerium für Verbraucherschutz, Ernährung, und Landwirtschaft*). Künast declared consumer safety the new top priority of the new ministry.

In May 2001, the Federal Government also introduced a TSE research policy designed to ensure that all relevant German research-funding institutions (at both federal and state level) adequately addressed research questions relating to TSE. An important part of that policy

in four countries and the European Community

was the establishment of the German TSE "research platform", initiated and predominantly funded by the Federal Ministry of Education and Research. Its task is to provide a communication and service network for all German TSE researchers, and both to inform the public about TSEs and to enable a dialogue between TSE scientists and the public.

In January 2002 a new bill was introduced requiring that there should be a strict institutional separation between risk communication and risk management on issues relating to food and food safety. The organization responsible for risk assessment and risk communication issues is the Federal Institute for Risk Assessment (*Bundesinstitut für Risikobewertung*), whilst the institution responsible for risk management is the Federal Institute for Consumer Protection and Food Safety (*Bundesamt für Verbraucherschutz und Lebensmittelsicherheit*).[17] Both institutions started work in November 2002.

▼ Italy

Italy is a parliamentary republic administratively divided into regions, provinces and districts. Regions are relatively autonomous territorial units with their own powers and functions. Each region exercises some of its administrative authority directly, but can also delegate several functions to the provinces and districts. Often policies are framed at the centre but responsibility for enforcement is delegated to local government.[18]

In Italy, the primary responsibility for all health issues (including both humans and farm animals) is taken by the Ministry of Health. BSE policy-making has thus primarily been the responsibility of the Ministry of Health. The Italian Ministry of Agriculture, which is responsible for sponsoring the farming and food industries, was not centrally involved in the management of the BSE problem, but nevertheless played an influential secondary role.

Prior to March 1996, beef consumption in Italy was the second highest after France, averaging an annual 26 kg per person between 1990 and 1995 (Eurostat, 1998). The country produced only two thirds of the beef it consumed, with about 6% of imported beef coming from the United Kingdom. Historically, and throughout the 1990s, Italian farmers used large amounts of animal feedstuffs containing meat and bone meal.

Until the first cases of BSE in imported animals appeared in 1994, and the events of March 1996, Italian policy focused on the formal translation of European directives into national measures. The sole but important exception was a 1989 ban on the import of British meat and bone meal for use in ruminant feedstuffs. As in Germany, BSE was primarily viewed as an external problem and not as a threat to Italian cattle. Thus no

---

[17] For a critical discussion of that approach see the Böschen et al. (2002) report to the Office of Technology Assessment of the German Parliament.
[18] The Italian chronology is based in part on a report by Estades et al.,(1999).

A chronology of BSE policy

domestic controls on the use of ruminant meat and bone meal in ruminant feed were introduced until the European Commission (EC) took the initiative in 1994, and no controls on bovine offal from domestic animals were put in place until common EU controls were introduced in 2000.

From November 2000 onwards, however, the situation changed dramatically. The discovery of BSE-infected cattle in France and Germany, and then the detection of the first cases in Italy some months later, created a high degree of concern amongst Italian consumers. During the second half of November 2000, beef purchases fell by almost 36% and remained at that level until mid-December. At the end of January 2001, sales of beef in Italy were 60–65% lower than the levels seen one year earlier.

• Italian policy prior to March 1996

When BSE first emerged in the United Kingdom, it aroused the interest of a small number of Italian scientists who had developed expertise in TSEs, but that interest was not generally shared by health or agricultural policy-makers in Rome. In general, BSE was not seen as being a threat to Italian cattle but only as a veterinary problem concerning imported animals. The aim of Italian policy was therefore to protect the country from British cattle and British feedstuffs.

Aside from a ban on imports of British meat and bone meal, introduced in November 1989, regulatory restrictions to reduce the risk from BSE were introduced by

the Italian Government as European Directives were adopted. After European Directive 90/200 was issued by the Commission, the Italian Government decided that all animals displaying antemortem clinical signals of BSE must be slaughtered separately and have their brains removed for analysis (Ministerial Decree No. 2683 of April 1990).

During 1991, however, key officials in the Italian Government became increasingly concerned about the risks posed by BSE. The Government responded by establishing a National Centre for Animal Encephalopathies and by recruiting two laboratories of the Higher Institute of Health to work on TSE research. In the early 1990s, therefore, the Italian Government began constructing an institutional framework to try to manage the risks posed by BSE.

Two animals in Italy were found to have BSE in 1994 but they came from a group of 50 animals that had been imported from the United Kingdom. All those cattle were slaughtered, the farmers compensated and tighter controls placed on herds containing animals imported from the United Kingdom. However, those two cases of BSE did not provoke much debate or concern.

• Italian policy after March 1996

In the wake of the British announcement of 20 March 1996, the Italian Government sought to reassure domestic consumers and consequently adopted more restrictive measures than those required under

in four countries and the European Community

European Commission legislation. For example, in April 1996, the Italian Government imposed restrictions on cattle and meat imports from France (Ministerial Decree No. 2666), and similar restrictions on imports from Switzerland in June (Ministerial Decree No. 4566).

In mid-December 2000, after the discovery of BSE in cattle in France and Germany and amid rising public concern, the Government appointed a Special Commissioner for BSE in order to coordinate the action of the ministries of health and of agriculture and of other public authorities concerned with the disease. At the end of December, systematic tests of cattle older than 30 months started. In January 2001, the first case of BSE was detected and, at the end of March 2001, when 60 000 tests had been performed, seven cases of BSE had been identified. This created what has been described as a "wave of panic" in the population.

Media coverage of BSE rose rapidly, and much of it was focused on the alleged shortcomings of the Italian policy-making and enforcement systems.

▼ Finland

In Finland, responsibility for policy relating to food-borne risks resides with the Ministry of Agriculture and Forestry (MAF). Once foodborne infection is suspected in humans, the responsibility for managing such an outbreak shifts to the Ministry of Social Affairs and Health (MSAF). Thus, responsibility for BSE

policy rests within MAF, while responsibility for vCJD surveillance is under the jurisdiction of MSAF.

The low prevalence of BSE in Finland is probably due to the country's comparative isolation, traditional farming practices, and high level of overall animal health, rather than to surveillance and control. In Finland, cattle are raised on small and isolated family farms, the average herd size is small and the grazing area per ruminant is large compared to EU averages. There is little trade in cattle, and no system exists for gathering cattle for markets.

Finnish policy on BSE, prior to 1994, was based on banning cattle imports from the United Kingdom and imports of meat and bone meal generally, and on surveillance of cattle that had already been imported. After joining the European Economic Area (EEA) (in 1994) and the EU (in 1995), measures to control BSE were largely driven by European Community requirements. In the years after Finland joined the EU, the country's surveillance systems assigned BSE only marginal importance compared to other challenges to animal health such as *Salmonella*.

The current arrangement for dealing with food and feed safety in Finland results from the restructuring of March 2001. BSE policy is overseen by MAF, whose Health and Food Department is responsible for general animal health and health policy. Risk assessment and risk management of foodstuffs are divided between two different institutions. The National Veterinary and Food Research Institute is responsible for risk assessment

A chronology of BSE policy

concerning animal health and food of animal origin, while the National Food Agency (NFA) is responsible for risk management regarding foodstuffs. The NFAs responsibilities include surveillance of food safety and quality from the farm to the dinner table. A third institution, the Plant Production Inspection Centre, is responsible for feed. While all of these institutions are within MAF's administrative responsibility, they are guided and coordinated by a working group for food control that also includes representatives of MSAF and of the Ministry of Trade and Industry.

Following the introduction of the rapid postmortem testing regime in 2001, Finland initially appeared not to have the same problems as had begun to occur in Germany, Italy and Spain, for example. In December 2001, however, the first case of BSE in a domestically reared cow was reported.

• Finnish policy prior to March 1996

Before Finland joined the EEA in 1994 and the EU in 1995, the importation of farm animals was subject to the consent of MAF. Levels of imports were very low.

Between 1980 and 1990, Finland imported almost 120 000 tonnes of meat and bone meal. The major source was the Netherlands, but others included Austria, Denmark, Germany, New Zealand and Sweden. However, the use of imported meat and bone meal in feed for ruminants was banned in 1990. This measure, along with a ban on imports of British cattle and a policy of monitoring already imported

cattle, was seen by the Government as prudent and sufficient.

Between 1980 and 2000, Finland imported between 919 and 1148 live cattle from countries in which BSE was known to be present. When the Government of Finland imposed a ban on the import of British cattle, it stated that the country contained only 84 cattle that had been imported directly from the United Kingdom (European Commission, 2002a,b).[19] It is known that some of these, including 11 cases from farms with established BSE cases in the same birth cohort, went into feed-chains or food-chains.

Domestically, however, little was done to monitor actively for BSE. Between 1990 and 1996, the number of cattle brains tested annually for BSE varied between 5 and 23, and this testing was based only on examination of reported suspects. Until 1995, it was lawful for farmers in Finland to use domestically produced ruminant protein in animal feed. Under those conditions, therefore, if BSE had entered Finland it might have been amplified domestically through the closed loop of the food-chain. That practice, banned within the EU in 1994, was prohibited when Finland joined the EU in 1995.

---

[19] Eurostat/UK recorded, however, that 127 cattle were exported from the United Kingdom to Finland during the period cited by the Government of Finland. The reason for the discrepancy between these two figures is not known (European Commission, 2002b).

in four countries and the European Community

• Finnish policy after March 1996

Since 1995 (when Finland became an EU member), all measures to control BSE have derived from European Commission requirements. Finnish officials who were interviewed said that until the discovery of BSE in Finland in December 2001, many in the Finnish administration assumed that the domestic measures required under European Commission rules were necessary only for legal and administrative reasons but were scientifically unnecessary and that they represented a disproportionately high cost.

Since March 1996, beef of British origin has been excluded from the food-chain in Finland. In 1996, all animals imported from the United Kingdom were ordered to be removed from the human and animal food-chains, examined in case of death, and destroyed when owners surrendered them. By 1997 the offspring of cattle imported from Britain had been tracked down and excluded from the food-chain. Since the beginning of 2001 special surveillance measures have been applied to all ruminants imported from countries in which BSE has been found. At the time of slaughter, their origin and age have to be reported. All ruminants over 20 months have to be tested.

Since 1998, EU legislation requires producers to report cases of cows over 20 months of age with suspected symptoms of BSE to municipal veterinarians (European Commission, 1998). In the same year, a national system for cattle identification was introduced that enabled information on the bovine products' country of origin to be provid-ed, as required under current Finnish legislation. Since then the number of BSE-screened cattle has been higher than in previous years (European Commission, 2002b).

The Commission's 1996 proposal for an EU-wide bovine offal ban, as noted previously, was not actually introduced until June 2000. Finland was not one of those few Member States that introduced their own ban in the interim. Furthermore, until the introduction of EU-wide controls in 2001, it remained lawful to feed ruminant proteins to non-ruminant farm animals. Finnish authorities allowed the feeding of cow fat to cattle until 2000, and pig fat was used in calf feeding until early 2001. Separate production lines for animal feeds containing meat and bone meal were not required until 2001.

Under European Commission rules, Finland started BSE screening in 2001. However, Finland was allowed an exception and was not required to screen all cattle slaughtered at the age of more than 30 months. During 2001, a total of 20 000 cows were to be tested for BSE. In addition, a sample of about 5000 healthy non-suspect cows were to be tested (European Commission, 2001).

In February 2001, a suspected case was provisionally identified but subsequent histopathological tests on that animal were all negative. The Ministry of Agriculture and Forestry in Helsinki did, however, report Finland's first (and so far only) case of BSE on 7 December 2001. The disease was detected in a dairy cow born in Finland in 1995. No meat or bone meal had reportedly been

A chronology of BSE policy

used in that herd for more than 20 years. No evidence of BSE was found in any of the other animals in that herd. The authorities presented the finding of this first case as proof that surveillance works, noting that the cow had been identified as a risk animal prior to slaughtering. To date, no conclusion has been reached about the source of the infection, although suspected sources include vegetable-based protein supplements contaminated by meat and bone meal or contaminated fat in milk-replacer feeds for calves.

The case has raised concern about animal feed in Finland, and attention has been drawn to the problem of identifying sources of feed, since according to the European Commission regulations only nutritional content is required to be reported. According to the media and to interviews with Finnish authorities in the aftermath of the first BSE case, it became evident that, even though countries such as Denmark had suspected that BSE could spread through the use of fat products, the Finnish authorities had considered such products to be safe.[20] They also considered the German decision to ban all animal-based feed for cows to be politically motivated. Continuing to allow feeding with animal fat was justified by the lack of evidence that it might be risky. While the European Commission had forbidden the use of animal proteins for feeding cows, the use of fats was considered safe.

---

[20] See for example *Helsingin Sanomat* 08.12.2001, 09.12.2002 and 19.12.2002 (http://helsinginsanomat.fi).

References

Anderson RM et al. (1996) Transmission dynamics and epidemiology of BSE in British cattle. *Nature*, 382:779–788.

Anon. (1989) Meat imports into the Federal Republic of Germany from the United Kingdom. Telex Message, 1989, *BSE Inquiry Year Book* No. 89/08.21/8.1. In: Phillips et al. (2000) op. cit.

Böschen S, Dressel K, Schneider M, Viehhöver W. (2002) Pro und Kontra der Trennung von Risikobewertung und Risikomanagement – Diskussionsstand in Deutschland und Europa. Im Rahmen des TA-Projekts "Strukturen der Organisation und Kommunikation im Bereich der Erforschung übertragbarer spongiformer Enzephalopathien. [Pros and cons of the separation between risk assessment and risk management – state of discussion in Germany and Europe. In the context of the technology assessment project: structures of the organisation and communication on the exploration field transmissible spongiform encephalopathies]. *TAB-Hintergrundbericht*, No. 10.

Bradley R (1988) BSE research project. Minute dated 19 July 1988 to WA Watson. *BSE Inquiry Year Book* Number 88/07.19/2.1–2.2. In: Phillips et al. (2000) op. cit.

Carvel J (1994) Shephard retaliates in German meat war. *Guardian*, 26 April, p.7.

Court of Auditors (2001) Special Report No 4/2001. *Official Journal of the European Communities*, 20.11.2001, C 324.

DEFRA (2002) *Statistics*. (http://www.defra.gov.uk/animalh/bse/statistics/incidence.html.)

Donnelly CA et al. (2002) Implications of BSE infection screening data for the scale of the British BSE epidemic and current European infection levels. *Proceedings of the Royal Society*, 269:2179–2190.

Estades J, Le Pape Y, de Looze M (1999) *BSE and the Italian national action system*. (http://www.grenoble.inra.fr/Docs/pub/A1999/BASEITA.pdf)

European Commission (1996) *Commission decision 96/239/EC total ban on dispatch of live cattle and all products from the UK.*

European Commission (1998) *Commission decision of 23 April*

in four countries and the European Community

1998 on epidemio-surveillance for transmissible spongiform encephalopathies and amending Decision 94/474/EC.

European Commission (1999) *Opinion of the Scientific Steering Committee on the human exposure risk (HER) via food with respect to BSE*. Adopted on 10 December 1999. (http://europa.eu.int/comm/food/fs/sc/ssc/out67_en.pdf.)

European Commission (2000a) *Commission Decision of 5 June 2000 amending Decision 98/272/EC on epidemio-surveillance for transmissible spongiform encephalopathies.*

European Commission (2000b) *Report on the assessment of the geographical BSE-risk (GBR) of Germany*, July 2000:36. (http://europa.eu.int/comm/food/fs/sc/ssc/out120_en.pdf.)

European Commission (2001) *Report of a mission carried out in Finland from 23/04/2001 to 27/04/2001 in order to evaluate the implementation of protection measures against bovine spongiform encephalopathy (BSE)*. DG/SANCO)/3283/2001. (http://europa.eu.int/comm/food/fs/inspections/vi/reports/finland/index_en.html.)

European Commission (2002a) *Opinion on the six BARB BSE cases in the UK since 1 August 1996*, 2001. Adopted by the SSC at its meeting of 29–30 November 2002:9. (http://europa.eu.int/comm/food/fs/sc/ssc/out237_en.pdf.)

European Commission (2002b) *Final report on the updated assessment of the geographical BSE-risk (GBR) of Finland*. (http://europa.eu.int/comm/food/fs/sc/ssc/out262_en.pdf.)

European Commission Food and Health Office (2001) *Draft report of a veterinary mission to Germany with regard to the implementation of Commission decisions 98/272/EC and 94/381/EC and Council Regulation 1760/2000/EC.*

European Parliament (1996) *Replies from the Commission to questions from the Committee Members, Temporary Committee of Inquiry into BSE*. Doc. PE 218.980, 18 September 1996:9–10.

European Parliament (1997) *Report on alleged contravention or maladministration in the implementation of Community law in relation to BSE. Part B. Work of the Committee of Inquiry and basic data*. Doc_EN\RR\319\319055 A4-0020/97B, 7 February 1997:27.

Eurostat (1998) Animal production. *Quarterly Statistics*, 2.

FAO (2001) *More than 30 countries have taken action on BSE, but more needs to be done.*. Food and Agriculture Organization of the United Nations Rome, Press Release 01/41, 21 June 2001. (http://www.fao.org/WAICENT/OIS/PRESS_NE/PRESSENG/2001/preno141.htm.)

Federal Health Office (1993) *Bericht und Fazit des Bundesgesundheitsamts zum Symposium "Übertragbare spongiforme Enzephalopathien". [Report and conclusions of the Federal Health Office regarding the symposium "transmissible spongiform encephalopathies"].*

Fleetwood A (1998) *Statement No. 127 to BSE Inquiry* 15. In: Phillips et al., 2000, op. cit., Disc 11.

FSA (2000) *Review of BSE controls, December 2000*. London, FSA.

Hansard (1996) 20 March 1996.

Kimberlin RH, Cole S, Walker CA (1987) Temporary and permanent modifications to a single strain of mouse scrapie on transmission to rats and hamsters. *Journal of General Virology*, 68:1875–1881.

Lawrence A (1998) *Statement No. 76 to BSE Inquiry*, para 135:24. In: Phillips et al., 2000, op. cit., Disc 11.

Ministry of Agriculture, Fisheries and Food (1990) Memorandum to House of Commons Select Committee on Agriculture. *Bovine Spongiform Encephalopathy (BSE)*, June 1990.

Office International des Epizooties (2002) *Number of reported cases of bovine spongiform encephalopathy (BSE) worldwide (excluding the United Kingdom)*. (http://www.oie.int/eng/info/en_esbmonde.htm.)

Phillips N, Bridgeman J, Ferguson-Smith M (2000) *The BSE Inquiry: Report: evidence and supporting papers of the inquiry into the emergence and identification of Bovine Spongiform Encephalopathy (BSE) and variant Creutzfeldt-Jakob Disease (vCJD) and the action taken in response to it up to 20 March 1996*. London, The Stationery Office. (http://www.bseinquiry.gov.uk/index.htm.)

Niederschrift über die Sitzung der Referenten der für das Veterinärwesen und Lebensmittelüberwachung zuständigen obersten Landesbehörden. [Speakers of the highest regional authorities responsible for veterinary issues and food surveillance.] Minutes of the meeting held on 5 August 1996:3.

Spongiform Encephalopathy Advisory Committee (2001) *Minutes of the 71st meeting held on 21 November 2001 at DEFRA.* (http://www.seac.gov.uk/papers/mins21-11-01.pdf.)

Chapter 3

Assessing public perception: issues and methods

Assessing public perception: issues and methods

Elizabeth Dowler, Judith Green, Martin Bauer, Giancarlo Gasperoni

Public perception of the relationship between food, risk and health has formed a critical element in the BSE and CJD affair. One of the criticisms of the Public Inquiry into the BSE situation (Phillips et al., 2000) was that the British Government had taken an outdated paternalistic attitude to public views, seeing the public as being in need of protection rather than generating informed debate (Klein, 2000). The necessity of taking public views into account was demonstrated by the dramatic drop in beef consumption in early 1996, and on subsequent occasions whenever particular events or circumstances occurred (and were announced officially or reported in the media) that fuelled anxieties about the safety of meat. Misjudging the public's expectations about information arguably led to a crisis of faith, not only in British food production but in the very processes of democratic decision-making (Eldridge et al., 1998). What people seem generally to think or believe influences their behaviour — and plays a vital role in shaping events. Policy-makers, especially those responsible for information policy, face significant challenges in assessing public perceptions and in shaping policy that takes information needs into account and responds adequately to key concerns.

This chapter reviews key issues in understanding public perceptions, and assesses various methods currently in use for examining them. In particular, it discusses the strengths and weaknesses of different methods, how costly and complex they are to implement, and the value of the information they provide for different policy actors. It is not concerned with methods for involving users in policy-making, but with those aiming to access existing views.

The term "public perception" is difficult to define. At one level, an instrumental or pragmatic definition is possible: public perception is simply the type of information obtained from a public opinion survey. That is, "public opinion" is merely the aggregate views of a group of people (usually a randomly selected sample) who are asked directly what they think about particular issues or events. Answers to structured questions can be recorded and analysed in simple, quantitative terms as a sort of "snapshot" of opinion at a given moment in time.

However, the relationship between replies given to opinion pollsters and any "real" opinion or view is contentious. There are clearly no direct ways to access the true beliefs of members of the public in all their complexity, and researchers are reliant on more or less valid methods for accessing them indirectly, through replies given to specific questions. There is a substantial literature on ways to refine questionnaires to minimize biases and assess validity (for example, see Woodward & Chambers, 1991; Petersen, 2000), but even the best designed opinion poll is restricted to gathering fairly superficial opinions.

More significantly, the "perceptions" accessed at one point in time from one individual are not necessarily representative of their views at other times, or in other contexts. Beliefs are not simply the result of linear knowledge acquisition. Perception involves understanding (or misunderstanding) and discernment, and includes an element of volition and action: people choose to "see" things in certain ways, and the social and cultural determinants of those choices differ with time and place. Further, many beliefs are the product of social interaction. The very act of voicing and discussing opinions leads to their development. Behaviour and practice are conditioned and shaped not only by beliefs but also by the reflexive processes of social interaction, through which behaviour is challenged or reinforced and modified by the views of others. Knowledge and experience operate within various social frameworks, including the nature and degree of people's trust in scientific experts and authority. This being the case, the process of capturing public perceptions and their concomitant outcomes through research has to be correspondingly complex.

One of the serious challenges facing governments, agencies and other policy actors is that they do not have the luxury of engaging in lengthy research to reach such in-depth understanding. They need reasonably reliable indicators of public perception and factors that affect public trust, along with methods for capturing and interpreting such indicators. These methods need to be affordable and to produce results within reasonably short time-frames.

This chapter reviews and comments on several methods currently available and being used, and discusses their potential value to policy-makers.

▾ Issues
• Perceptions of health and risk in industrialized societies

Risk is one of the key areas of public perception on which policy-makers need information. Public perception of risk is a topic of considerable interest and urgency in the public policy arena throughout the industrialized world. In academic circles, the expansion of consumer and risk literature is cited as evidence of the growing crises of late modernity (Beck, 1992; Adam, 1995). Because the public increasingly mistrusts the ability of governments or international agencies to manage the social, physical, natural and technological environments, a sense of fragmentation and the growth of pluralist extremes (particularly political ones) is said to be increasing. Over recent decades, research and debate have addressed these issues from a number of perspectives (for examples, see Douglas & Wildavsky, 1982; Giddens, 1990; Beck, 1992; Green, 1997; Lupton, 1999; Millstone & van Zwanenberg, 2000).

This growth in mistrust is as true of food as it is of many other aspects of modern life. As Caplan (2000) puts it, "eating has become a risky business". It is claimed that anxieties of various kinds about food have intensified in recent years, despite the evident sophistication of the food system experienced by most European consumers every day, and the improvements to the reliability and safety of the modern food supply (see, for instance, Frewer, Howard & Shepherd, 1998; Miles & Frewer, 2001; Frewer & Salter, 2002). Anxieties about food risks typify the contemporary "riskiness" of modern life described by Beck (1992): its very "everyday" nature means that everyone is potentially exposed to hidden or undetectable threats to health and safety (Draper & Green, 2002).

Assessing public perception:

Since risk detection increasingly relies on expert assessment, and its management on professional monitoring and regulation, ordinary people are largely excluded from the process, except in the management of domestic hygiene (Green, Draper & Dowler, 2003). What Beck calls the "scientization" of risk (Beck, 1992:170) contributes to public mistrust: the ever more sophisticated food system relies on processes that may inherently increase risk (such as pesticide residues in foods or biotechnological manipulation of crops). Furthermore, the success of the modern food system in providing a secure abundance of varied, high-quality foodstuffs has resulted in increasing consumer expectations, including those of quality and safety.

As Beardsworth & Keil (1997:171) point out, the levels of seriousness that consumers ascribe to such hazards "may be very different from those calculated by scientists, who may perceive a rather different hierarchy of risks". Whether they are responsible for household food purchasing and preparation or not, all consumers have to eat: all are thus involved in balancing diverse risks against other sets of benefits, including less tangible aspects of cultural and social identity, as well as taste, pleasure and convenience. Their perception of "food safety" may include a wide variety of elements such as purity (constructed as avoidance of adulteration), hygiene (avoidance of contamination) and healthiness (avoidance of ill health). Indeed, to an increasing number of consumers, "healthy food" includes the notion of a sustainable food system that not only minimizes risks to individuals but also to the natural environment, and to social

and economic well-being (Tansey & Worsley, 1995; Marsden et al., 2000; Mepham, 2000; Lang et al., 2001; McMichael, 2001). Unfortunately, these perceptions and how they translate to behaviour are imperfectly understood: as a result, the cultural, social and economic dimensions of food choice, as well as wider issues of trust (in government, in producers and farmers, in the food system), tend to be ignored in food-related research and policy response (Caplan, 1997).

Public responses to problems and occasional food safety crises have often been simplified in policy perceptions to "public misunderstanding of science" or mistrust in "experts", and to failures of communication — a communication that is constructed as one-way and instrumental (McKee et al., 1996). The literature on public perception of risk in food as part of environmental health suggests that critical debates in other fields have not penetrated this area — notably the debate about *whose* perceptions, voices and priorities should be taken into account in problem identification and measurement, participation and policy response.

• Perceptions and beliefs: a "lay epidemiology"?

A potentially useful advance in current thinking about the dislocation between public and expert assessments of risk is the development of research on what has been termed "lay epidemiology" (Davison et al., 1991). Lay epidemiology investigates public belief systems about risk vulnerability from the perspective that public perceptions are not irrational or ignorant and in need of correction by further information; rather, they are seen as coherent

issues and methods

and rational in terms of the social and cultural contexts within which they are held. In studies of issues such as heart disease (Davison et al., 1991), immunization policy (Rogers & Pilgrim, 1995) and accidents (Green, 1997), qualitative research has identified a logic in lay beliefs that in fact mirrors that of the experts. Although individual perceptions of risk may appear at a superficial level to be opposed to expert opinion, the underlying rationale may be very similar. There is evidence that the public is sophisticated in its understanding of both the concept of population risk and the limits to using population-based knowledge (derived from a variety of research techniques) to inform individual-level risk assessments. These findings may be generalizable to the issue of food safety.

There is also a symbolic element to lay epidemiology, in terms of what Sperber (1990) has identified as an "epidemiology of beliefs". In addition to monitoring the progress of a disease process in relation to infectious or toxic agents (such as those that cause BSE or CJD), it can be argued that there is a need to monitor the parallel progress of the "symbolic environment" — an environment of perceptions and beliefs — in which the various actors operate.

Public perceptions on issues like food safety are conditioned by a wider environment of public beliefs. An example is perceptions of the trustworthiness of scientific experts or government, both to give appropriate and accurate information (e.g. about a disease and how it can be avoided) and to implement systems to prevent or reduce negative effects. Trust in public institutions is one of the factors that influences assessments of risks (Freudenburg, 1993), and has been described as the major mediator of uncertainty in modern societies (Giddens, 1991). In terms of individual opinions, public perceptions may or may not coincide with the latest scientific advice. They reflect the particular characteristics both of the belief (e.g. some beliefs spread more easily than others) and of the people who hold them (e.g. some people are more susceptible to certain sorts of belief).

Symbolic representations spread widely because it is their core elements, associations and metaphorical imagery that make up beliefs. They help to familiarize the public with unfamiliar threats, and render concrete and objectify otherwise abstract concepts into a topic about which people can talk and make decisions. In practical terms, the two main functions of symbolic representations in social life are to permit familiarity and to enable communication (Farr & Moscovici, 1984; Bauer & Gaskell, 1999).

Representations of this kind are part of the public sphere within which government (international, national and local), producers, distributors and consumers go about their business. At one level, representations circulate in informal conversations, such as in local cafes or bars or any kind of gathering where the relevant issue (in this case, BSE or CJD) can become a topic of conversation. At another level, representations circulate in the mass media, which for many people are an important source of information on remote topics that affect people indirectly or hypothetically (see Chapter 6).

Assessing public perception:

• Who needs to know and why?

Critical questions in this discussion are why such surveillance needs to be done, and who is interested in such information and why? In principle, there are a number of reasons for policy-makers at various levels to investigate public perceptions of risk. These include objectives such as:

• determining public priorities for policy action (needs assessment);

• assessing views of the impact of current policy (policy evaluation);

• assessing views of various policy options (policy formation);

• determining the effectiveness of information about policy (public understanding); and

• devising successful communication strategies (policy implementation).

These elements reflect different needs for information at different stages in the policy process and among different policy actors. Clearly, the methods for producing any of this information must be appropriate to each need.

National (as well as regional and local) governments want to predict popular perceptions for several reasons. Positive incentives include the prospect of improving governance and managing policy responses more effectively (for instance, to avoid "scares" escalating into "crises"). More contentiously, it is possible that less constructive political motives sometimes exist, such as helping to avoid culpability or shift responsibility. Lomas (1997), for instance, suggests that consulting users can be used to mitigate responsibility for difficult policy decisions. Even

without conscious "spinning" (i.e. interpreting a statement or event in a way that will influence public opinion), research results will inevitably be used to further different actors' agendas. Describing the uses to which a survey of clients of maternity services was put, Martin (1990:164) notes that "each group with an interest in the survey's findings was looking to it to produce data to support their own views". She describes how decision-makers in the health service used the results to vindicate a decision to close one unit, while a users' group interpreted the results as indicating the need to maintain all local services.

International bodies, such as the European Commission or the FAO/WHO Codex Alimentarius Commission, have mandates to regulate product safety throughout the food system, and therefore may have an interest in the public's perceptions of food safety standards, and their monitoring and implementation. The European Commission is actively establishing a new European Food Safety Authority (EFSA) that will be responsible for advising the Commission and all Member States on a wide range of food safety issues. Given that the evidence presented in this study suggests that there are significant differences within and between Member States, it may be especially important for the EFSA to develop sophisticated ways of monitoring and engaging with public beliefs, attitudes and aspirations. This would involve a change of roles since, like national governments, international public health bodies' surveillance regarding food has usually focused on the short term and the immediate (outbreaks of infection and contamination) rather than links to

issues and methods

longer-term hazards such as chronic or non-infectious disease (Shetty & James, 1997; Lang & Rayner, 2001).

It may be particularly important to take public perceptions into account when policy decisions have to be made on criteria that are political or value-driven rather than technical. The allocation of scarce resources in health care is one example that has attracted considerable debate (Lomas, 1997; Lenaghan, 1999), as the public have increasingly been canvassed by governments wanting both legitimacy for value judgements about health-care rationing and credibility for the decisions taken.

It is widely accepted that trade and sectoral economic concerns have generally underpinned most food-policy deliberations (see, for example, Cannon, 1988; Tansey & Worsley, 1995; Humphrys, 2001; Lang et al., 2001). Ample evidence is presented in this book that most policy-makers regard the public's reactions as significant only when people refuse to purchase commodities whose trade guarantees jobs and national economic stability. Thus, attempts to emphasize (or introduce to debate) food as an issue of public health, as opposed to one of economics, have met with resistance — in practice if not on paper — in Europe (Lang, 1999; Lang & Rayner, 2001).

In practice, as this book illustrates, most government institutions in fact use "communication strategies" largely to reassure and maintain confidence in product quality and safety. Moreover, as well as constructing the public according to what it buys, surveillance methods are not usually seen as two-way: what and who is measured is decided by professionals, who also determine the uses to which information is put. The process is largely extractive, so that the public, from whom information is obtained, often by contracted professionals using quantitative survey methods, are passive providers rather than actively engaged in expressing their concerns (Chambers, 1997, among many). The FSA in the United Kingdom has employed a range of strategies in recent years to consult the public, although as yet the impact on policy practice has not been documented (see the FSA web site for examples at http://www.food.gov.uk). Few communication strategies appear to recognize the complex assessment processes employed by individual members of the public, and which may affect their judgements and purchasing behaviour in diverse ways.

• Constructing the public: consumers or citizens?

The tendency to equate "the public" with "consumers" brings up a significant and controversial issue, in which a political concept is conflated with an economic one — arguably to the detriment of a political process built on ideas about citizenship. There is considerable concern that the citizen is being redefined as a purchaser whose "ballots ... help create and maintain the trading areas, shopping centres, products, stores and the like" (Dickinson & Hollander, 1991). Such a tendency is clearly an over-simplification, which constructs the public as no more than a collection of individual economic agents making choices, with quantifiable consequences. Those who have money with which to make purchases, or a means of exchange, can participate in a marketplace.

Assessing public perception:

A public composed of citizens, on the other hand, is more complex. As Gabriel & Lang (1995:174) argue:

> ... the idea of citizen implies mutuality and control as well as a balance of rights and duties .... Citizens are active members of communities, at once listened to, but also prepared to defer to the will of the majority. Citizens have to argue their views and engage with the views of others. In as much as they can make choices, citizens have a sense of superior responsibility. As a citizen, one must confront the implications of one's choices, their meaning and their moral value. ... citizenship has at its core a 'bond'.

In this interpretation, citizens are recognized as members of overlapping communities with networks of loyalties and communication, in which beliefs, attitudes and practices revolve and mesh in complex ways.

This concept of citizenship should carry strong resonance for governments or agencies keen to understand and engage with public perceptions about food and risk. Economic indicators of purchase (consumption) cannot easily be interpreted to take account of these apparently intangible factors, which can nonetheless have powerful effects on apparently straightforward behavioural outcomes. Stability in the marketplace cannot simply be interpreted as evidence of public confidence or trust. If they are viewed as heterogenous citizens, the public will be assigned an engaged and potentially more active role in risk assessment and management.

The relationship between the state and the public (the latter constructed either as citizens or as consumers) has been highly contested in recent decades. The phenomenon known as "consumer power" has become a battleground, with one side seeing it as a basis for asserting collective values and the other as a support for privatization of formerly public services such as energy or water utilities (Gabriel & Lang, 1995). Tellingly, the tendency for information and communication activities to focus either on value-for-money initiatives or on consumer complaints or advice reveal a preoccupation with the interests of individual consumers rather than reflecting the wider interests of the public.

Yet the conflation of citizens and consumers is not complete, and arguably the distinctions are re-emerging in the new millennium. The BSE/CJD crisis itself may have contributed to the resurgence of ideas about collective, as opposed to individual, responsibilities. The concerns of large numbers of people about the risks presented by food, together with the opacity of increasingly complex food systems, have reinforced the notion that many parts of everyday life cannot simply be left to the market to run, driven by the decisions of consumers acting individually according to the laws of supply and demand. As agents of the nation state, governments have duties and responsibilities to citizens to ensure a safe and healthy food supply. These are usually implemented through regulation and enforcement. In recent years, the relationship between such statutory

issues and methods

duties and the private-sector retail providers has evolved with such increasing complexity that the benefits to consumers are ever harder to establish (Marsden et al., 2000).

• **Representing the public: by "bodies" or by research**
However "the public" is interpreted, some means has to be used to represent its perceptions, preferences and concerns. In practice, policy-makers have only imperfect indicators of what are essentially private views, derived from the public accounts people provide.

Representation by "bodies" means that the public is directly represented by specific individuals who participate in a publicly accountable decision-making group such as a parliament or government, or a commission or task force. The latter type of group usually focuses on a specific issue with a given time limit. Political representation has a different time dimension: politicians are usually elected for a lengthy period, which means that voters are endorsing their decision-making ability for several years, even though there might be individual decisions with which constituents are unhappy. Equally, public representation bodies, such as a consumer council, may make particular decisions, or support positions, that do not accord with the views of all consumers. However, both types of "body" should be open to public scrutiny and acceptance or rejection, on a regular basis.

The legitimacy of all such bodies to represent public perceptions is open to challenge along several lines. Even when a range of stakeholder groups are included on a commission or task force, the choice of person or institu-

tion to represent different interests can be contentious, as there may be several competing organizations. A variety of questions can and should be asked: Whose interests are represented by those with power? Whose voices and interests are excluded? To what extent do those being represented feel that their views are fully and accurately expressed? What means do they have to redress any imbalances? (For discussion and case studies of such issues, see the recent publication by the English National Consumer Council (2002) on promoting effective consumer involvement in decision-making and policy-making.)

Public opinion can also be represented through research, using methods such as those described in this book (surveys, focus groups, media content analysis, or interpretation of behavioural outcome data such as expenditure patterns or votes). Such representation, particularly by survey or focus group, can be almost immediate and very issue-specific. Its legitimacy as a basis for decision-making can be challenged on grounds of the time-bounded nature of responses that are made, as well as methodological aspects of the research instruments used (their scientific probity, reliability and validity). However, unless every member of the public is to be personally consulted on every issue at stake (an unattainable ideal: individuals cannot get involved in all issues that affect them, nor do they always want to), the views of both the general public as a whole, or of defined groups within it, have to be represented in some way in order to influence government decision-making processes. The two forms of representation outlined here complement each other and should be kept in balance.

Assessing public perception:

• Information as an input to policy-making processes

There are basic technical difficulties in constructing an appropriate evidence base for defining problems or evaluating interventions in complex areas such as public health. These issues are widely discussed in the literature. For instance, Joffe & Mindell (2002:137), in offering a framework for the information needed to assess the health impact of complex interventions, argue that providing:

> ... an evidence base is a far from trivial exercise. It needs to use the best available evidence, bringing together authoritative reviews (where available) and research papers from a variety of disciplines. It also needs to include qualitative research, and evidence from the specific policy areas such as transport or fiscal policy as well as in the health sciences.

These commentators insist that even complex interventions in public health, which of necessity involve social policy decisions, are in fact amenable to systematic review and experimental design.

In this they are taking a stand within a powerful contemporary debate about the nature of public policy-making, and the use of evidence within it (Packwood, 2002). The discussion so far has been predicated on the assumption that information about public perceptions is not only needed to inform rational policy-making processes, but is provided so that it will be used. The basis for this assumption is the popular and enduring problem-solving

model, in which dispassionate civil servants use research and information either to fill an identified knowledge gap in the policy process or to establish an evidence base for future decision-making. This assumption, while convenient, has frequently been contested (Lindblom, 1959; Hogwood & Gunn, 1984; MacRae, 1991; Fisher, 1998).

Within public health, as in other arenas, there has been considerable debate over the role of evidence of different kinds in decision-making (examples include: Walt, 1994; Berridge & Thom, 1996; Macintyre & Petticrew, 2000). For instance, Elliott & Popay (2000) argue that the problem-solving model does not explain or inform policy-making as it is in fact practised, or does so only incompletely. In their examination of policy-making by local health authorities in the United Kingdom, they demonstrate that research plays a more subtle and less central role than the problem-solving model implies. In their study, Elliott & Popay (2000:467) report:

> ...research played a variety of parts, ranging from providing perspectives and indeed 'answers' to immediate policy questions, illuminating wider policy issues, developing new purchasing roles and negotiating relationships with users and providers. The 'developmental' aspects of the research process were particularly striking .... Some aimed to build ongoing 'dialogical' relationships with researchers to reflect on practice as well as develop policy ... [though these were] often goals to aspire to rather than an accurate reflection of practice.

issues and methods

... this need to weigh up different interests and the value judgements involved in bringing evidence to bear on policy are fundamental aspects of policy-makers' jobs not accounted for by the problem-solving model.

Understanding how research really feeds into policy is critical to rethinking how mechanisms for incorporating public perceptions can be devised in order to improve planning and policy capacities (see, for example, Macintyre et al., 2001; Percy-Smith et al., 2002).

▾ Methods
• Numbers versus narratives: quantitative and qualitative methods

In the research described in this book, the study team used a multi-strategy approach, integrating quantitative and qualitative methods within the large, single project. Most technical discussions of social research methods begin with a distinction between quantitative and qualitative research. While there is some debate in the social science community about the validity of the distinction, it remains a standard way of thinking about investigation into social reality. Much has been made of the differences or parallels between the two approaches (or modes of enquiry), of the need for understanding and respect between adherents of the two traditions, and of the need to explore common ground and usage (e.g. Brannen, 1992; Hammersley, 1996).

It is important to understand that the differences between the two approaches go deeper than the fact that one emphasizes measurement and the other does not.

Bryman (2001), among many others, notes that quantitative and qualitative enquiry are generally accepted as having different epistemological and ontological bases. For example, qualitative research tends to be inductive and more concerned with the generation of theories than with testing them. In contrast, quantitative research has a deductive orientation. Quantitative methods are rooted in the empiricist tradition and apply the ostensibly objective and value-free methods used in the natural sciences to the study of social realities. Qualitative methods are described as "interpretivist" in their emphasis on understanding individuals' social reality, and the intentions, motives, beliefs and social rules and values that infuse this with meaning. This is also referred to as an "insider" (or "EMIC") perspective. Practitioners of qualitative research (and researchers) do not assume it to be value-free. It is carried out from a different ontological position — that of constructionism. This position not only emphasizes the constant state of change in social phenomena, but also holds that the categories used to understand both the natural and social world are themselves social products. In other words, these categories do not have "built-in essences" but may vary depending on where, when, and by whom they are studied.

The following sections of this chapter discuss three methods of social research that can be useful in gauging public perceptions: focus groups, surveys, and content analysis. A final method, the use of outcomes as indirect indicators of public perceptions, is also touched on briefly. Examples from a range of policy fields are pro-

Assessing public perception:

vided to illustrate how the kinds of data produced can be utilized by policy-makers. The empirical chapters in this book demonstrate the potential for using similar findings in the field of food safety policy.

The strengths and weaknesses of each method are examined briefly, along with practical considerations such as their cost and the ease with which they can be "contracted-out" to private service-providers. Examples drawn from the United Kingdom are provided to illustrate how and why each method has been used. A summary of the characteristics of each method is provided in Table 3.1 at the end of this chapter. While considering their differences, it should also be borne in mind that there are also important similarities. In all quantitative and many qualitative methods, the quality of the data obtained depends on key technical factors such as structure and procedures for sampling, the framing and ordering of questions, analytical frameworks and interpretative rigour. Above all, it should be remembered that the aims of any given inquiry must inform the choice of method — and that the best solution may be to use a mix of methods, each accessing public perceptions via different means. That was, in fact, the approach taken in this investigation into public perceptions of risk and BSE/CJD.

• Focus groups

Originally devised as a market research tool for identifying trends or analysing customer satisfaction, focus groups are prime examples of qualitative research. They have been widely used in recent years as a method for accessing public perception by policy-makers on issues as diverse as users' feelings about vaccination information (Evans et al., 2001), acceptability of HIV health promotion materials (Kitzinger, 1990) and risks from the nuclear industry (Waterton & Wynne, 1999).

A focus group typically brings together between six and twelve participants who are representative of the target group whose attitudes, beliefs and perceptions need to be investigated. Professional facilitators lead the participants through a carefully planned agenda of research questions. The participants may be recruited using random selection (in order to gain representation of a cross-section of the general population) or purposively (in order to access the views of specific segments of the population). Depending on the purpose of the research, groups may be either homogenous or heterogenous in terms of some key social, economic or demographic characteristics. Homogenous groups are used to maximize access to the ways in which members of the public may communicate in more naturalistic settings, whereas heterogenous groups bring together a range of people precisely in order to explore differences. There are a number of manuals on how to run focus groups for research purposes (for example, see Krueger & Casey, 2000) and there is a growing social science literature on the methodology (Barbour & Kitzinger, 1999; Bloor et al., 2001).

Among the strengths of focus groups as a research method is that the group discussion format allows access to the ways in which knowledge and opinions are formed and expressed in social contexts (Kitzinger, 1994). Their

issues and methods

informal structure and setting, as well as the skills of the focus group facilitators, encourage participation by people whose voices might not otherwise be heard. The method provides detailed information — sometimes called "thick description" — about non-obvious beliefs and opinions, and about the background of attitudinal judgements. It is very useful for investigating belief structures and for understanding the symbolic basis of attitudes and nuances between different population segments. However, policy-makers using this method's results must guard against the temptation to over-generalize the findings from such small groups to larger populations.

There is some evidence that focus group methods may be less likely to access socially uncomfortable or deviant views than methods using confidential questionnaires. For example, Staley (2000:34) found that Londoners asked about financing adult education for refugees were more likely to express racist views in an anonymous self-completed questionnaire than in a discussion setting. However, using homogenous groups for sensitive issues may encourage the expression of "private" views (Farquhar & Das, 1999). Working with existing community groups also provides a useful way of accessing the views of hard-to-reach groups, whose voices are often marginal to policy-making.

In cost terms, focus groups are relatively inexpensive, although their unit costs (the cost of interviewing each participant and processing that information) are very high compared to the more mechanized quantitative methods. Firms specializing in market or social research sell this service.

Waterton & Wynne's (1999) study of public attitudes to the nuclear industry in north-west England provides a useful example of how focus groups can be used to develop a sophisticated understanding of community perceptions. In this case, the local authority was interested in community views about the proposed development of a local nuclear power plant. Focus groups were commissioned to provide a complement to the opinion polls. The focus groups revealed a far more complex attitude to risk than the polls, which had suggested that the community held simplistic and stable views. Among other findings, the focus groups showed that concerns about the nuclear industry were bound up with the community members' sense of identity as "locals" and as being resilient to risks. This identity was constructed in the face of potential stigmatization from people outside the community who might see them as risk "victims" and otherwise vulnerable. In comparing the two sets of results, the researchers found that attitudes to risks were "relational" (expressed in relation to particular social contexts), developed through the ongoing process of social interaction, and were influenced by relationships of trust (notably trust in the nuclear power plant, which was a significant employer in the area).

The same study illustrates one potential weakness of focus groups as a method for informing policy: decision-makers often find the results of focus groups difficult to use, or even to believe. Waterton & Wynne describe the

Assessing public perception:

difficulties of conveying focus group findings to the local authority in ways that were easily understood and provided clear choices for action. In general, research that reflects the complexity, ambiguity and developmental nature of public views is difficult to present in easily digestible formats for decision-makers, and deriving the "messages" for information strategies can be contentious.

• Surveys of public perceptions

Surveys of public perceptions (often referred to as opinion polling) use standard quantitative survey methods to give a rapid answer to straightforward questions, based on people's immediate answers to questions put face-to-face, on paper questionnaires, or over the telephone. Questions are designed so that answers are easily categorized and quantified (May, 2001). Standardized procedures are used to reduce bias and produce valid and replicable (reliable) results that can be generalized. There is an ongoing debate over whether such survey methods actually capture the full dimensions of public opinion. In recent years, many public opinion companies have reinforced their surveys with qualitative studies, using methods such as focus groups or semi-structured interviews to investigate in-depth feelings and motivations.

The strengths of surveys lie in their efficiency, consistency, comparability over time, generalizibility (with appropriate sampling) and ease of analysis. They are an efficient method, in that the data gathered seem to be precisely what commissioners want, and they can be relatively cheap and simple to administer. In most industrial-

ized countries, a number of companies carry out regular polls of random samples of households, and policymakers can simply add a bank of questions to these surveys. Some surveys (the European Commission's Eurobarometer surveys are prime examples) are carried out and published on a regular basis. They provide answers, repeatable if necessary, within a reasonably short time-scale, and their data are readily available and relatively inexpensive for secondary analysis. Based on structured and closed questions, they can be easily analysed and their results presented in straightforward ways for decision-makers (EUROPA, undated).

These strengths are offset by a number of weaknesses inherent to the methodology. As they reflect data based on individuals' answers to specific, relatively simple questions, they lack depth and may disproportionately access "public" views (i.e. those perceived by the interviewee to be acceptable to their peers or mainstream opinion) rather than more private or considered beliefs or attitudes. By focusing on topics of interest to those who have commissioned the surveys, the questions extract responses that in practice may distort the relative significance of those issues for respondents themselves. In addition, such results cannot be assumed to be reliable indicators or predictors of behaviour: people may give answers to questions (honestly or otherwise) that are not in fact consistent with everyday behaviour; their answers may rather reflect hopes, aspirations or intentions. The validity of public opinion surveys therefore depends on how closely the indicators chosen really measure (or represent) the concept they are designed to gauge (Bryman,

issues and methods

2001) and whether those who have commissioned the surveys actually need information on what people think or are using these as proxy indicators of likely behaviour.

As with focus groups, surveys are services for which a market exists, with a wide variety of specialist firms to choose from.

A recent example of the use of public opinion surveys to inform public policy was the Cabinet Office's "People's Panel" in the United Kingdom, commissioned from the market research firm MORI (MORI, 1998). A panel of 5000 people representative of the population of each region was recruited and used for a number of surveys on attitudes to public services, including comparative surveys on satisfaction with services. Although it has discontinued the panels, the Cabinet Office is on record as considering this to be a successful initiative that has improved the commitment of government agencies both to consulting users and to including public voices in policy development. A review of the panels by the Office of National Statistics suggests that the approach stimulated consumer research and provided "a high level feel for public opinion on a number of issues", but also noted some weaknesses, notably the high attrition rate in respondents and the finding that some members of the public "saw the Panel as symbolic rather than genuinely useful".

• Content analysis of mass media coverage
The term "content analysis" actually brings a multitude of procedures together to classify units of text for the purpose of comparing their presence or absence, their

comparative frequencies, and their co-occurrence. The basic features of content analysis include: (a) systematic sampling from a population of texts to allow for an inference from the sample to the population, (b) the development of a coding frame, (c) the coding process by which text units are classified according to agreed rules and definitions, and (d) various measures to ensure the reliability of the coding process since, in most cases, this work is conducted by several coders. The method's strength is in longitudinal comparison within and across different contexts, and over time.

Classic discussions of content analysis have stressed its "objective" character (Berelson, 1952; Holsti, 1969; Krippendorff, 1980) in contrast to the subjectivity of hermeneutical text interpretation. More recent thinking proposes that the value of content analysis lies not in its objectivity per se but in its "systematicity" and its capacity to objectify the interpretative process for the purpose of public accountability (Bauer, 2000). It is also a hybrid within the qualitative versus quantitative debate. Although ultimately content analysis aims at a quantitative description of text materials, its coding procedures require qualitative reasoning to identify non-trivial text differences. The methodological axiom of "no quantification without qualification" is particularly important in the conduct of any content analysis.

Content analysis of mass media faces two inference challenges. The first is generalizing from a sample of material to the whole corpus of media coverage on an issue, over a period of time. Carefully controlled sampling

Assessing public perception:

procedures, usually probability or random sampling, have to be used to represent the corpus of a text, without critical loss of information. The second inference problem is in interpretation beyond the text material, to be able to say something about its particular producers, readers or even the cultural context of producer-readers — the *Zeitgeist* or public opinion (Holsti, 1969). The apparent constant feedback and interaction between text producers and readers are used to support the argument that content analysis of mass media coverage does in fact represent reasonably well the changing culture of a society over time (i.e. can be generalized). Inference from texts to specific readers or specific producers is more difficult if not impossible to support (Bauer, 2000).

Unlike other social science methods, content analysis is mostly carried out by academic researchers, since few private companies carry out such work. The costs involved in this form of research are initially high, but once the initial preparatory stages are completed the cost per unit of analysis is low. Overall, its costs fall in between those of the focus group and those of the sample survey.

A recent study of images of infant feeding in the British media provides an example of how content analysis has been used to inform policy-making (Henderson et al., 2000). Taking a one-month sample of television programmes and newspaper articles in the United Kingdom, the researchers identified different cultural portrayals of breastfeeding and bottle-feeding. Breastfeeding was portrayed less often, was associated with middle-class or celebrity families, and was more likely to be linked to problems with feeding. Content analysis revealed no mention of the health benefits of breastfeeding. In contrast, bottle-feeding was portrayed as normal and unproblematic, and was associated with ordinary families. Although studies such as this cannot shed light on public perceptions (in this instance, of the relative benefits of breastfeeding and bottle-feeding), they provide essential information for policy-makers, such as those concerned with health education, on the cultural contexts within which women make infant feeding choices.

• Behavioural indicators: food consumption and expenditure patterns

A final potential source of information about public perceptions regarding food is found in the analysis of behavioural or so-called "outcome" data. Examples include indicators of consumption (household expenditure surveys, household food consumption surveys, etc.) and sales figures from the food industry. Presented as time-series, these have been used as proxy markers to investigate the impact of particular events such as food scares on purchasing behaviour, or to mark the development of longer-term trends.

This approach has several practical advantages, particularly if the data are readily available at a reasonably low price. National statistical institutions often mount annual surveys of household expenditure where purchases of different commodities are differentiated. They also sometimes run annual surveys of household food consumption (what is eaten, rather than what is purchased). These data

issues and methods

are usually in the public domain, as well as in published summary formats, and can be re-analysed to examine responses differentiated by socioeconomic, demographic or geographical groups. Data collected by retailers, or by other commercial organizations are not so readily obtained if they are market sensitive, and may be costly.

However, there are also clear difficulties about using such secondary analysis to infer public perceptions about particular food commodities. Aside from the practical question of accessibility of datasets (which may be further complicated by bad documentation, technological problems or the above-mentioned proprietary factors), such analyses must be cautious about what methods were employed to collect the data in the first place, and the fact that operational definitions used in the original research design might not adequately fit the secondary research goals. There may be many reasons why behavioural or other "outcome" data do or do not change, other than what people believe and/or consciously think. As discussed above, behaviour does not necessarily follow perception.

▼ Conclusions

There has been considerable development of methods designed to access public views in order to inform policy. The resultant data have the potential to inform decision-makers about public risk perceptions and public priorities for policy-making in the areas of risk management and risk information.

There are strengths and weaknesses in each of the approaches discussed above. Also, the appropriateness of a particular method depends on which stage in the policy process the public perception data are intended to inform (e.g. while defining the questions at the beginning of the process, or while writing detailed directives at the end) and on the nature of the particular decision being taken. Taking public perceptions into account can, in principle, improve the effectiveness of government policy, increase the public's faith in the policy-making process and ensure that information about risks resonates with public concern. In practice, however, there is limited evidence that public perceptions are incorporated into policy in any meaningful or consistent way.

This chapter has outlined several widely used methods for examining public perceptions. The following chapters explore in detail the information derived from focus groups, public opinion surveys and media content analysis in this study of the BSE/CJD crisis.

Table 3.1. Strengths and weaknesses of methods of social research: focus groups,

	Cost (estimates)	Strengths/weaknesses
Focus group	• relatively cheap, but with high unit costs • € 1500–5 000 per group, depending on recruiting needs • a study with 5 groups could cost € 7500–25 000	**Strengths:** • investigates belief structures and symbolic basis of attitudes • provides detailed descriptions from different segments of the population • high validity, and thus good for conceptual or theoretical generalization **Weaknesses:** • low reliability, and thus little basis for empirical generalization • can be difficult to provide accessible analysis for policy-makers depending on circumstances
Sample survey	• can be relatively cheap depending on quality of survey • low unit costs for question and interviews • € 500–3000 per item, depending on the quality of sample • a survey with 20 items could cost € 10 000–60 000, plus costs of further analysis	**Strengths:** • relatively simple to administer, obtain direct answers to commissioner's questions • high reliability and thus allows empirical generalization or inferences about whole populations • distribution of opinions and attitudes in a population • structured comparison of subgroups **Weaknesses:** • low validity, and thus poor for conceptual generalization • client has little control over data collection process • highly inferential from sample to population • access "public" rather than private views • may not be good indicators or predictors of actual behaviour
Content analysis	• mid-range in total cost • high initial costs (including sampling of materials and development of coding process) • very low unit costs	**Strengths:** • potential to track historical development of beliefs and ideas as presented in media • can do retrospective analysis • provides baseline **Weaknesses:** • large coordination effort in comparative research • reliability of empirical generalization • ambiguous inference: to producers, audience, and context
Outcomes data	• relatively inexpensive unless data are proprietary	**Strengths:** • potential to be used as a proxy marker, though can also be used to condone poor policy practice **Weaknesses:** • caution needed in evaluating quality of original data and its validity for the secondary research purposes • may not be valid indicator of public perceptions

surveys and content analysis

Time horizons	Practicalities
• cross-sectional • real-time data collection only, but can be used in panel design such as in citizens' panels	• can be put to tender, or done entirely or in part by researchers • large market of contractors, but researchers more likely to produce full detailed analysis
• mainly cross-sectional data • repeat measures possible • real-time data collection only	• can easily be put to tender • highly competitive market of contractors
• mainly longitudinal and cross-sectional • reconstructive data collection	• limited market of contractors means work must mainly be done by researchers themselves
• cross-sectional • needs controls for long-term trends	• many national governments collect suitable data on regular basis • limited market of contractors for reanalysis

References

Adam J (1995) *Risk.* London, University College London Press.

Barbour R, Kitzinger J, eds. (1999) *Developing focus group research: politics, theory and practice.* London, Sage.

Bauer MW (2000) Classical content analysis: a review. In: Bauer MW, Gaskell G, eds. *Qualitative analysis with text, image and sound.* London, Sage:131–151.

Bauer MW, Gaskell G (1999) Towards a paradigm for research on social representations. *Journal for the Theory of Social Behaviour,* 29:163–186.

Beardsworth A, Keil T (1997) *Sociology on the menu: an invitation to the study of food and society.* London, Routledge.

Beck U (1992) *Risk society: towards a new modernity.* London, Sage.

Berelson B (1952) *Content analysis in communication research.* Glencoe, IL, Free Press.

Berridge V, Thom B (1996) Research and policy: what determines the relationship? *Policy Studies,* 17:23–34.

Bloor M, Frankland J, Thomas M, Robson K (2001) *Focus groups in social research.* London, Sage.

Brannen J (1992) *Mixing methods: qualitative and quantitative research.* Aldershot, Avebury.

Bryman A (2001) *Social research methods.* Oxford, Oxford University Press.

Cannon G (1988) *The politics of food.* London, Century.

Caplan P, ed. (1997) *Food, health and identity.* London, Routledge.

Caplan P (2000) Eating British beef with confidence: a consideration of consumers' responses to BSE in Britain. In: Caplan P. *Risk revisited.* London, Pluto Press.

Chambers R (1997) *Whose reality counts?* London, Intermediate Technology Publications.

Cragg A, Gilbert R (2000) *Public attitudes to food safety. Report to the Food Standards Agency.* London, Cragg Ross Dawson Ltd. (http://www.food.gov.uk/multimedia/pdfs/qualitativerep.pdf.)

Cragg Ross Dawson (2002) *FSA Public Attitudes to GM. Debrief notes on qualitative research.* Prepared for COI Research Unit, London, on behalf of FSA London. (http://www.food.gov.uk/multimedia/pdfs/gmfocusgroupreport.pdf.)

Davison C, Davey Smith G, Frankel S (1991) Lay epidemiology and the prevention paradox: the implications for coronary candidacy for health education. *Sociology of Health and Illness,* 13:1–19.

Assessing public perception:

Dickinson R, Hollander SC (1991) Consumer votes. *Journal of Business Research*, 23:9–20.

Douglas M, Wildavsky A (1982) *Risk and culture: an essay on the selection of technological and environmental dangers.* Berkeley, CA, University of California Press.

Draper A, Green J (2002) Food safety and consumers: risk and choice. *Social Policy and Administration*, 36:610–625.

Eldridge J (1998) The re-emergence of BSE: the impact on public beliefs and behaviour. *Risk and Human Behaviour Newsletter*, 3:6–10.

Elliott H, Popay J (2000) How are policy makers using evidence? Models of research utilisation and local NHS policy making. *Journal of Epidemiology and Community Health*, 54:461–468.

EUROPA (undated) *Methodology – instrument description.* (http://europa.eu.int/comm/public_opinion/description_en.htm.)

Evans M et al. (2001) Parents' perspectives on the MMR immunisation: a focus group study. *British Journal of General Practice*, 51:904–910.

Farquhar C, Das R (1999) Are focus groups suitable for 'sensitive' topics? In: Barbour R, Kitzinger J, eds. *Developing focus group research.* London, Sage.

Farr R, Moscovici S, eds. (1984) *Social representations.* Cambridge, Cambridge University Press.

Fisher F (1998) Beyond empiricism: policy inquiry in postpositivist perspective. *Policy Studies Journal*, 26:129–146.

Frewer L J, Howard C, Shepherd R (1998) Understanding public attitudes to technology. *Journal of Risk Research*, 1:221–235.

Frewer L J, Salter B (2002) Public attitudes, scientific advice and the politics of regulatory policy: the case of BSE. *Science and Public Policy*, 29:137–145.

Freudenburg WR (1993) Risk and recreancy: Weber, the division of labour and the rationality of risk perception. *Social Forces*, 71:909–932.

Gabriel Y, Lang T (1995) *The unmanageable consumer: contemporary consumption and its fragmentation.* London, Sage.

Giddens A (1990) *The consequences of modernity.* Cambridge, Polity Press.

Giddens A (1991) *Modernity and self identity: self and society in the modern age.* Cambridge, Polity Press.

Green J (1997) *Risk and misfortune: the social construction of accidents.* London, UCL Press.

Green J, Draper A, Dowler E (2003) Short cuts to safety: risk and "rules of thumb" in accounts of food choice. *Health, Risk and Society*, 5:33–52.

Hammersley M (1996) The relationship between qualitative and quantitative research: paradigm loyalty versus methodological eclecticism. In: Richardson JTE, ed. *Handbook of research methods for psychology and the social sciences.* Leicester, BPS Books.

Henderson L, Kitzinger J, Green J (2000) Representing infant feeding: content analysis of British media portrayals of bottle and breast feeding. *British Medical Journal*, 321:1196–1198.

Hogwood BW, Gunn LA (1984) *Policy analysis for the real world.* Oxford, Oxford University Press.

Holsti OR (1969) *Content analysis for the social sciences and humanities.* Reading, MA, Addison-Wesley.

Humphrys J (2001) *The great food gamble.* London, Hodder & Stoughton.

Joffe M, Mindell J (2002) A framework for the evidence base to support health impact assessment. *Journal of Epidemiology and Community Health*, 56:132–138.

Kitzinger J (1990) Audience understandings of AIDS messages: a discussion of methods. *Sociology of Health and Illness*, 12:319-335.

Kitzinger J (1994) The methodology of focus groups: the importance of interaction between participants. *Sociology of Health and Illness*, 16:103–121.

Klein R (2000) The politics of risk: the case of BSE. *British Medical Journal*, 21:1091–1092.

Krueger R, Casey MA (2000) *Focus groups: a practical guide for applied research*, 3rd ed. Thousand Oaks, Sage.

issues and methods

Krippendorff K (1980) *Content analysis: an introduction to its methodology.* London, Sage.

Lang T (1999) Food and nutrition. In: Weil O, McKee M, Brodin M, Oberle D, eds. *Priorities for public health action in the European Union.* Brussels, European Commission:38–156.

Lang T, Rayner G, eds. (2001) *Why health is the key to the future of food and farming. Joint submission to the Policy Commission on the Future of Food and Farming in the UK.* (http://www.city.ac.uk/ihs/hmfp/foodpolicy/publications/pdf)

Lang T, Barling D, Caraher M (2001) Food, social policy and the environment: towards a new model. *Social Policy and Administration,* 35:538–558.

Lenaghan J (1999) Involving the public in rationing decisions: the experience of citizens juries. *Health Policy,* 49:45-61.

Lindblom CE (1959) The science of 'muddling through'. *Public Administration Review,* 19: 79–88.

Lomas J (1997) Reluctant rationers: public input into health care priorities. *Journal of Health Services Research and Policy,* 2:103–111.

Lupton D (1999) *Risk.* London, Routledge.

McKee M, Lang T, Roberts J (1996) Deregulating health: policy lessons from the BSE affair. *Journal of the Royal Society of Medicine,* 89:424–426.

McMichael P (2001) The impact of globalisation, free trade and technology on food and nutrition in the new millennium. *Proceedings of the Nutrition Society,* 60:215–220.

Macintyre S, Petticrew M (2000) Good intentions and received wisdom are not enough. *Journal of Epidemiology and Community Health,* 54:802–803.

Macintyre S et al. (2001) Using evidence to inform health policy: a case study. *British Medical Journal,* 322:222–225.

MacRae D (1991) Policy analysis and knowledge use. *Policy Sciences,* 24:28–40.

Marsden T, Flynn A, Harrison M (2000) *Consuming interests: the social provision of foods.* London, UCL Press.

Martin C (1990) How do you count maternal satisfaction? A user-commissioned survey of maternity services. In: Roberts H, ed. *Women's health counts.* London, Routledge.

May T (2001) *Social research: issues, methods and process,* 3rd ed. Buckingham, Open University Press.

Mepham TB (2000) The role of food ethics in food policy. *Proceedings of the Nutrition Society,* 59:609–618.

Miles S, Frewer LJ (2001) Investigating specific concerns about different food hazards. *Food Quality and Preference,* 12:47–61.

Millstone E, van Zwanenberg P (2000) A crisis of trust: for science, scientists or institutions? *Nature Medicine,* 6:1307–1308.

Mori (1998) *Technical report on the People's Panel main stage. Research study conducted for the Cabinet Office.* London, Cabinet Office.

National Consumer Council (2002) *Involving consumers - everyone benefits.* London, National Consumer Council (http://www.ncc.org.uk.)

Packwood A (2002) Evidence-based policy: rhetoric and reality. *Social Policy & Society,* 1:267–272.

Percy-Smith J et al. (2002) *Promoting change through research: the impact of research in local government.* York, York Publishing Services for the Joseph Rowntree Foundation.

Petersen RA (2000) *Constructing effective questionnaires.* London, Sage.

Phillips N, Bridgeman J, Ferguson-Smith M (2000) *The BSE Inquiry: Report evidence and supporting papers of the inquiry into the emergence and identification of Bovine Spongiform Encephalopathy (BSE) and variant Creutzfeldt-Jakob Disease (vCJD) and the action taken in response to it up to 20 March 1996.* London, The Stationery Office. (http://www.bseinquiry.gov.uk/report/index/htm)

Rogers A, Pilgrim D (1995) The risk of resistance: perspectives on mass childhood immunisation programmes. In: Gabe J, ed. *Medicine, health and risk.* Oxford, Blackwell.

Rychetnik L, Frommer M, Hawe P, Shiell A (2002) Criteria for evaluating evidence on public health interventions. *Journal of Epidemiology and Community Health*, 56:119-127.

Shetty PS, James WPT (1997) Determinants of disease: Nutrition. In: Detels R, Holland W, McEwan J, Omenn G, eds. *The Oxford textbook of public health*. 3rd ed. Oxford, Oxford University Press.

Sperber D (1990) The epidemiology of beliefs. In: Fraser C, Gaskell G, eds. *The social psychology of widespread beliefs*. Oxford, Clarendon Press:25–43.

Staley K (2000) *Voices, values and health: involving the public in moral decisions*. London, King's Fund.

Tansey G (1999) *Trade, intellectual property, food and biodiversity. Key issues and options for the 1999 review of Article 27.3(b) of the TRIPS Agreement*. (http://www.biotech-info.net/TRIPS.pdf.)

Tansey G, Worsley T (1995) *The food system: a guide*. London, Earthscan.

Walt G (1994) *Health policy: an introduction to process and power*. London, Zed Books, and Johannesburg, Witwatersrand University Press.

Waterton C, Wynne B (1999) Can focus groups access community views? In: Barbour R, Kitzinger J, eds. *Developing focus group research*. London, Sage.

Woodward CA, Chambers LW (1991) *Guide to questionnaire construction and questionnaire writing*. Ottawa, Canadian Public Health Association.

Chapter 4

Risk and trust: determinants of public perception

Risk and trust: determinants of public perception

Alizon Draper, Judith Green, Elizabeth Dowler, Giolo Fele, Vera Hagenhoff, Maria Rusanen, Timo Rusanen

▾ Introduction

The aims of this component of the study were to investigate consumer perceptions of BSE- and CJD-related risk, and more specifically to describe:

- how these are socially constructed;
- if and how social setting has an impact

on perceptions of risk and on trust in government and other information sources; and

- the impact of these perceptions on consumer behaviour.

BSE is only one of a number of food "scares" that have occurred in Europe during the last decade (others include *Listeria* in soft cheese, *Salmonella* in eggs and chickens and *Escherichia coli* food poisoning), although arguably none of these has produced quite the policy and public response that BSE has provoked. The reaction of the public to these food scares has been seen by some government officials and scientists as an over-reaction, and one that is not justified by the objective threat to health posed by these particular risks. This indicates a divergence, between risk as measured and assessed by official experts and scientists and risk as perceived and understood by the public. Although attention has been called to the need to communicate risk more effectively (for example, see Marmot, 1996), the huge public reaction to these food scares, and to BSE in particular, cannot be attributed simply to the misunderstanding of science by the public.

The acknowledgement that public perceptions are at variance with risk as assessed by technical experts is the starting point of most risk perception and communication studies. There is now a very large body of academic literature on risk perception in which public perceptions of the risks associated with a range of hazards, such as nuclear power, environmental pollution, road accidents and HIV/AIDS, have been examined. Much of this research is based upon organizational theory, psychometrics and cognitive psychology. It focuses on how lay people judge the comparative probability of risky situations or activities by assessing aspects of these situations that might determine these judgements, such as whether the risk is voluntary or involuntary. While providing information on how people may rank different types of risk and their relative salience, such studies provide little insight into what can be called the "semantics of risk"; they cannot illuminate the deeper reasoning and contextual understanding that inform and shape peoples' responses to risk or the role of social, cultural, economic and political factors in shaping these. Therefore, a theoretical approach drawn from sociology, anthropology and political science was used in this component of the study, and particularly the approaches to the study of risk as developed by Douglas (1986), Giddens (1991) and Beck (1992).

This part of the study used qualitative research methods — specifically focus group discussions — to compare and analyse how consumer perceptions of food and BSE/CJD-related risk were framed within the four countries.

▾ Methodology

• Data collection and analysis

The qualitative research method used in this study was the focus group discussion. The strength of this research method is that the group discussion format allows access to how knowledge and opinions are formed and expressed in social contexts (Kitzinger, 1994). The discussions were conducted using a common protocol that was piloted in the four countries and then revised on the basis of comments received. Natural groups (defined as those who either socialize or have some prior social relationship with each other outside the research setting, for instance via work, school or church) were used as much as possible. Their use permitted enhanced understanding of how risk is constructed and communicated in naturalistic social situations.

All discussions were taped (with the prior consent of participants) and transcribed. The analysis of transcripts was carried out inductively following the principles of grounded analysis. Such an approach involved a close reading of the focus group transcripts, aimed at providing a detailed description and analysis. The advantage of this approach is that it enabled identification both of the underlying factors that shaped people's attitudes to food risks and the contextual nature of these attitudes. Rather than searching for illustrative examples of pre-existing models of risk attitudes, the analysis protocol was designed to facilitate the development of more grounded models, which reflected the ways in which people conceptualized and managed risk in everyday life. The first stage of analysis was thus a process of "fracturing" the data to explore the basic dimensions of how participants discuss food choice, food safety and food risks. Once this had been delineated, the study then identified how perceptions of BSE and media accounts of it fitted into more general conceptions of food. The transcripts from all four countries were coded into extracts relating to these thematic headings using a shared analytical framework. This was based on the analysis of first transcripts from the United Kingdom and summaries from other countries.

The next stage of analysis entailed examining the transcripts in relation to questions such as: Which dimensions of food safety were relevant, and in which contexts? How did participants use notions of food risk and safety in their accounts? Were there differences between groups (for instance by country or life stage) in terms of which dimensions were salient? How were these concepts and dimensions related to each other? These themes and concepts were used to code or index the transcripts to collect incidences of each theme or concept from across the data set.

The study also examined how these accounts were used in discussions. For instance, in the United

Risk and trust:

Kingdom focus groups, examples of "sources of safety knowledge" linked to dramatic changes in behaviour were largely those of personal experience. Although most participants were "routinely sceptical" in the abstract about expert opinion, they did in fact draw upon several "expert" sources to justify behaviour and provide evidence for views.

The results of this "grounded analysis" were then used to address key project questions, and to identify how public perceptions of BSE were shaped by the contexts in which they were constructed. The final step was a comparative approach, looking at how these themes and concepts were used across the groups and countries and how they shed light on public perceptions of BSE.

• Sample characteristics

Purposive sampling was used to recruit participants from the following four population groups:
  • family food purchasers: peer groups of parents with primary responsibility for buying food for a family;
  • adolescents: peer groups of young people between 14 and 16 years of age;
  • single consumers: young people between 20 and 25 years of age; and
  • people aged 55 years and over.

These groups were chosen to reflect different life stages and, within these, differing responsibilities in relation to food purchasing and preparation within the household: those who are dependent upon others, those who are independent and responsible only for themselves, and those with responsibility for others. As stated above, where possible, natural groups of people were recruited.

In total, 36 focus group discussions were held across the four countries. Table 4.1 below summarizes these by country, population group and fieldwork locations.

Table 4.1. Focus group summary

Country & location	Adolescents: 14–16 year-olds
Finland Kuopio	●
Germany Kiel Eckernförde	● ●
Italy Bologna Naples Trento	● ●●
United Kingdom London and environs Coventry and environs	● ●●●

● = 1 focus group discussion   ●● = 2 focus group

determinants of public perception

The different fieldwork locations in each country were selected according to locally appropriate selection criteria and to reflect local regional differences.

Finland
- Kuopio: a large town of approximately 85 000 people in eastern Finland.

Germany
- Kiel: a town of approximately 230 000 people, the capital of Schleswig-Holstein, a largely rural state.

20–25 year-olds	Family food purchasers	55+ year-olds

discussions ●●● = 3 focus group discussions

- Eckernförde: a town of approximately 23 500 people near Kiel.

Italy
- Bologna: a medium-sized city of approximately 390 000 people, the capital of a wealthy region in northern Italy.
- Naples: a large city of approximately 1 million inhabitants in southern Italy.
- Trento: a small city of approximately 100 000 in north-eastern Italy, in a mountainous region whose economy is largely dependent upon agriculture and tourism.

United Kingdom
- London and environs: British capital located in the south-east, a region characterized by higher than average levels of income and education.
- Coventry and environs: a city of approximately 300 000 in the Midlands area of the United Kingdom, which is characterized by low employment.

• Recruitment procedures
Participants were invited to come to discuss the topic "Choosing safe foods". An incentive was offered of approximately €10–25, in the form of either a store voucher or cash. They were informed that the discussions would take approximately two hours in total. A variety of recruitment strategies were used in the different countries reflecting local circumstances:
- Finland: recruited through social networks wherever possible.

• Germany: newspaper notices (targeting family food purchasers, young singles and people aged 55+); telephone recruiting (family food purchasers and people aged 55+); leaflets distributed in supermarkets (young singles); personal communication (young singles and adolescents).

• Italy: social networks and market research company; and

• United Kingdom: social networks (London and two groups of adolescents in the Midlands); professional recruitment company (Coventry and young singles in London).

▾ Findings
• Rules for assessing food safety and risk
In the course of discussions, participants from all countries used complex sets of "rules of thumb" to assess the relative safety or riskiness of food items. These rules allowed people to make practical decisions about food choice in a context of considerable public information about food safety.

Many of these everyday rules consisted of either dichotomies of safe versus unsafe, or scales or degrees of safety. In these dichotomies, "safety" was mostly subsumed under several characteristics and articulated as a contrast of opposites. Safe food was thus variously equated with the natural, the organic, the fresh, the pure, the home-made and the traditional, as opposed to unsafe food that was associated with the chemical, the synthetic (or artificial), the commercial and the modern. In this way, safety was bundled with other food characteristics (such as nutritional value, or moral worth) and choosing food from one side of the opposing categories was a shortcut to a "safe" choice. The following comments illustrate the way in which "safe" is tied up with other characteristics, such as being organic, not being ready-made, and not being frozen.

Finland

I absolutely prefer organic meat, though I have doubts about fish because of the farmed rainbow trout. You're not always sure whether you know the whole truth.

Italy

I place fish, fruit and vegetables and dairy products first in terms of food safety, and also because I prefer them and because they are less tampered with than meat and poultry.

(Single, Naples).

United Kingdom

... but I didn't, never have bought and she [daughter] has never liked hamburgers and all the frozen foods which are the things I might have worried more about, you know, if you were buying ready-made lasagne and hamburgers ... [that] was perhaps the beginning of my disenchantment with supermarkets possibly and wanting to use local shops more ...

(Family food purchaser, London).

determinants of public perception

Conversely "unsafe" was associated with the opposing characteristics.

Finland
I am ambivalent about convenience food as all sorts of things have been added. I oppose them in principle, but I also use them.
Germany
Why does food contain so many additives? If it is fresh you do not need them — it is alarming!
(Older citizen).

The contrast between known versus unknown origins was a recurrent and salient theme in all countries, with knowledge of provenance an important factor in creating trust in food. Indeed, provenance was for many participants the major criterion upon which safety was assessed. Food, and meat in particular, bought from a known source such as a small local butcher or a known farmer, was seen in many groups as being more trustworthy than meat bought from large supermarkets.

Finland
The shop assistant told me that all the beef sold in Finland is Finnish. But they don't know everything and they are biased [since they know people prefer Finnish beef] but I trust their frankness.
United Kingdom
I think it's a matter of trust. I have a butcher. He is a very good butcher ... I trust the meat I buy off him and all his beef is definitely

from BSE-free herds ... therefore I am very happy to eat it. I would not be so happy buying beef at a supermarket even if that was stated ... again it comes back to trust. (Older citizen, rural).

As these quotes illustrate, purchasing food of known provenance was one strategy for risk reduction, in that local food from local retailers was cited as preferable to that of unknown provenance.

Provenance is related to transparency. The origins of food were ideally not only known, but also visible and obvious. For this reason, minced meat and canned foods were common examples of potentially "risky" items because they might "hide" foodstuffs classified as inedible.

Finland
If you buy some kind of canned tuna you never know what kind of muck there is inside.
United Kingdom
A. Minced meat is the worst because it contains all bits of bone and bits of brain.
B. All minced meat is so dodgy. Everything has got bits of hoof and hair in it, you can't really...
(Adolescent, London).

Scales of safety were also drawn and these were often based on geographical origin. Thus, foods of local origin were perceived as safer than those of more distant origin, on a graded scale that begins with home-produced (i.e. in a home garden) and moves through local or regional production to national and finally to imported foods. For those to whom it was available, home produce was cited as the most safe (with occasional disadvantages!).

Finland

We eat only berries that we have picked ourselves. I think fruits and berries contain an awful lot of preservatives.

Italy

For vegetables and fruit we bought an enormous plot of land which we cultivate as far as we can. It does have its disadvantages, however, as sometimes my husband comes home with the car full of basil!

(Homemaker, Trento).

United Kingdom

We probably all agree then that if we grew the vegetables ourselves without any pesticides and things ... at least I would assume that if I grew them in my own garden and if I had got my own seed presumably, always assuming that the seed we buy is safe, one would assume that if we grew it ourselves, I would assume, that I knew that I hadn't put any chemicals on it, so I would assume that my runner beans and my tomatoes and my friend's reared in her greenhouse and she then gives them to me and then I go on with the process, I would assume that they were safe to eat. That would be my definition.

(Older citizen, rural).

In the middle were foods from the region or "home" part of the country.

Germany

I think beef from Schleswig-Holstein is somewhat safer.

(Adolescent, Kiel).

In contrast, foods that had travelled the greatest distance were at the other end of the spectrum, and seen as most suspect and potentially risky.

Italy

The food's kept in the refrigerators: you don't know what happens to it!

(Adolescent, Trento).

United Kingdom

You know when they have to ship things in from faraway countries, they have to pump them with so much rubbish to keep them fresh all the time ... with tomatoes they have to pump them with fish genes to make them frost free.

(Adolescent, London).

These scales of safety were reflections in part not just of practical concerns about food risks (such as the risks of long-distance transport or the preservatives needed to transport food) but also of symbolic boundaries of "otherness". Food classification is a key marker of cultural boundaries, and the focus group discussions reflected the way in which discourses on safety are often utilized to convey national identities and sometimes stereotypes (often chauvinistic) of others.

determinants of public perception

Finland

I think Finnish food is safe, apart from some issues concerning fish. Compared to foreign food I think it is quite safe.

Germany

I have little trust [in food security systems outside Germany] ... because the general public is of different mentalities ... the further south you go, the less strict they are. That's the way it is.

(Family food purchaser, Eckernförde).

Among some of the younger groups there appeared to be less dietary chauvinism; meat from one African country was seen as not safe, whereas certain European countries, were seen as producing safer products.

United Kingdom

A. Germany has got a better reputation than Britain ...

B. I lived there. You go into a shop ... everything is very clean but ... all places vary ...

C. That is what they are famous for.

Question: So you would have more faith in the safety of a German sausage than the British ones?

Yes.

(Adolescent, London).

This quote shows that aesthetics — specifically the "clean" appearance of both the food and the food venues, such as shops and restaurants — was also an important theme and a useful rule of thumb for informing safe choice. For organic produce, however, this rule was inverted: the irregular and dirty appearance of food was taken as an indicator of its authenticity and superiority, and there was suspicion of uniformity.

United Kingdom

I go to a market but for about three years now it has been selling tomatoes that are always the same size, all the same colour, always ripe, right through the winter. Those are genetically modified tomatoes.

(Older citizen, rural).

• **Techniques of risk assessment and risk reduction**

As the data presented above show, "safety" as a discourse covered a number of different arenas for participants. These included factors related to location of origin (production, transit, preparation, storage), time-scales (immediate threats of infection through to long-term impacts on health) and different cultural frameworks for assessment (health, morality, ecology). For the majority of participants, the issue of safety had to be rooted in specific contexts, with meaningful characteristics of food, in order to influence decisions to buy or consume. As the focus groups progressed and participants talked about their own food choices and behaviour, the strategies used to manage risk or maintain confidence became apparent. In great part these flowed from the rules described above, but also involved other techniques and strategies.

Risk and trust:

The implementation of the practical rules of thumb described above enabled risks to be assessed quickly and in a routine, unremarked way. Specific risks such as BSE were also compared with other sources of risk, both in food and in other areas, to make a calculation of relative risk.

United Kingdom
A. I didn't stop buying beef ... I looked at the risks and I thought they were so infinitesimal compared to other risks that I decided I probably wasn't at risk, but it's extremely difficult for us as consumers ... to assess risk because we have so little training in that and so little information on which to base our judgement.
B. Also by the time we know the whole truth, the chances of getting [the disease] have really passed hasn't they?
(Older citizen, rural).

Aesthetic data, derived from visual and other sensory data, were important elements in risk assessment. This included inspection of both products and venues (shops, restaurants, cafes, etc.) to see if they looked or smelt "safe" or "unsafe". Interestingly, "unsafe" was often articulated as "unclean" or "unhygienic", as these quotes illustrate.

Finland
I found those pieces of beef so rough and jagged so I thought, this is the mad cow meat, and I threw it away. I lost my appetite and now I don't buy beef.

Germany
The person behind the meat counter always has her handkerchief up her sleeve. It makes me sick. Then I think of her, she touching my cold meat, and I prefer to buy pre-packed meat from the supermarket.
(Adolescent, Kiel).

On the other hand, "safe" was often associated with rather nostalgic smells, especially in Italy, as well as hygiene and cleanliness.

Italy
The pastures of Trentino ... go and drink the milk the cows produce there and smell the fragrance!
(Elderly citizen, Trento).

The foods perceived as most risky were those that could not be inspected through sensory methods, such as minced meat (commonly cited as a particularly risky food), and where ingredients could be "hidden". Thus, aesthetic appearance was recognized as not always a comprehensive guide to all potential food risks. Indeed, a theme could be discerned of suspicion of overly clean vegetables or eggs.

Italy
I feel more confident if eggs are dirty outside, rather than nice and clean.
(Single, Bologna).

In Germany, many participants and particularly adolescents and younger people felt greater confi-

determinants of public perception

dence in pre-packaged and frozen meats than in fresh meat because of their associations with cleanliness and hygiene. This was also true for baby food in both Germany and the United Kingdom. A consumer belief that food manufacturers would take particular care in preparation of foods intended for infants meant that these pre-prepared foods were often seen as particularly safe.

> Germany
> [Baby food manufacturers] — they are so trustworthy.
> (Family food purchaser, Kiel).

The sense that there were different arenas of safety also limited people's faith in single methods of assessment. For instance, participants noted progress in reducing risk of infectious disease and improvements in food safety, but also felt that these may present other risks that are as yet undetermined.

> United Kingdom
> There is always the argument too that we are becoming less resistant to bugs because we are using antibacterial handwashes and [other antibacterial products], that we are reducing bacteria that would have been good for us, that when we were young we probably had ... a "peck of dirt a day" attitude.
> (Family food purchaser, London).
> Finland
> It has been changed [food safety after

Finland joined the EU in 1995] but it is difficult to say whether things are better. Perhaps it is 60% positive but there are also negative things: products may have long expiry dates, but is there any basis for setting them?

The sense of nostalgia for the past was not just associated with "safe" food. It was also associated with mixed feelings about recent change and the consequences of entry into the EU, and the implications of this for the regulation of foods. These quotes from Finland illustrate this sense of change.

> When I was a child, we didn't have these symptoms, these epidemics. Now that there is large-scale farming, the same product is consumed by a large number of people.

> In the past there was much more time for the cattle. If one wished one could take care of them and wash them, so that they felt better. I think a cow feels better when it is cleaner. There is no time for something like that with those huge units.

> My friends in the country tell me about the many kinds of tests that the farmers themselves have to make now, such as testing the milk. In the past, such careful testing of so many factors didn't happen.

Risk and trust:

Strategies for risk reduction included choosing to buy food with known provenance or from known sources, such as a local butcher. Knowledge of provenance and trust were often cited as aids to decision-making while shopping.

Finland
There are many kinds of eggs available. You don't need to buy eggs from battery hens, you can buy organic eggs. It would be nice to know more about the conditions under which hens are kept.
Germany
I prefer that the farm sells directly to the consumers, so you can buy directly from the farmer.
(Family food purchaser, Kiel).

Although few people reported having reduced their meat consumption, either partially or totally, in response to BSE, some participants took care only to buy meat of national origin or to avoid British meat if buying meat from other countries.

Finland
If there is Finnish meat in the shop I will buy it. it is the origin that is important. We have not yet bought any imported meat.
Italy
I avoid meat from Great Britain. If I see the words "Great Britain" on meat I don't buy it.
(Family food purchaser, Trento).

United Kingdom
If I am buying mince or something, if I buy it in the supermarket I make sure I buy the best, farm-assured British beef ... rather than the cheap stuff, not that I ever bought it before but I would specially make sure.
(Family food purchaser, rural).

In Finland participants reported reducing beef consumption, but this was explained as being for reasons of health (to reduce fat consumption and hence cardiovascular disease risk) rather than because of BSE.

The utilization of "rules of thumb" to typify certain groups of food (such as organic, fresh, locally produced) as relatively safe was more common than abandoning beef as a strategy for choosing safe foods. Domestic hygiene practices were also seen as important, particularly in Germany and the United Kingdom. These include practices regarding the storage, preparation and cooking of food (e.g. peeling fruit and vegetables before consumption) and also kitchen hygiene.

United Kingdom
A. The only thing that I have become more aware of is food preparation and keeping surfaces cleaner than I used to maybe. I think that is because I watched something on television, a Watchdog thing [consumer protection group], about all these

determinants of public perception

wonderful antibacterial agents that you can get are actually rubbish. I was avidly buying all these things and really getting into all my extra-clean chopping boards, and this bit of research they had done [showed] that it was actually ... the cleaning that you did rather than the products that you used that was important, and that buying all these expensive products did nothing. And it really took me by surprise and made me actually think about what I was actually doing and not just buying things which I knew.
B. But it's comforting to know a quick spray ... is fine, rather than actually a good scrub.
C. Like my gran did, used to boil up her dishcloths every day or every few days.
D. That's right.
(Family food purchasers, London).

• Bulwarks against uncertainty
Participants' strategies for assessing and managing risk in everyday life included certain factors that acted as bulwarks against uncertainty. These included knowledge of the provenance of a food, a factor that emerged in all countries as important in establishing peoples' confidence. For many, labelling and certification systems (e.g. date stamps) were a potential source of confidence and used as a "shortcut" to safety.

United Kingdom
But with eggs, which are just as much a

[potential] killer as meat or poultry could be, you can develop infection from these things. You can't tell from looking at an egg, so therefore dating is very important in eggs and they are dated.
(Older citizen, rural).

However participants in all countries expressed some cynicism about the trustworthiness of organic product certifications.

Finland
I once made a mistake and bought organic meat. At that time "the organic industry" was a novelty. The shopkeeper asked me to see whether I could tell the difference between the organic meat and ordinary meat. The next time I saw him I said the only difference I could find was the price!

Germany
I have my doubts about organic food. A lot of farmers use pesticides, the pesticides pollute the organic farmers' fields, and the product isn't organic after all.
(Older citizen, Eckernförde).

An interesting contrast emerged in trust in different levels of regulation. Although geographical distance was associated with least trust in the safety of food in all countries, in Italy and the United Kingdom distance was often associated with most trust in the reliability of monitoring or certification systems

Risk and trust:

— and more trust was placed in supra-national regulation and agencies such as the EU and WHO.

United Kingdom
The EU will make a stop to things, I think it will make things safer because they are going to stop dodgy things going on. I mean if they are passing laws and stuff, then they are going to be stopping a lot of things. (Adolescent, Midlands).

These were perceived to be more trustworthy than national governments, and as being separate from the vested interests of producers and politicians. However, Finnish and German participants were more likely to highlight the negative effects of membership of international bodies, either because the sheer scale made regulation difficult or because of a "levelling down" of regulations.

Finland
It is a very negative thing that we try to make everything so large-scale in agri-culture [due to the EU membership in 1995]. Agriculture products are grown ever faster, or calves are fed feeds that make them grow faster. I think that is negative, although I think surveillance is better now.
Germany
I fear that, now that we are in Europe, more and more laws and their implementation are being scrapped because we have to fit in a little too much with others. (Older citizen, Eckernförde).

Some made a distinction between the existence of trusted regulations and the limited ability to enforce them.

Germany
I think the law is probably all right but people find loopholes and ways round it. That's the terrible thing, and it leads to confusion. (Adolescent).

A key bulwark against uncertainty was what could be called "fatalism": a sense that it was impossible to either attend to all potential risks or account for their implications. "Trust" was an element making a fatalistic attitude possible. This does not reflect a lack of concern necessarily, but rather a recogni-tion that one cannot respond as a consumer to all potential influences on decisions, so some have to be taken in a routine or non-reflective way.

Finland
In that respect one can go shopping without undue concern, without stopping to wonder "what if this" or "what if that". That would be hysterical behaviour.
Germany
One has to accept it, otherwise one wouldn't eat anything! (Older citizen, Eckernförde).
United Kingdom
But this has gone on for centuries. We've been eating salt for centuries and only recently have been told that too much is bad for us. So I think what you have to do in principle is to eat what seems to be safe

determinants of public perception

and if nothing goes wrong be thankful for it.
(Older citizen, rural).
Italy
Because I think there's something in every-
thing, yet we've still got to eat. I've reached
the stage where I don't give a damn.
(Elderly citizen, Bologna).

• Sources of safety knowledge

Most participants found it difficult to cite specific
information sources. However, in the stories they
told about food decisions, there was considerable
evidence of the kinds of information sources that
were used to inform, justify and change behaviour.
For many of those for whom food safety was a
salient issue, personal experience emerged as the
most important source of knowledge. These experiences were various and included encounters with
meal moths and salmonella, concern about *Listeria*
while pregnant, and allergies.

Other sources cited included family and friends,
radio, newspapers, television, school and food
retailers. However, the degree of trust placed in
these sources varied and few were explicitly cited in
relation to decision-making. Schools were not cited
as a major source of safety knowledge, and information received there was likely to come in an ad
hoc way from particular teachers rather than as
curriculum-based safety education.

As discussed below, the key characteristics of

trusted information sources were that they were
perceived to have no vested interests or that their
interests were known. In the United Kingdom, participants perceived supermarkets to have strong
material interests, but felt they would not mislead
customers through fear of losing profits.

One source that was discussed in more depth by
the focus groups was information on food labels.
Participants, particularly in Italy, saw food labels as
a positive change for consumers in that they provide
information (including safety information) that was
not previously available.
> Italy
> I pay close attention to labels and I'd like a
> quality source mark on everything, that
> would please me greatly, at least I'd feel a
> bit more protected.
> (Family food purchaser, Trento).

However, there were problems noted with size of
writing and the difficulty in understanding some
technical information, such as "E" numbers, and
uncertainty (see above) over how trustworthy organic
labelling was. In Germany, participants reported that
overuse of quality labels by manufacturers and
retailers led to declining trust in their usefulness.
> Germany
> On [one supermarket's] products, for exam-
> ple, you find the DLG [German Agricultural
> Society] award on every second product.
> (Man, 25 years).

• Contexts for using safety rules

Given that safety was not a key concern for many participants, the implementation of personal safety rules was often contingent on social context. Food was consumed not just for nutritional value. It also has social and cultural functions, which both shape the meaning of "safety" and also potentially constrain the utilization of more personalized safety rules.

> United Kingdom
> Basically I don't really worry about [safety] anyway but I do tend to buy, you know, real meat, company meat or organic meat if I am buying it for the family. But I would have no qualms about eating any of these things if I was in a restaurant or a pub, I would eat it.
> (Family food purchaser, London).

In accounting for their behaviour, many participants recognized the complex ways in which beliefs about food safety, ideal accounts of behaviour and real influences on food choice interacted.

> Germany
> We don't eat much meat — about three times a week. If we do, we eat poultry, although this is the worst meat; we like it very much.
> (Woman, 37 years).

The meaning of "natural" emerged as an important example of this kind of complexity. Although many participants from all groups identified natural foods (those with least processing before they reach the kitchen) as healthiest, there are also elements of trust in technology as a means of ensuring safety. This was particularly true in the case of baby food: some participants had more trust in mass-produced baby foods than in home-cooked ones. Many in Germany, especially adolescents and young single people, also felt more confident about processed foods. Interestingly, foodstuffs can also be "too close" to nature — some family food purchasers identified free-range chickens and pigs as potential risks because "you didn't know where they had been".

> United Kingdom
> One of my concerns about chickens and pigs is that they are omnivorous ... you don't know what a pig or a chicken has eaten before it is killed. It's not that they are going to poison you at that point, it's how happy you feel about what has entered your food-chain in terms of what is going through your system, and free range chickens will eat disgusting things, because they're free range, you'll find them on top of manure heaps.
> (Family food purchaser, rural).

Thus these rules of thumb for food categorization were useful shortcuts to making and justifying decisions about food choices. However, they were necessarily complex and contingent: firstly, because the constraints of real life might limit how

determinants of public perception

far safety could be a concern; secondly, because rules could conflict by categorizing foods as both safe in terms of one dimension (e.g. natural and organic) and unsafe in another (e.g. not refined enough for a baby).

• Safety as a part of — or traded against — other concerns
Except for German participants, safety was not an explicit concern in buying and preparing food. Safety was mostly subsumed within other concerns related to food such as taste and pleasure, health and nutrition, socializing and hospitality, convenience and kinship. These concerns both included safety or implicitly had a higher priority when choosing food.

Finland
Thinking of other kinds of products, what about pastry? Rarely do you stop and think about [the safety of] pastry.
Italy
If you like something, you eat it.
You can find something unhealthy in everything you eat. You can't think about it too much.
(Adolescent, Trento).
United Kingdom
But there is nobody at your elbow when you go shopping is there, saying buy this, buy that. I just go and if I like it I buy it. I don't think about a radio report or a newspaper report to buy it, I just buy it if I like it.
(Older citizen, Coventry).

The exception was the cost of food. Here safety was seen as a quality of food explicitly opposed to cost, with low cost perceived to be an almost inevitable trade-off against both quality and safety.

United Kingdom
I have a big problem really with fast food because ... it's not so much food safety, there probably is [safety], but they get their burgers so cheaply. You think what corners are they cutting to get that burger?
(Adolescent, London).

Cost, however, was cited as an important issue for many groups affecting food purchases.

Italy
I think about prices, not about poisons.
(Single, Bologna).
Germany
But organic meat is far too expensive! We can't afford that.
(Older citizen, Kiel).

• Trust in experts
In all countries, participants expressed what might be called a "routine scepticism" of government and other figures of expertise, such as scientists and figures in the media. The one significant exception to this was the trust placed in their politicians by the Finnish participants. Otherwise the British, German and Italian participants were largely distrustful and scathing about their politicians.

Risk and trust:

Germany
Politicians are always ambiguous. They waffle their way around a subject. Therefore they are not to be trusted.
(Single, Kiel).
United Kingdom
I think anything said by any politician you take with a pinch of salt, don't you?
(Family food purchaser, London).

Much routine scepticism was also expressed about the media and journalists, although some distinction was made between different types of journalists. In Italy, for instance, scientific journalists were seen as more trustworthy and credible because their accounts were based on "research data". Some in the United Kingdom felt that the "broadsheet" newspapers were more trustworthy than the tabloids, and in Germany regional newspapers were rated as more trustworthy sources than national newspapers.

Scientists were trusted as long as they were perceived to be independent.
Germany
Scientists work for themselves and want to be the best, to publish and to maintain their status.
Italy
Experts are all very well, but I'd trust those who are not in the economic loop and who act not their own interests but in those

of the consumer.
(Adolescent, Trento).
Italy
... if a foreign scientist said something I'd believe it. Why foreign? Because foreigners are impartial.
(Single, Naples).

Some participants viewed supermarkets with a degree of suspicion and cynicism but, as mentioned above, felt that these businesses would not risk selling unsafe products for fear of damaging profits.
Germany
The supermarkets would lose all their customers if they weren't trustworthy.
(Adolescent, Kiel).
United Kingdom
If we knew where it [the source of a food scare] was, it would probably put people off buying there because of what happened. They don't want to lose their profits, so they have to keep certain standards.
(Adolescent, Midlands).

For many groups, trusted sources were primarily those perceived to have no vested interests, such as consumer organizations, which were the category most often mentioned explicitly in all countries. Implicitly, "local" was also an important dimension of trust, with familiarity, personal experience and known sources being trusted. Thus small local retailers were trusted. Also others who shared the

determinants of public perception

characteristics of known sources were trusted by extension — for instance, organic shops or market traders.

One issue for many British and Italian participants was "experts" whose views are contradictory. Although some accepted the ambiguities of scientific knowledge, others saw such contradictions as undermining their faith in scientific expertise.

Finnish and German participants reported more trust in their national systems, and indeed were concerned that the European controls would be less stringent than existing national ones. Interestingly, however, the EU was cited by participants in both Italy and the United Kingdom as — potentially — a more trustworthy source of regulation and enforcement than their own national systems.

> Italy
> You can trust the European Union, because it serves the interests of several countries rather than just one, there are various safeguards and it is organized.
> (Adolescent, Trento).

• Responsibility for safety

Various levels and types of responsibility for safety emerged in the discussions. On an individual level, most participants were concerned about presenting themselves as responsible food handlers, whereas "others" were potentially risky.

> United Kingdom
> A. I think also you would have to educate the general public. They buy meat, they put it into the back of the car, and may not go home for three or four hours, that sort of thing. Should get them to have cool boxes ... But an awful lot of people buy meat, sausage rolls, such like and just leave them there, and go on a picnic and still leave them there and if they are not eaten they eat them at home afterwards.
> B. A lot of food poisoning ... is due to lack of care by the consumer.
> (Older citizen, rural).

For family food purchasers in all countries, responsibility for children was clearly important. It was cited as a key factor in changing food purchasing or preparation behaviour, and for being more explicit about responsibility for safety.

> United Kingdom
> And I think probably being at home more as well ... preparing more food than I used to, so you are certainly a lot more conscious of doing things properly than I was before. I never knew whether the dishcloth had been there for a week or two or three months before because I just didn't have time to think about it, whereas now I am probably more aware.
> (Family food purchaser, London).
> Italy
> We try to eat as simply as possible, perhaps because I've been a mother

Risk and trust:

now for a year and a half.
(Family food purchaser, Trento).

In general, participants described themselves as primarily responsible for dealing with food risks within the domestic domain — for preparing food hygienically and cooking safely. This responsibility extended to controlling the entry of risks into the home, for instance by not choosing food past its "sell by" date or by selecting healthy foodstuffs. However, they expected official agencies to provide a "safety net", with regulations and monitoring to ensure the safe production and distribution of food (see below).

The study deliberately included adolescents because they are on the brink of assuming responsibility for their own food consumption. In general, they saw parents as the party primarily responsible for food safety, and trusted them to do this.

> United Kingdom
> My mum is cooking [Christmas dinner] and I trust her.
> (Adolescent, Midlands).
> Italy
> I trust my mother. I don't go out and do the shopping or say "Mama, but did you look to see where the meat came from?"
> (Adolescent, Bologna).

For some though, parents were seen as unscientific in their approach, and potentially "risky" food handlers.

United Kingdom
I rearrange our fridge in my dad's house. They will go shopping, they will just throw it all in and go off and do whatever, and I go in and I think really I would put that chicken down there, and maybe move that there. I don't know, it's just as I am finding something to eat, I will just move it a little bit, or think that is a bit old and chuck it away. (Adolescent, London).

If participants saw themselves, or their immediate family, as having primary responsibility for safety within the home, they were clear that the state had a legitimate role in ensuring that food is safe and not compromised by "vested interests". It was recognized, though, that balancing safety with other interests (such as economic ones) was as delicate at the national level as it was in the domestic sphere. As participants noted, many people want cheap food, but cheapness involves an inevitable trade-off with safety. The role of government was to ensure that regulations protected the consumer, and that they were enforced. Although little trust was placed in politicians as an information source, national governments were seen as having an important role in food safety — in establishing and enforcing appropriate legislation.

▾ Discussion

The information presented above shows the complexity of public constructions of food safety and risk,

determinants of public perception

and that people use sophisticated strategies to assess the riskiness of food. These strategies and shortcuts permit the "routinization" of food choices and the management of uncertainty in everyday life.

Safety per se was not, though, a major concern for respondents and provided a limited framework for making decisions about food. When asked directly about the risks in food, participants reported concern; but in more open discussion, levels of concern about food risk emerged as relatively low. Only in discussions of cost did safety emerge as an explicit issue — and here it was seen as clearly incompatible with cheapness; if food was cheap, a corner must have been cut somewhere. The data also show that the concept of safety itself was framed in many different ways. "Safety" in its various definitions was not the only conceptual framework for buying, preparing and consuming food, but competed with other frameworks constructed around such concerns as price, pleasure, socializing and convenience.

While there are few other qualitative studies with which to compare these findings, there is nonetheless some evidence that the findings are typical of consumers in other industrialized countries, revealing a rational approach to risk assessment and one that incorporates other concerns in food choice. Sellerberg's study in Sweden (1991) argued that people constructed "strategies of confidence"

to establish their trust in food against a background of uncertainty and conflicting advice. In the United Kingdom, Macintyre et al. (1998) found knowledge of provenance and national identity to be important for people in judging the safety of food. People balanced and weighed up competing criteria (e.g. preference versus healthiness) in selecting food. Also in the United Kingdom, Caplan (2000) found that people constructed dichotomies of safety, such as knowledge and confidence versus ignorance and risk, and that social relations were important in creating trust (it matters not only to know where the beef comes from, but to know the person it is bought from). Like the British participants in this study, the rural Australians in Lupton's (2000) study cited frameworks other than safety as being most salient in choosing food, in this case those of "health" and "balance".

The fieldwork for this study was conducted from 1999 onwards. Few people in any country cited BSE as a cause of behavioural change. This, and the fact that food safety and BSE emerged as major concerns in only one country (Germany), make it important to underline the fact that the study was not carried out while an actual "crisis" was happening. It is likely that different findings would have emerged if this had been the case. Such a conclusion is reinforced by the findings of Eldridge et al. (1998), who compared the views of consumers in 1992 — i.e. in the wake of the first "media panic" about BSE — with their views four years later. They found consumers to be more aware and more concerned in 1996, and many claimed to have changed their consumption patterns.

As the consumption data presented in Chapter 5 show, in the United Kingdom at least there was a sharp decline in beef consumption in 1996, but subsequently consumption levels returned to pre-1996 levels. This suggests that levels of public concern about BSE and other food-related risks may have a "decay function", in that media attention foregrounds and perhaps fosters concern, but once this ceases public concern "decays". Because the data for this study were collected during a "non-crisis" period, they cannot be used to assess the role of the media in influencing public concerns; they only show that trust in media sources was variable, with differentiation between the type of newspaper and journalist. Macintyre et al. (1998), however, did specifically examine public reactions to mass media messages about food scares. They found that personal experience was important in mediating people's responses to messages in the media; experience of food poisoning by self or a known other was the principal factor in causing behavioural change and actually seeking out information from the media. Many, however, were also cynical about the media and felt that they (the media) had their own agenda.

▾ Conclusions

The qualitative methods used in this study reveal the complex nature of perceptions about safety and risk. Accounts provided in open discussion, rather than in response to closed questions, suggest that food safety was not a major preoccupation of most participants, at least at times when there were no "live" food scares (i.e. receiving wide media coverage).

Key findings about common issues across the four countries include the following.

• In an environment that was increasingly rich in information, participants used complex strategies to apply their perceptions of food safety. The key strategy was the adoption of rules of thumb to assess the relative safety of food items. Rules of thumb may cluster a variety of qualities such as provenance, healthiness and nutritional value, as well as safety per se.

• Implementation of rules of thumb was very much contingent upon social context. The concept of safety itself was not a unitary concept: it had many meanings for participants and it was through these that it was discussed and negotiated.

• Concerns about safety also competed with other food discourses, such as taste, cost and pleasure.

• BSE was just one of many concerns about food, and it was not reported to have had a marked long-term impact on food choices in any country.

• "Provenance" was a major concern for all participants, who had greater trust in food from known sources.

• Participants saw consumer organizations as

determinants of public perception

their main allies, and perceived them as the sources of information least likely to be contaminated by vested interests.

Key findings about differences between countries were:
- food safety was not a major concern for participants except in Germany, where they expressed relatively high levels of concern about both food safety and BSE;
- Finnish participants placed a high degree of trust in politicians, in contrast to participants from other countries; and
- in Italy and the United Kingdom, participants perceived the EU to be a potentially trustworthy source of controls for food safety; in Germany and Finland, participants had more faith in national systems.

For policy questions, this study suggests that focus group discussions are a useful method of enquiry when decision-makers need a detailed understanding of not only the content of public opinion, but also (a) how it is formed and (b) how it is voiced in everyday social interaction. Focus group discussions can also suggest issues that information should take into account, and identify those segments of the population most concerned about food risk. (The value of focus groups in the policy process is further discussed in Chapter 10.)

References

Beck U (1992) *Risk society: towards a new modernity*. London, Sage.

Caplan P (2000) Eating British beef with confidence: a consideration of consumers' responses to BSE in Britain. In: Caplan P, ed. *Risk revisited*. London, Pluto Press:184–203.

Douglas M (1986) *Risk acceptability according to the social sciences*. London, Routledge & Kegan Paul.

Eldridge J, Kitzinger J, Philo G, Reilly J (1998) The re-emergence of BSE: the impact on public beliefs and behaviour. *Risk and Human Behaviour Newsletter*, 3:6–10.

Giddens A (1991) *Modernity and self identity: self and society in the late modern age*. London, Polity Press.

Kitzinger J (1994) The methodology of focus groups: the importance of interaction between research participants. *Sociology of Health and Illness*, 16:103–121.

Lupton D (2000) The heart of the meal: food preferences and habits among rural Australian couples. *Sociology of Health and Illness*, 22:94–109.

Macintyre S, Reilly J, Miller D, Eldridge J (1998) Food choice, food scare, and health: the role of the media. In: Murcott A, ed. *The nation's diet: the social science of food choice*. London & New York, Longman:228–249.

Marmot M (1996) From alcohol and breast cancer to beef and BSE – improving our communication of risk. *American Journal of Public Health*, 86:921–923.

Sellerberg A-M (1991) In food we trust? Vitally necessary confidence – and unfamiliar ways of attaining it. In: Fürst El, Prättälä R, Ekström M, Holm L, Kjaernes U, eds. *Palatable worlds*. Oslo, Solum Forlag:193–201.

Sample surveys of public perceptions and opinion

5

Sample surveys of public perceptions and opinion

Giancarlo Gasperoni, Alizon Draper, Vera Hagenhoff, Maria Rusanen, Timo Rusanen

This chapter discusses the findings generated by second-ary analysis of information collected in sample surveys. In particular, efforts were made to identify and obtain survey information for the following reasons:

- existing data sets could provide valuable information on risk perception and trust;
- the usefulness of surveys to assess perceptions and trust could be compared with that of other techniques (such as focus group discussions), in order to better understand the potential of different ways of incorporating perceptions into communi-cation strategies; and
- to explore whether publicly available information on public perceptions and trust had been taken into account or could have been put to better use.

The study acquired, reviewed and re-analysed data regarding:

- public knowledge and awareness of food safety issues (exposure to mass media coverage, degree of reception, sources of information);
- how individuals perceived food scares and their implications;
- if and how they modified their behaviour in different spheres of everyday life (especially eating and purchasing habits);
- public trust in institutional communication, food producers and distributors, scientists, health officials, and other figures with interests in the general public's attitudes; and
- behaviour regarding food consumption, especially of meat.

▼ Conceptual considerations

The sample survey is arguably the most widespread tool for gathering information in social research. In general terms, sample surveys have the following features:

- the unit of analysis is the individual;
- sampling techniques are used to select respon-dents;
- data are collected through the administration of questions (usually from a standardized script) to individual respondents and the recording of (usually predetermined) answers;
- the survey is administered by a group of inter-viewers, who are trained to follow the interview script and record the answers consistently and accurately;
- collected information is stored in a computerized data matrix; and
- statistical analysis techniques are used to obtain frequency distributions and other more complex results.

Mass surveys have a variety of strengths allowing for robust data cross-tabulation, i.e. the explor-ation of relationships among operationally defined variables. As may be inferred from the previously mentioned features of surveys, data collection typi-cally involves a large number of interviewees; due to standardization, responses are comparable; analysis can be performed quickly; and findings can be effectively summarized (in easy-to-understand tables and graphs) for communication purposes.

At the same time, their limitations and weaknesses must be understood in order to assess the real benefits offered by this technique in the target area of study.

Surveys evolved over a period in which so-called "quantitative methods" were dominant in social research, and so they are often attached to some typical assumptions of those methods. It is assumed, for instance, that results obtained on a relatively small sample can be generalized to the larger population from which that sample was drawn; that just about anything can be "measured"; that there is no significant interaction among subjects and research tools; and so on. Today no one embraces such positivist assumptions, and the distortions and errors to which surveys are prone are widely acknowledged in the literature.

• Questions about questionnaires

It has long been known (Payne, 1951; Sudman & Bradburn, 1974; Schuman & Presser, 1981) that survey results may vary according to factors such as the order in which questions or response categories are presented, the total number of predetermined responses administered to respondents, the number of answers subjects are allowed to give, and the presence or absence of "don't know", "none of the above" or "other" categories. The choice of certain words rather than others can be very important. For example, "forbidding" something is not quite the opposite of "allowing" it, and not "liking" something is different from "disliking" it. Similarly, the terms "voluntary pregnancy termination", "abortion" and "fetus murder" may designate the same surgical procedure, but certainly do not elicit the same reactions among interviewees. It is also recognized that respondents may adopt strategic behaviours based on their perception or anticipation of the researchers' expectations or goals, resulting in data "tainted" by social desirability, response sets, and other sources of bias.

While survey techniques permit researchers to ask questions on practically any topic, they usually concentrate on asking people to express judgements, share viewpoints on social and political issues, and evaluate facts, situations or persons. Surveys do not permit a researcher to observe behaviour; at best they record respondents' stated behaviour, which may or may not coincide with actual conduct. In general, the cognitive claims of surveys are further weakened when they deal with topics such as "attitudes", "values", "opinions", "perceptions", "representations" and so on. Such topics are of particular interest to social researchers, for the following reasons: attitudes are assumed to be a product of social environments in which respondents live; the attitudes may be of social relevance; and attitudes contribute to determining social behaviour.

Nevertheless, despite the complex makeup of attitudes and their heuristic potential, surveys often

Sample surveys of

use operational definitions that, in focusing on respondents' degree of favour, agreement, etc., ignore other important features of these attitudes. Those features may include the malleability of these attitudes (i.e. the ease with which they may change), their empirical weight (the degree to which attitudes influence actual behaviour), the salience of these objects in respondents' lives, subjects' awareness of their own attitudes, and so on.

• Sampling issues

A major source of potential distortion concerns sampling difficulties. Sample survey findings tend to be generalized to the general population on the basis of inferential statistics. This assumes that samples are "representative" and/or "randomly drawn". Such assumptions, however, are increasingly untenable due to the sizeable incidence of "non-response", i.e. prospective interviewees who, for some reason, interviewers cannot contact or who simply refuse to participate in surveys. People who are well-educated, are young, live alone and/or belong to ethnic minorities are generally more difficult to contact for interview purposes, and this difficulty is growing with greater sensitivity to privacy rights. People who are socially isolated, marginal or detached tend to be more prone to refusing interviews (Goyder, 1987).

The exclusion of such "non-respondents" is usually dealt with either by interviewee replacement in the data collection stage or by differential case-weighting in the data analysis stage. Neither strategy can remedy the fact that non-respondents are not a random and/or representative subset of a target sample, that a target sample and an achieved sample are different, that the reasons for which this difference exists are probably related to the issue being investigated, and that an achieved sample usually does not meet the criteria required for sample-to-population generalization of results on the basis of inferential statistics.

• Evolution of data collection techniques

Sample surveys are also changing from the standpoint of questionnaire administration techniques. An increasing proportion of surveys are based on telephone (and, in more recent years, web-based) interviews, whereas face-to-face personal interviewing is declining. Due to its economic convenience, telephone (usually computer-assisted) interviewing has rendered survey studies easier, faster and more widespread, but it also places serious limits on the type of questions that can be asked (no lengthy wording, no long lists), the visual aids that can be used, the length of the questionnaire and the quality of interviewer—respondent interaction (hindered by the spatial and social distance separating the two subjects). The increasing role of technological components in interviewing processes may aggravate these problems.

• Secondary analysis

The findings illustrated in the rest of this chapter

public perceptions and opinion

were generated through secondary analysis, and this has specific implications for the conclusions that can be drawn from them. Secondary survey analysis may be defined as the extraction of knowledge about topics that are in some way different from the topics that were the focus of the original surveys. Although it offers many practical advantages (especially as regards overall costs for conducting research), secondary analysis also involves several types of additional difficulty. Examples include:

• accessibility of data sets, which may involve further problems such as bad documentation, software incompatibility or political sensitivity;

• availability of knowledge about the methods employed;

• combination of studies using different techniques (for sampling, interviewing, weighting, etc.);

• the fact that operational definitions and available items might not adequately fit research goals; and

• the need to engage not in pre-arrangement of data collection (as in an original survey) but rather in a re-arrangement of previously collected data.

Within the realm of secondary analysis, it has been said that "one must take what one can find" and "we must make the most of what we have" (Hyman, 1972: 23 and 18; see also Kiecolt & Nathan, 1985). Secondary analysis of survey data and execution of original surveys are thus two very different

approaches to social research in general and risk perception in particular. Evaluating the usefulness of the latter on the basis of results obtained with the former is fraught with risk.

For all these reasons, it is usually extremely difficult to claim that findings drawn from different surveys can be readily compared: two studies rarely share the same question/answer wordings, questionnaire structures, sampling frames, nonresponse incidence, questionnaire administration techniques, and so on. So-called longitudinal studies — based on repeated cross-sectional surveys or, better yet, panel surveys (in which the sample members do not change over time) — usually guarantee a greater degree of uniformity in data collection procedures. They therefore give a greater degree of comparability and, in particular, the opportunity to study social change. Such studies are relatively costly and consequently rare. The Eurobarometer surveys are an example of repeated cross-sectional surveys (see below), in which some effort goes into periodically administering the same items in order to trace the transformation of frequency distributions over time. This chapter contains some examples of the results that may ensue from such repeated cross-sectional surveys. However, in general, Eurobarometer surveys are dedicated to a vast array of topics so that item repetition is relatively infrequent and restricted to a few topics (often focusing on the perception of EU institutions).

Sample surveys of

• **Surveys as a social phenomenon**

Besides being a research technique, surveys are a major social phenomenon, itself worthy of study. Surveys exercise a good deal of appeal in part because they resemble a hallmark of democracy (i.e. elections: they share the use of the term "poll") and they claim to "measure" something called "public opinion". Much has been written about the meaning of "public opinion", the dangers of associating survey findings and public opinion (Blumer, 1948; Bourdieu, 1973; Price, 1992), the abuse of surveys as "pseudo-events" by mass media (more engaged in newsmaking than newsgathering) and the consequent risk of impoverishment of public debate and political participation. The fact remains that survey findings not only provide knowledge about a social phenomenon but often provide an efficacious means of disseminating such knowledge. Mass media are apt to circulate "news" presented in this form and readers/viewers are likely to pay more attention to it. In other words, "survey findings" may also constitute an effective tool in (rather than for) a communication policy.

▾ **Sources of data**

National project participants in the United Kingdom, Germany, Italy and Finland were instructed to search and identify sample surveys concerning target issues. The target issues were understood to be:

• specific reactions within the public to "mad cow disease", CJD and related issues and events;

• specific reactions within public opinion to other food scares and related events;

• attitudes toward food safety in general;

• meat-eating behaviour; and

• trust in institutional and media sources and information sources in general.

Once the surveys on the target issues had been identified, the participants were to collect basic information on those surveys' availability, obtain their findings, find out about the availability of the data sets of the identified surveys and (if freely available) obtain them too.

• **Country-specific studies and data sources**

In the United Kingdom and, to a lesser degree, in Germany, there have been many BSE-related studies. Studies have been much less numerous in Italy and particularly so in Finland. This reflects, among other things, the differing seriousness of the BSE situation (or the perception of seriousness) in the four countries involved in the study, at least in the period analysed (up to 1998). It may also reflect the differing research traditions and resources available for social research centres. The analysis in this study focused more on the international sources of data, which permitted a minimal degree of comparability across countries.

United Kingdom. Survey studies on BSE and CJD are relatively plentiful, owing to the fact that the specific animal health issue emerged in the United

public perceptions and opinion

Kingdom much earlier and became a more significant public health issue there than elsewhere. Many surveys were identified on food safety and trust in the United Kingdom that had been carried out by market research or opinion polling firms, and government-commissioned research and academic studies were identified as well. Unfortunately, the available research appears to have been generally commissioned on an ad hoc basis (in response to particular incidents) and offers only inconstant coverage of food safety issues. It was not possible to compile an exhaustive list of these surveys, particularly in relation to market research; there is no central index or database of market research, and individual companies appear to archive their work erratically, if at all. Most of the market research identified by this study dates only from the last few years. It was difficult to gain more than general details regarding sampling, questionnaires and findings. Market research data sets available for further analysis were both limited and costly. The government-commissioned surveys identified were much more accessible and could be obtained at a reasonable cost from the University of Essex Data Archive. These data sets include quantitative data on meat consumption, for instance from the National Food Survey in the United Kingdom. Academic research proved surprisingly limited, with only a few attitudinal surveys identified in the literature. Many of these were based on theoretical models drawn from social psychology, such as the theory of reasoned action.

Germany. In addition to commercial market research, in Germany it was possible to access academic research studies regarding food safety in general, meat consumption and even BSE/CJD. As in the United Kingdom, market research, opinion polls, government-commissioned research and academic research were all carried out on these topics on a relatively large scale in the latter half of the 1990s. This wealth of data does not stem from recent BSE/CJD panics, but seems rather to be rooted in well-entrenched research traditions promoted by the agricultural sector and a well-developed agricultural science sector in higher education. Marketing research centres (*Lebensmittelpraxis*, CMA-Mafo) conducted the most intensive studies, but also the most costly as regards data access. Academic research is well represented by the *Institut für Agrarpolitik und Marktforschung* at the University of Giessen, the *Agrarwissenschaftlichen Fakultät* at the University of Hohenheim, and the *Institut für Agraroekonomie* at the University of Kiel. Academic studies, which are more accessible, focus on a wide variety of topics, including nutritional knowledge, food/meat/beef consumption patterns, quality image and, more specifically, awareness of BSE, the impact of BSE on consumer attitudes and behaviour, and factors determining mistrust in food.

Italy. Contacts with the major Italian commercial and non-commercial survey research agencies

Sample surveys of

revealed only two sample surveys of the general population. These were carried out in March 1996, when "mad cow disease" became a newsworthy item in national media coverage, and the findings about the disease had been made public. It was not possible to recover the original data set for either survey. Other research agencies claimed to have conducted sample surveys on these topics but stated that the research was private, so that neither the data nor the findings (nor, indeed, the nature — and certainly not the names — of the companies or organizations who commissioned the studies) could be divulged.[1] Many research institutes contacted claimed that they had conducted no polls or surveys on the specific topic of BSE/CJD or in general on food scares. The *Istituto Studi Ricerche e Informazioni sul Mercato Agricolo* (ISMEA), a research institute that is ultimately responsible to the Ministry of Agricultural Resources, commissioned a survey study concerning the BSE situation in 1996 and a later survey study concerning public perceptions of the "chicken dioxin" crisis originating in Belgium.

Finland. There have been almost no studies conducted on BSE in Finland, reflecting its status as

one of Europe's "BSE-free" countries until 2001. Food and Farm Facts Ltd. (*Elintarviketieto*), of the Gallup group, has conducted yearly surveys on small samples (500 interviewees) since 1997; the data, property of Information Services for the Meat Industry, are not publicly available. Two large Finnish newspapers, *Turun Sanomat* and *Aamulehti*, published limited survey data collected (only in December 2000) by Taloustutkimus, a Finnish market research and opinion polling firm.

• International studies and data sources
Finding international sources involving all four countries in this study was particularly crucial. Available national-level studies, relatively plentiful in the United Kingdom and Germany, were rather rare in Italy and especially Finland. The Eurobarometer studies have been the major source.

The "Standard Eurobarometer" was established in 1974. It consists of a survey of about 1000 representative face-to-face interviews per European Community (later Union) member country, carried out between two and five times per year. Reports are published twice yearly. The Eurobarometer provides regular monitoring of social and political attitudes in the European populations. Crucially, Eurobarometer data are available for purposes of secondary analysis. The following Eurobarometer data sets were acquired for statistical re-analysis.
  • Eurobarometer 35.1: Consumer behaviour in the Single European Market

---

[1] Informally, it was acknowledged that such studies were paid for by the meat industry and/or the pharmaceutical industry.

public perceptions and opinion

- Eurobarometer 37.1: Consumer behaviour towards food products and labelling
- Eurobarometer 38.0: Consumer behaviour and safety of products and services
- Eurobarometer 39.1: Consumer behaviour in the Single European Market
- Eurobarometer 44.1: Consumer behaviour towards food products and labelling
- Eurobarometer 47.0: Consumer protection
- Eurobarometer 49: Safety and labelling of food products
- Eurobarometer 50.0 (various topics) + 50.1: Consumer behaviour toward food products and labelling
- Eurobarometer 51.0: Trust in national and European institutions
- Eurobarometer 52.0: Trust in national and European institutions.

The data set for Eurobarometer 43.1bis was also acquired and slated for re-analysis, but items relevant to this study were found to be missing from the publicly available data set. Data for Finland were collected only after its admission to the EU (in January 1995; thus for this study, data from Eurobarometer 44.1 were used).

Another international source was the EU Project on Quality Policy and Consumer Behaviour (QPCB), coordinated by Tilman Becker of the *Institut für Agrarpolitik und Landwirtschaftliche Marktlehre*, University of Hohenheim. The project,

which started in 1996 and ended in January 1998, dealt with the increased importance of quality products in the food sector and the coordination of national regulations regarding food production and food marketing in Europe. The data were collected in spring 1997 through telephone surveys of 500 households in six EU countries: Germany, Ireland, Italy, Spain, Sweden and the United Kingdom. The survey targeted individuals responsible for household food shopping, and thus women accounted for the great majority of respondents. Results are documented in the *Summary report on consumer behaviour towards meat in Germany, Ireland, Italy, Spain, Sweden and the United Kingdom* (Becker, Benner & Glitsch, 1998) and in *Quality policy and consumer behaviour in the European Union* (Becker, 2000). The two publications highlight both the differences and the similarities found between the participating countries.

▾ Research findings
• Changes in meat consumption
This section briefly presents findings about changes in meat consumption in Europe and in the four countries involved in this study. However, considerable caution must be used in interpreting changes in food consumption as evidence of a response to a specific phenomenon (such as BSE) or as an indicator of perception of risk. In any country, long-term trends can be discerned that are determined not by one but by many interwoven factors: these include changes in the population's

Sample surveys of

demographic make-up, income levels, control and structure of food production and distribution, and general diet and health concerns. Food consumption data (routinely collected by many governments) may accurately mirror short-term changes in levels of concern determined by crises. However, disentangling short-term changes (such as those caused by BSE or other food scares) from long-term trends (such as the decades-long decline in beef consumption in Germany and the United Kingdom) is

practically impossible.[2] Even more caution is needed when using survey data (such as those drawn from Eurobarometer or the QPCB) recording stated rather than observed behaviour.
However, there are some potentially useful findings to be considered in the surveys reviewed in this

[2] This decline is documented in the food balance sheets produced by FAO (see http://apps.fao.org/page/collections).

Table 5.1. Frequency of purchase of selected meat products, selected countries

Meat product/frequency of purchase	EU		United Kingdom		Germany		Italy		Finland	
Cooked meat, pâtés, salamis, etc.	Late 1995	Late 1998	Late 1995	Late 1998	Late 1995	Late 1998	Late 1995	Late 1998	Late 1995	Late 1998
Once a week or more	67.3	69.2	63.6	66.1	77.6	82.5	66.3	67.1	79.7	67.3
Less often	25.7	24.1	25.9	22.6	18.7	14.7	28.0	27.1	17.1	27.6
Never	6.4	6.0	9.9	10.4	3.1	2.5	5.1	5.1	3.2	4.7
Don't know	0.6	0.6	0.6	0.9	0.6	0.4	0.5	0.7	0.0	0.5
Total	100	100	100	100	100	100	100	100	100	100
Meat or poultry	Late 1995	Late 1998	Late 1995	Late 1998	Late 1995	Late 1998	Late 1995	Late 1998	Late 1995	Late 1998
Once a week or more	81.3	81.9	88.4	86.6	68.6	70.5	83.3	84.0	68.8	65.6
Less often	15.8	15.2	9.1	9.4	27.4	26.9	13.5	12.7	28.1	30.7
Never	2.3	2.3	2.2	3.3	3.0	2.3	2.6	2.3	3.2	3.3
Don't know	0.6	0.6	0.2	0.7	1.0	0.3	0.7	1.0	0.0	0.5
Total	100	100	100	100	100	100	100	100	100	100

(Eurobarometers 44.1: November–December 1995 and 50.1: November–December 1998, percentage values)

public perceptions and opinion

study. A question about consumption of two meat-product groups — "cooked meat, pâtés, salamis, etc." and "meat or poultry" — was administered a few months before the March 1996 BSE crisis, in Eurobarometer 44.1 (November–December 1995), and again some three years later in 50.1 (November–December 1998). As shown in Table 5.1, purchasing levels seem to have remained stable at the European level. In late 1995, 67% of respondents purchased "cooked meats, etc." and 81% purchased "meat or poultry" at least weekly, compared to 69% and 82%, respectively, in late 1998. This suggests that, if there was any reduction in beef consumption (as there certainly was, albeit to different degrees and for different lengths of time in each country) it was compensated for by increased purchases of alternative meats.

If specific countries are examined, a somewhat different picture emerges. In Germany, for instance, meat purchases (and, one may assume, consumption) became more frequent in the three-year interval considered, whereas in Finland there was a reduction, especially in cooked meat purchases. In general, meat purchases were more frequent in households with children and in families with higher socioeconomic status.

The QPCB study in the spring of 1997 asked family food purchasers to assess changes in their household's consumption of meat, which was broken down into three distinct categories: beef, pork and chicken. The three categories present very different profiles, as can be seen in Figure 5.1.

- **Beef**. In each of the three countries involved in both the QPCB study and the present study (United Kingdom, Germany, Italy), about half of all respondents said that there had been no change in quantities consumed with respect to five years earlier. However, practically all of the remaining respondents (from 39% in Italy to 51% in Germany) said that there had been a reduction in consumption. In Italy, a minority of 10% of food purchasers nevertheless stated that beef consumption had actually grown over time.

- **Pork**. A strong majority of respondents reported no change in quantities consumed. The net change was negative in all three countries, however, in that the percentage of food purchasers reporting a decline in consumption was two to four times greater than the percentage reporting consumption increases. The reduction was greatest in Germany.

- **Chicken**. More than half of all respondents reported no change in their household's consumption of chicken in the 1992–1997 period. Among the remaining respondents, there was a strong increase, with the number of respondents reporting an increase being between two-and-a-half and five times greater than the number reporting declining consumption.

These findings seem to confirm that many families' "meat portfolio" has changed content over the

Sample surveys of

years. To some degree, of course, this is probably dependent on factors having nothing to do with the BSE scare. The question, therefore, is: which factors may have contributed to determining these changes? The next section examines findings concerning of food safety. (This chapter examines only sample survey findings; the same general topic is explored in other parts of this study, especially through focus groups: see Chapter 4.)

- **Public concern and perception of risks to food safety**

Safety of products in general and food in particular

At the beginning of the 1990s, the great majority of European consumers were concerned about product safety in general. As can be seen in Table 5.2, over 70% of EU citizens stated that they were either "very" or "somewhat" concerned about the safety of consumer products and services. In no

Figure 5.1. Change in chicken, pork and beef consumption 1992–1997, selected countries

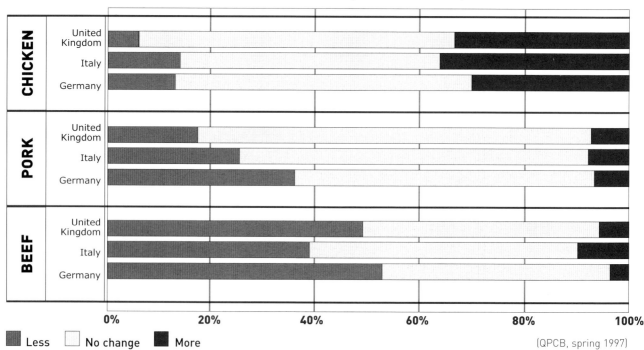

Less   No change   More

(QPCB, spring 1997)

public perceptions and opinion

country was the level of concern thus defined lower than the 50% threshold, with the exception of Denmark. Nevertheless, there was much variability across countries. Considering only the countries involved in this study, an extraordinarily high level of concern is seen in the United Kingdom (86% of respondents at least "somewhat" concerned), an average level of concern among Italians (70%) and a particularly low level in Germany (51%). Germany, along with Denmark and Belgium, expressed (in 1992) relatively low levels of unease due to product safety, with 40%–60% of respondents stating that they were either "not very" or even "not at all" concerned.

Product safety is a general concept that includes food safety, but also includes other types of concern that have nothing to do with food products. This obvious consideration probably explains why, in later Eurobarometers, the question asked in Table 5.2 was refined to take into account many different types of product categories.

Eurobarometer 47, administered at the beginning of 1997 (almost one year after the first "mad cow disease" crisis in the United Kingdom), contained two questions about food safety. In the first, respondents were asked to indicate which, among 13 product and service

Table 5.2. Concerns about product safety, selected countries

Response distributions to the question: "In general, do you feel very concerned, somewhat concerned, not very concerned, or not at all concerned about the safety of products and services for consumers?"

Degree of concern	EU	United Kingdom	Germany	Italy
Very	27.7	45.9	12.5	20.0
Somewhat	43.0	39.9	39.0	50.4
Not very	20.9	11.8	34.8	21.9
Not at all	6.7	2.1	11.1	5.1
Don't know	1.7	0.3	2.6	2.5
Total	100	100	100	100
Very + somewhat	70.7	85.8	51.5	70.4

(Eurobarometer 38.0: September–October 1992, percentage values)

Sample surveys of

categories, evoked particular concern as regards safety.

Table 5.3 shows that, at the European level (15 countries), 68% of respondents chose the "food" category. This, along with "medicines", was the only category selected by over half of all subjects.[3] All four of the countries in this study present levels of concern that were below the European average:

Germany 67%, Italy 61%, United Kingdom 54% and Finland 39%. Finland was by far the least concerned about food safety: electrical appliances caused more concern than food (or medicines, for

---

[3] This overall pattern presented many exceptions at the national level. For example, Denmark, France and Luxembourg expressed particularly high levels of concern about food safety whereas other countries, such as Austria and Portugal, were more at ease.

Table 5.3. Concerns about specific types of products, selected countries

Response distributions to the question "Which of the following do you feel particularly concerned about, as regards the safety of products and services for consumers" (several answers possible)?

Product or service types / Percentage feeling "concerned"	EU	United Kingdom	Germany	Italy	Finland
Food	67.9	54.2	66.7	61.3	39.3
Medicines	67.3	60.7	59.1	63.5	42.2
Cleaning products	37.9	40.0	31.5	21.4	29.0
Electrical appliances	32.7	41.1	10.5	19.3	53.7
Public transport	30.1	31.6	11.5	29.3	6.8
Toys	29.9	50.5	11.9	12.0	26.3
Cars	28.7	28.6	8.5	15.3	5.2
Planes	26.8	21.5	26.7	24.6	14.9
Public places	25.8	21.8	12.8	19.0	6.2
Cosmetic products	25.6	21.3	27.7	20.0	22.4
Restaurants	20.9	20.8	8.3	13.1	6.9
Sports events	20.1	17.8	13.4	20.3	5.5
Hotels	12.7	14.0	4.4	6.7	4.8
None	7.6	11.8	9.9	5.9	10.6
Don't know	3.2	2.0	5.4	3.2	5.3

(Eurobarometer 47.0: January–February 1997; categories ordered in terms of decreasing concern at EU level, percentage values)

public perceptions and opinion

that matter). In the United Kingdom, citizens expressed almost as high a degree of anxiety about toy safety as they did about food safety.

Analysed at the level of subsets within national populations, each country presented different profiles in their concerns about food. In Italy, for example, concern for food safety was higher among respondents belonging to households with no children, having higher socioeconomic status, and residing in central regions. In the United Kingdom, such concern was higher among individuals with high socioeconomic status, but also (unlike Italy) in households with children, as well as in non-metropolitan parts of England. In Finland there was a gender difference absent in the other three countries: women were much more concerned about food safety than men. In Germany there was no signifi-

cant variation among subgroups.

The national response profiles can be further refined by taking into account each population's tendency to express concern in general.[4] Table 5.4 lists the percentage of respondents that indicated food to be a source of particular safety concern, the average percentage of subjects indicating concern for each product/service category, and the difference between these two values. The fact that

---

[4] An example for illustrative purposes: France has proportionally more citizens who claim to be concerned about food safety than other countries, but French citizens are, on average, more concerned about safety in all product/service categories than other Europeans. This means France's higher level of concern for food safety may depend not so much on the specificity of its population's perception of food, as on its general perception of product/service safety.

Table 5.4. Concern about food in particular and products/services in general, selected countries

Geographical area / Percentage feeling "concerned"	Concern for food safety in particular	Concern about product/ service safety in general[a]	Difference: "food" - "general"
Germany	66.7	22.5	+44.2
Italy	61.3	25.1	+36.2
European Union	67.9	32.8	+35.1
United Kingdom	54.2	32.6	+21.6
Finland	39.3	20.2	+19.1

[a] Mean percentage across all product/service categories in Table 5.3.   (Eurobarometer 47.0: January–February 1997, percentage values)

Sample surveys of

in each country these differences were largely positive confirms that food was everywhere a source of worry to a much greater degree than other product categories. But the degree of additional concern felt in relation to food varies widely across countries. In particular, the populations in Germany and Italy were most concerned about food safety, vis-à-vis safety of other products and services. This conclusion deserves a closer look: for example,

Germany's percentage of food-concerned citizens (66.7%) was similar to the European average (67.9%), but this hides the fact that Germans were on the whole less concerned about general product safety (22.5%) than Europeans as a whole (32.8%). This means their concern for food safety was relatively high. The populations of Finland and the United Kingdom appeared unconcerned with food in relative terms: food was a source of worry to a

Table 5.5. Concern about food and products/services in respondents' own country, selected countries

Response distributions to the question: "For each of the following products and services, do you think that those offered in (your country) are generally safe, or not?"

Product or service types / Percentage responding "safe"	EU	United Kingdom	Germany	Italy	Finland
Food	52.1	68.1	28.7	44.8	85.9
Cosmetic products	53.1	73.4	46.7	44.5	68.4
Sports events	54.0	72.2	54.1	44.4	87.4
Cleaning products	55.3	65.2	46.7	48.4	72.2
Planes	60.7	80.6	56.3	45.8	86.7
Public places	61.6	76.7	59.8	49.0	89.3
Public transport	62.3	73.0	66.1	41.5	89.7
Medicines	62.9	76.6	45.0	45.9	84.0
Toys	64.1	68.9	63.6	61.8	72.9
Hotels	66.9	80.6	70.5	57.4	87.1
Restaurants	67.0	79.0	68.3	55.4	84.3
Cars	71.2	77.2	75.4	62.0	86.1
Electrical appliances	73.7	83.7	73.7	57.0	70.8

(Eurobarometer 47.0: January–February 1997; categories ordered in terms of increasing perception of safety; percentage values)

public perceptions and opinion

higher-than-average degree, but less so than in other countries.

A second question in Eurobarometer 47 offered respondents the same range of thirteen product/service categories and asked whether they were generally safe in the interviewees' country of residence. The food category was once again, at European level, the category that least evoked an image of safety (Table 5.5). Little more than half of all respondents (52%) felt that food in their home country was safe. Finland was again the country that appeared to be least concerned about food safety: 86% of the population felt their food was "safe". The United Kingdom was also relatively unconcerned, with 68% of subjects responding that their country's food was safe. At the other extreme, Italy and Germany (along with Greece) were

the only EU countries in which less than half the population believed that their food was "safe".

In most of the countries in this study, the perception of food as being safe was greater among individuals with higher household incomes. In some (but not all) countries there were significant geographical differences: in the United Kingdom, those living in London felt less safe than other British citizens; in Italy, those living in the north felt safer. In both of these countries, perceptions of safety were higher among older members of the population, whereas in Finland the opposite was true.

In Table 5.6, the greatest difference between the percentage of people who felt that food was safe and the average percentage of people who felt that all the product/service categories in the questionnaire

Table 5.6. Relationship of food and product/service safety in respondents' own country, selected countries

Geographical area / Percentage responding "safe"	Food in own country	Products and services in general[a]	Difference: "food" – "general"
Germany	28.7	58.1	-29.4
European Union	52.1	61.9	- 9.8
United Kingdom	68.1	75.0	- 6.9
Italy	44.8	50.6	- 5.8
Finland	85.9	81.9	+ 4.0

[a] Mean percentage across all product/service categories in Table 5.5.   (Eurobarometer 47.0: January–February 1997, percentage values)

Sample surveys of

were safe was seen among German respondents. This means that food was perceived as particularly unsafe compared to the other product categories. At the other extreme, in Finland, food was perceived to be safer, on average, than other product categories.

Meat safety

Eurobarometers 47 and 49 offer an opportunity to assess public perceptions of the safety of a food product that is especially relevant for BSE and CJD risk: fresh meat. In Eurobarometer 47, interviewees were requested to evaluate the improvement (or worsening) in quality of a set of food products over time, including fresh meat. As Table 5.7 shows, at the European level, about 30% of respondents

claimed that meat quality had been improving, whereas 43% felt that it had been getting worse, with a net "balance" of -12.5 percentage points. In Germany and Italy, respondents expressed perceptions of the evolution of fresh meat quality that were more negative than the European average. In Finland and the United Kingdom, negative responses tended to counterbalance positive ones. Finland's profile was characterized by the highest incidence of respondents (44%) who stated that meat quality was neither improving nor worsening. In Finland and Germany, perceptions of the evolution of meat quality were more or less stable across population subgroups. In Italy, the conviction that the quality of fresh meat had improved

Table 5.7. Improvement or worsening in meat quality, selected countries

Response distributions to the question: "Some people think that the quality of food products sold in (your country) is improving, whilst others think it is getting worse. For each of the following products sold in (your country), please tell me if you think its quality is tending to improve or tending to get worse."

Geographical area	Tending to improve	Tending to get worse	Neither improving nor getting worse	Don't know	Total	Difference: "improve" – "get worse"
Germany	22.0	58.5	12.9	6.6	100	-36.5
Italy	26.7	42.2	25.2	5.9	100	-15.5
European Union	30.1	42.6	22.0	5.3	100	-12.5
Finland	22.9	28.0	43.9	5.1	100	- 5.1
United Kingdom	30.7	29.4	32.2	7.7	100	+ 1.3

(Eurobarometer 47.0: January–February 1997; percentage values referring to the product category "fresh meat")

public perceptions and opinion

was more frequent among those living in the north, middle-aged individuals, and people with higher incomes. In the United Kingdom, that belief was more frequent among people living outside London (and, in general, among people living in the other constituent countries of the United Kingdom apart from England), as well as among women, older people and richer individuals.

A little more than a year later, in April–May 1998, Eurobarometer 49 asked Europeans whether they thought fresh meat was "safe" or "not safe", thus tapping a conceptual dimension that can reasonably be presumed to relate to quality. As can be seen in Table 5.8, approximately 60% of the interviewees said that they felt fresh meat to be safe — a percentage slightly higher than the 52% who, a little more than a year earlier in Eurobarometer 47 (Tables 5.5 and 5.6), believed that food in general was safe.

The differences among European countries were pronounced. At one extreme was Germany, where only 34% of respondents said that they felt meat to be safe; at the other was Italy, where those satisfied with meat safety amounted to 85%. Finland was similar to Italy, with 81% responding "safe". The United Kingdom was close to the European average, with 67% of respondents saying that they felt their meat to be safe. Once again, Finland and Germany differed from Italy and the United Kingdom, with a lower level of variability across population subgroups (although in Finland men seemed more satisfied with the safety of meat than women). In the United Kingdom, those living in London again seemed much less satisfied than other citizens; men, childless households and individuals with higher incomes were more comfortable with meat safety than other subgroups. In Italy, on the other hand, women and households

Table 5.8. Perception of the safety of fresh meat, selected countries

Response category	EU	United Kingdom	Germany	Italy	Finland
Safe	60.4	67.1	34.3	84.6	81.2
Not safe	33.6	23.2	57.4	10.1	14.6
Don't know	6.0	9.7	8.2	5.3	4.2
Total	100	100	100	100	100

(Eurobarometer 49.0: April–May 1998, percentage values)

Sample surveys of

with children were more comfortable with their meat. Table 5.9 compares the percentages of respondents stating that food was safe in January–February 1997 and that meat was safe in March–April 1998. The questions were worded differently, and administered in different questionnaire contexts to different samples of people, so caution should be used in interpreting the findings. Nevertheless, the table gives some sense of how perceptions of meat safety fit within the wider context of perceptions of food safety. The last column of the table is equal to the difference, in percentage points, between the number of respondents who believed that fresh meat was safe and those who believed that food in general was safe. A positive value means that respondents, on average, feel that meat was a relatively safe food category (compared to food in general), whereas a negative value means that meat was perceived as relatively unsafe.

Italy stands out as a country in which respondents expressed an extremely high degree of confidence in fresh meat. In Finland, Germany and the United Kingdom the differences were close to 0, indicating that perceptions of safety in food and in meat were basically the same.

Factors affecting perception of food quality
The findings reported above shed some light on perceptions of food safety in general and meat safety in particular in the second half of the 1990s. However, these findings say nothing about why a particular food or meat product was considered to be safe or unsafe. For this, the study looked at questions first administered a few months before the March 1996 BSE crisis in Eurobarometer 44.1

Table 5.9. Perception of food safety versus meat safety

Geographical area	Fresh meat is "safe" (EB 49)	Food is "safe" (EB 47)	Difference: "fresh meat"– "food"
Finland	81.2	85.9	-4.7
United Kingdom	67.1	68.1	-1.0
Germany	34.3	28.7	+5.6
European Union	60.4	52.1	+8.3
Italy	84.6	44.8	+39.8

(Eurobarometers 47.0: January–February 1997 and 49.0: March–April 1998, percentage values)

public perceptions and opinion

(November–December 1995) and again some three years later in Eurobarometer 50.1 (November–December 1998).The question focused on factors determining perceptions of food quality in general and decisions relating to the purchase of meat and poultry.

Table 5.10 shows that the ranking of factors determining the perception of food quality changed, at the European level, over the three-year period. The

most important factors in 1995 were the conditions of hygiene in which a food product was made or produced, "tastiness" of the food, "appetising" appearance and "natural taste". Surprisingly, the importance of the first of these factors declined noticeably over time, whereas the second and the third grew slightly more relevant.

Country-specific differences were sometimes quite

Table 5.10. Most important factors in determining the quality of a food product, selected countries, 1995–1998

Factors determining food product quality	EU		United Kingdom		Germany		Italy		Finland	
	Late 1995	Late 1998	Late 1995	Late 1998	Late 1995	Late 1998	Late 1995	Late 1998	Late 1995	Late 1998
Strict hygiene conditions	41.1	31.5	46.1	32.4	40.0	30.8	47.1	35.7	39.3	34.5
Is tasty/has a good taste	38.8	43.5	43.4	55.2	38.0	43.7	31.9	32.6	56.3	57.3
Looks appetising	35.4	37.3	45.3	49.8	38.8	39.6	16.5	17.4	22.7	25.8
Keeps its natural taste	35.3	35.0	32.8	32.9	27.2	26.7	35.4	34.2	28.7	25.6
Is checked by a public body	26.6	23.6	16.7	12.1	37.0	31.4	27.3	23.2	30.1	21.5
Carries a quality label	25.3	27.7	20.4	22.3	25.0	31.1	29.8	28.9	25.0	17.7
Well-known reputable brand name	24.8	26.8	40.0	33.0	17.8	22.0	35.6	40.3	14.9	16.7
Is made/produced in (your country)	23.8	22.5	18.5	14.8	28.9	26.2	14.7	17.5	59.6	63.4
Comes from specific countries or areas	15.0	15.7	7.1	6.3	22.1	27.1	15.6	13.7	7.3	13.1
Is more expensive than the average	3.8	2.8	4.1	2.8	3.5	2.7	3.6	2.9	1.5	1.7
Don't know	1.8	1.5	1.7	2.2	3.3	1.0	1.6	2.8	0.7	2.0
Something else	0.9	1.5	1.2	1.9	0.9	1.8	1.0	1.1	0.9	1.5

(Eurobarometers 44.1 and 50.1; several answers possible, percentage values)

Sample surveys of

marked. For example, Finns and Britons placed more of a premium on "tastiness", Germans and Britons valued a food's appearance, and Italians stressed natural taste. Reputable brand names were valued to a greater degree by Italians and Britons. At the European level as a whole, and in each of the four countries as well, the call for con-

trols performed by public bodies seems to have diminished between 1995 and 1998.

Table 5.11 ranks the factors that influenced household decisions regarding the purchase of meat and poultry. The "look of the product" — defined by aspects such as colour, smell, freshness and consistency — was by

Table 5.11. Factors influencing family decisions to buy meat and poultry, selected countries, 1995–1998

Factors influencing decisions to buy meat and poultry	EU		United Kingdom		Germany		Italy		Finland	
	Late 1995	Late 1998	Late 1995	Late 1998	Late 1995	Late 1998	Late 1995	Late 1998	Late 1995	Late 1998
Look of the product (colour, smell, freshness, consistency)	66.3	66.4	78.8	73.3	47.9	57.6	69.2	67.3	65.4	57.4
Not too high a price	32.1	30.0	44.6	42.5	23.8	37.4	22.1	17.7	47.8	31.6
Area or country where the product was made or produced	25.4	28.3	20.1	22.2	36.5	45.7	20.1	16.5	49.0	60.7
Type of outlet selling it	24.2	24.6	34.4	26.3	17.4	25.8	31.7	26.3	7.9	9.7
Quality label	23.9	26.7	15.3	22.8	19.3	27.4	18.6	14.7	30.0	32.2
Date stamps	12.5	13.7	5.0	10.9	12.1	15.7	8.1	8.3	7.7	10.5
Brand	11.1	12.7	10.1	13.4	18.7	18.4	11.0	10.8	9.7	14.1
Designation of origin	9.8	10.5	4.8	3.6	21.4	23.3	7.5	5.7	13.2	1.7
Its traditional character	7.9	8.5	8.2	8.9	5.7	7.5	10.6	9.0	20.3	16.0
Not too low a price	3.4	3.2	3.5	3.2	2.4	3.0	4.8	4.3	0.8	1.1
Nothing		0.5		0.3		0.2		0.5		0.3
Something else	1.5	1.5	1.2	1.5	1.3	1.0	1.2	2.8	0.2	1.3
Don't know	8.5	2.4	4.7	3.6	24.2	1.5	3.8	3.4	6.1	6.8

(Eurobarometers 44.1 and 50.0/50.1; several answers possible, percentage values)

public perceptions and opinion

far the most important factor, and indeed the only one mentioned consistently by the majority of respondents. Four other factors were mentioned by a sizeable minority (one quarter or one third of interviewees): price, area or country of production, type of sales outlet, and the presence of a quality label on the product. Origin and quality labels slightly increased in importance over time, which may indicate a greater sensitivity to "quality" considerations.

Once again, differences were apparent between countries. Italians assigned less importance to price, but more to outlet type; Finns and Germans were more influenced than others by the area or country of production; Germans depended on quality labels to a greater degree than others; Finns were much more concerned than others about where meat and poultry came from, etc.

The QPCB study was not totally consistent with these Eurobarometer findings. One example of results that differed can be seen in Table 5.12, which lists (in order of descending priority) the features named by food purchasers when asked to specify what helped them to evaluate "quality in the shop" for beef (i.e. the characteristics of a beef product or its packaging that can be directly examined by the consumer). The "look of the product" — its colour, leanness, marbling — was reported to be less important than place of purchase or place of origin in most countries, and price was not a priority. It should be noted

Table 5.12. Helpfulness of visible characteristics in purchasing beef, selected countries (characteristics ordered in terms of descending priority)

Helpfulness of characteristics	United Kingdom	Germany	Italy
1	Colour, leanness	Origin, place of purchase	Colour, place of purchase
2	Place of purchase, marbling, label	Leanness, colour	Origin
3	Price, origin	Marbling, label	Marbling, label, leanness
4		Price	Price

(QPCB, spring 1997)

Sample surveys of

that, besides methodological differences (sampling frame, etc.), the two sets of results also relate to different objects: food quality in general for the Eurobarometer and beef quality for the QPCB project. This illustrates the point argued above: it is difficult, in secondary analyses, to compare findings drawn from different surveys.

Factors affecting perception of food and meat safety
Eurobarometer 49 (March–April 1998) asked potential consumers what factors they thought determined the safety of food products. The response distributions present a high degree of dispersion, and even the most frequently cited items barely achieve a majority of answers at the European level.

Table 5.13 indicates that the main factors that respondents associated with safety in a food product were: complete absence of pesticides; complete absence of hormones; and evidence that the food was produced according to controls imposed by

Table 5.13. Factors determining safety of a food product, selected countries

Factors determining food-product safety	EU	United Kingdom	Germany	Italy	Finland
100% free from pesticides	56.4	56.3	58.0	63.5	46.4
100% free from hormones	53.9	48.7	55.1	49.0	53.7
Product controls undertaken by authorized bodies	49.1	39.7	50.5	51.9	55.7
100% free from additives	35.7	33.5	33.5	43.9	30.6
Only contains permitted preservatives	34.5	35.4	37.7	28.3	53.5
Only contains permitted additives	32.8	34.4	41.5	17.6	56.2
Suitable packaging	28.5	27.0	27.6	23.7	23.3
100% free from preservatives	28.1	19.5	28.3	34.9	19.8
Scientists' limits on amounts of pesticides/hormones	20.5	26.3	18.1	12.6	17.0
None	0.9	1.0	1.4	0.5	0.3
Other	0.6	0.6	0.6	1.3	0.5
Don't know	5.3	7.0	6.0	3.3	3.0

(Eurobarometer 49.0: April–May 1998, several answers possible, percentage values)

public perceptions and opinion

authorized bodies. The absence of additives and preservatives was also important.

As seen earlier in Table 5.11, the "type of outlet" selling a food product was a relatively important factor in purchasing decisions. This indicates that quality and safety perceptions are influenced by where food is bought. Table 5.14 lists the outlets where consumers believed the safest foods could be found. The distribution of responses was surprisingly polarized: almost half of all respondents seemed to have great confidence in supermarkets, hypermarkets and large stores (representing the "industrial" or "big business" dimension of food production and distribution); but just as many respondents seemed to trust farmers and small producers (who represent the "local" or "small business" dimension).

This balance between "big" and "small" distribution at the European level does not always hold at the national level. "Big" stores were greatly preferred by British people, for instance, while small producers were preferred by Germans. In many countries where "farmers and small producers" were not mentioned often, "small grocers or corner shops" were frequently cited: this suggests that national response distributions might have been influenced by specific features of national retail structures. This is in part confirmed by the fact that supermarkets were preferred to a greater degree in metropolitan regions (Northern

Table 5.14. Sources of safe food products, selected countries

Response distributions to the question: "In your opinion where do you find the safest food products?"

Sources of safe food	EU	United Kingdom	Germany	Italy	Finland
Super/hypermarkets or large stores	46.5	78.3	21.8	47.1	53.5
Farmers/small producers	45.5	23.9	62.3	44.6	61.5
Markets	23.7	9.1	28.1	9.8	29.6
Small grocers or corner shops	19.5	17.3	10.1	16.9	34.2
Somewhere else	2.5	2.0	1.8	4.1	1.3
Nowhere	6.2	2.1	11.6	7.4	0.8
Don't know	6.6	6.2	8.3	7.2	3.2

(Eurobarometer 49.0: April–May 1998; several answers possible, percentage values)

Sample surveys of

Table 5.15. Concerns about beef, selected countries (concerns ordered in terms of descending priority)

Rating of concerns	United Kingdom	Germany	Italy
1	Salmonella, antibiotics, BSE, hormones	BSE, hormones, antibiotics	Hormones, BSE, antibiotics, salmonella
2	Fat/cholesterol	Salmonella	Fat/cholesterol
3		Fat/cholesterol	

(QPCB, spring 1997)

Table 5.16. Helpfulness of safety indicators regarding beef, selected countries (indicators ordered in terms of descending priority)

Helpfulness of indicators	United Kingdom	Germany	Italy
1	Freshness	Country of origin, freshness	Feed
2	Label, feed	Feed	Freshness
3	Origin, organic	Organic, producer, label	Origin, label, organic
4	Price	Price	Price
5	Producer		

(QPCB, spring 1997)

public perceptions and opinion

Italy, London, Uusimaa, West Germany).The QPCB survey included a few questions specifically concerning the safety of beef. Table 5.15 shows that the chief concerns were the use of hormones and antibiotics and the risk of contracting salmonella. Also, BSE was perceived as a major source of risk. These concerns do not seem to match up well with the "safety indicators" suggested by the sample food purchasers in Table 5.16: freshness was an important indicator of safety, but obviously this is no guarantee against the risks implied by hormones, antibiotics or salmonella.

• The question of trust
Trust in information sources

At the beginning of the 1990s, European consumers felt that they were, for the most part, not very well informed about food safety. In particular, in the only specific — albeit partial — reference to "mad cow disease" in Eurobarometer data (mentioned in the reference to "diseases in animals bred for human consumption", 1992, Table 5.17), Denmark, Italy and the Netherlands were then the only EU countries in which more than 20% of the population felt they had enough

Table 5.17. Sufficiency of information about food risks, selected countries

Response distributions to the question: "Do you feel that people are sufficiently informed or not about each of the following situations?"

Situations / response category	EU	United Kingdom	Germany	Italy
Pollution in food				
Yes	21.7	17.0	20.4	27.8
No	73.3	79.9	73.6	65.6
Don't know	4.9	3.1	5.9	6.6
Total	100	100	100	100
Diseases in animals bred for human consumption (e.g. mad cow disease)				
Yes	18.9	18.1	16.6	23.4
No	73.3	79.1	74.8	63.9
Don't know	7.8	2.8	8.6	12.7
Total	100	100	100	100

(Eurobarometer 38.0: September–October 1992, percentage values)

Sample surveys of

Table 5.18. Truthfulness of information sources, selected countries

Response distributions to the question: "Do the following people or organizations tell you the whole truth, only part of the truth or no truth at all about the safety of food products?"

Degree of truth	Producers	Small grocers	Stall-holders	Supermarkets
EU				
Whole truth	11.8	19.2	16.0	18.1
Only part of the truth	68.6	59.5	56.7	58.6
No truth at all	14.0	12.2	19.6	16.6
Don't know	5.7	9.1	7.6	6.6
Total	100	100	100	100
United Kingdom				
Whole truth	10.5	18.5	8.1	31.4
Only part of the truth	77.5	61.0	52.7	57.8
No truth at all	6.4	10.4	30.3	6.6
Don't know	5.7	10.2	8.9	4.2
Total	100	100	100	100
Germany				
Whole truth	7.7	19.4	23.5	8.6
Only part of the truth	61.7	53.4	51.8	59.3
No truth at all	24.0	13.8	15.5	23.5
Don't know	6.5	13.5	9.3	8.5
Total	100	100	100	100
Italy				
Whole truth	9.8	12.4	8.4	20.7
Only part of the truth	65.9	60.4	55.8	54.9
No truth at all	17.8	18.9	26.3	15.2
Don't know	6.5	8.4	9.5	9.2
Total	100	100	100	100
Finland				
Whole truth	26.3	23.0.	22.5	18.8
Only part of the truth	67.6	69.0	62.4	67.1
No truth at all	1.9	3.8	8.5	8.5
Don't know	4.2	4.2	6.6	5.6
Total	100	100	100	100

(Eurobarometer 49.0: April–May 1998, percentage values)

public perceptions and opinion

Consumer organizations	Public bodies	European institutions
51.9	26.0	21.1
34.4	51.2	47.8
6.0	11.7	12.4
7.6	11.2	18.6
100	100	100
47.7	25.5	19.4
38.8	55.8	51.0
4.9	7.4	9.4
8.6	11.3	20.2
100	100	100
54.9	25.7	16.5
29.3	47.5	46.5
7.9	12.0	16.6
7.8	14.8	20.4
100	100	100
47.3	21.3	25.1
35.4	51.2	42.4
7.0	14.9	10.2
10.3	12.6	22.4
100	100	100
53.3	39.9	16.0
36.4	48.4	55.4
1.9	3.3	9.9
8.4	8.5	18.8
100	100	100

information. This Eurobarometer was performed in 1992, well before "BSE" became a household word, especially outside the United Kingdom and cattle-breeding circles. In the United Kingdom, as can be seen in Table 5.17, the demand for more information relating to food pollution (i.e. contamination) or disease among animals bred for human consumption was only slightly higher than the European average.

In 1998, Eurobarometer 49 asked respondents to rank the credibility of several potential information sources — producers, small grocers, stall-holders, supermarkets, consumer organizations, public bodies and European institutions — regarding the information they provided about food safety. Consumer organizations were by far the most frequently mentioned as trustworthy, as can be seen in Table 5.18. At the European level, just over half of all respondents felt that consumer organizations told the "whole truth" about food safety, but 34% said that even consumer organizations were only partly credible (and an additional 6% lent them no credence at all). Public bodies and European institutions fared only slightly better than the other sources, some of which might have been perceived to have direct economic interests in not being totally honest about food safety. Finns appeared to have more trust in sources such as producers, small grocers, stall-holders, and especially public bodies (which 40% of Finnish respondents described as telling the "whole truth"). This may help explain why Finns were generally less concerned about food safety compared to other European populations. In 1997, Eurobarometer 47 also explored consumer

113

Sample surveys of

Table 5.19. Perceived bias of information sources, selected countries

Response distributions to the question: "Do you think that the information on the quality of food products provided by each of the following sources is generally more in the interest of consumers, more in the interest of industry or neutral?"

Information biased towards:	Teachers and lecturers	Scientists	Public authorities	Government agencies	European Commission
EU					
Consumers	36.2	23.2	24.1	14.5	18.9
Industry	12.2	38.4	39.0	49.5	40.9
Neutral	36.2	25.6	22.1	19.4	20.9
Don't know	15.4	12.8	14.7	16.6	19.3
Total	100	100	100	100	100
United Kingdom					
Consumers	29.5	18.4	25.5	12.0	13.8
Industry	11.5	44.7	39.4	55.4	41.3
Neutral	37.7	20.6	17.5	14.3	18.0
Don't know	21.3	16.3	17.6	18.3	26.9
Total	100	100	100	100	100
Germany					
Consumers	29.8	22.2	27.2	9.6	11.5
Industry	12.9	36.8	34.3	59.5	52.3
Neutral	41.4	29.5	24.6	16.1	19.5
Don't know	15.9	11.5	13.9	14.8	16.7
Total	100	100	100	100	100
Italy					
Consumers	43.5	32.0	19.1	12.5	28.7
Industry	10.5	33.6	46.9	50.2	32.6
Neutral	31.7	21.7	18.0	17.4	21.0
Don't know	14.3	12.7	16.0	19.9	17.6
Total	100	100	100	100	100
Finland					
Consumers	23.8	9.9	16.8	12.2	10.8
Industry	20.1	31.9	33.6	40.8	42.3
Neutral	41.6	44.1	32.7	30.0	22.5
Don't know	14.5	14.1	16.8	16.9	24.4
Total	100	100	100	100	100

(Eurobarometer 47.0: January–February 1997; percentage values)

public perceptions and opinion

Producer groups	Political parties	Trade unions	Shops/ supermarkets	Radio & television	Press
23.9	12.3	35.6	37.2	37.3	36.2
55.2	45.5	25.9	40.6	24.6	21.5
9.0	22.6	20.1	12.1	25.4	27.6
11.9	19.5	18.3	10.1	12.7	14.7
100	100	100	100	100	100
22.2	9.1	22.6	45.6	45.0	39.8
50.1	48.7	38.5	30.6	16.5	16.8
10.3	20.3	18.1	12.0	23.7	26.9
17.3	21.9	20.8	11.8	14.8	16.5
100	100	100	100	100	100
16.1	11.6	42.5	29.6	35.6	36.2
70.7	52.2	20.4	50.9	23.5	19.2
5.5	18.9	20.9	11.1	30.1	32.1
7.7	17.3	16.2	8.3	10.8	12.5
100	100	100	100	100	100
25.8	9.9	33.0	27.5	24.0	21.4
54.5	49.4	31.8	47.6	40.8	38.2
8.4	19.5	16.6	14.1	21.0	23.0
11.4	21.2	18.6	10.8	14.2	17.3
100	100	100	100	100	100
26.4	13.7	41.1	33.8	29.6	29.1
49.1	43.9	25.2	42.7	21.1	20.2
11.3	16.0	15.9	11.3	33.3	32.9
13.2	26.4	17.8	12.2	16.0	17.8
100	100	100	100	100	100

Sample surveys of

trust in information sources about food quality. One question invited respondents to assess whether a range of information sources — almost completely different from the range used in Eurobarometer 49 — were biased more in the interest of consumers or the food industry, or were neutral. As can be seen in Table 5.19, teachers and lecturers, trade unions, radio and television and the press were perceived as being by far the most consumer-oriented, or at least neutral, sources at the European level. Teachers and lecturers

were considered to be acting in the interest of industry only by a small majority of respondents. Trade unions, radio and television and the press were perceived as being biased towards industry by at least one in four interviewees, but those who believed that they acted in the interest of consumers were even more numerous. Government agencies and political parties were considered to be pro-industry to the same degree as producer groups. Shopkeepers and supermarkets were considered to be much more partial towards con-

Table 5.20. Perceived truthfulness of information sources about food quality, selected countries

Response distributions to the question: "Could you tell me which sources you think tell the truth about the quality of food products?" (several answers possible)

Information sources	EU	United Kingdom	Germany	Italy	Finland
Scientists	35.8	30.9	34.3	35.7	42.4
Teachers and lecturers	32.7	33.1	25.2	27.7	28.2
Radio and television	21.5	25.4	28.1	7.7	25.0
The press	21.1	17.6	30.3	6.5	20.2
Trade unions	13.5	11.7	17.4	8.1	9.2
Producer groups	13.3	11.3	10.2	14.3	15.7
Public authorities	12.3	12.1	15.9	4.9	21.0
Shops/supermarkets	10.8	18.8	6.3	5.7	9.3
European Commission	10.5	7.7	5.5	14.6	8.0
Government agencies	6.7	5.6	3.0	3.3	14.1
Political parties	3.0	2.9	2.6	1.7	2.4
Nobody	16.2	14.4	19.4	15.9	9.8
Don't know	13.3	12.0	11.4	17.5	14.8

(Eurobarometer 47.0: January–February 1997, percentage values)

public perceptions and opinion

sumers than any other of these actors, including scientists. Finns again distinguished themselves in that they assigned neutral behaviour to most actors to a greater degree than other Europeans. Italians trusted the European Commission more than other populations, but trusted radio, television and the press much less. British respondents were the most trusting of the media, but also the most suspicious of scientists.

A related question ranked which of the sources listed in Table 5.19 told "the truth about the quality of food products". As can be seen in Table 5.20, the results present a high degree of variability. Even though each interviewee could give several answers (and on average gave 2.1 responses), only one information source — scientists — was cited by at least one third of respondents. This is different from the finding in Table 5.19, which indicated that just over one third of

respondents (38.4%) at European level viewed scientists as a source whose information was biased towards the interests of industry. It is likely that views about scientists were highly polarized: some people do not trust them, whereas those who do trust them believe in them to a great degree.

If the scientists anomaly is excepted, the other results are consistent with the data reported in Table 5.19, in that the most trustworthy sources were perceived to be teachers and lecturers, radio and television, and the press. Almost 30% of all respondents said that they did not trust any of the actors, or did not know whom to trust.

The QPCB survey also included a question about trust in various sources of information about meat. Table 5.21 provides an indication that meat retailers were the most trusted sources of information.

Table 5.21. Most trusted sources of information about meat, selected countries (sources ordered in terms of descending priority)

Level of trust in sources	United Kingdom	Germany	Italy
1	Supermarket butchers	Independent retailers/ butchers	Independent retailers/ butchers
2	Independent retailers/ butchers	Supermarket butchers	Supermarket butchers
3	Own opinion	Consumer groups	Department of Health
4	Newspapers	Magazines	Friends
5	Government	Reports	Consumer groups
6	Labelling	Friends	Reports

(QPCB, spring 1997)

Sample surveys of

Among meat retailers, more trust was placed in independent butchers in some countries, whereas in the United Kingdom supermarket butchers were deemed to be more trustworthy (this is consistent with the findings in Table 5.18). Press sources such as newspapers and magazines, if mentioned at all, were ranked relatively low.

• Trust in food safety controls
Eurobarometer 49 included two questions on the role of "controls" and on the authorities responsible for such controls in determining consumer

perceptions of food product safety. One question focused on when food products were considered "safe", the other on when they were considered "unsafe".

Table 5.22 shows that in all countries, albeit in varying degrees, controls at the national level (presumably by public authorities) were mentioned by a majority of respondents, and more frequently than any other type of control. Support for national controls was especially high in Finland. European-level controls were cited by 43% of all

Table 5.22. Trust in food safety controls

Response distributions to the question: "Personally, when do you consider a food product to be safe?"

Types of safety controls	EU	United Kingdom	Germany	Italy	Finland
National controls	66.0	54.4	64.7	63.2	77.6
European controls	42.9	27.7	45.4	45.4	30.6
Controls undertaken by the producers themselves	32.6	37.4	37.3	32.2	26.0
Control procedures undertaken by shopkeepers' associations	30.1	30.7	48.5	16.8	38.4
Controls undertaken by large retailers	29.2	42.0	33.5	23.2	35.5
Other	3.6	3.7	2.5	5.8	1.8
Never	3.1	2.6	5.2	3.7	0.4
Don't know	5.1	8.0	4.3	4.7	2.7

(Eurobarometer 49.0: April–May 1998; several answers possible, percentage values)

public perceptions and opinion

respondents, but within different countries support for European checks was extremely variable, ranging from 27.7% of respondents in the United Kingdom to over 45% in Germany. At the other end of the scale, shopkeepers' associations and large retailers were mentioned by a relatively small proportion of respondents.

Role of the EU

The results reported above suggest that most people did not feel a compelling need for the EU to be involved in guaranteeing product safety. Nevertheless, Eurobarometers, for obvious institutional reasons, have explored this topic in some detail. In three consecutive surveys, performed in 1998 and 1999, European citizens were asked whether or not "protecting consumers and guaranteeing the quality

of products" should be an EU priority. As shown in Table 5.23, not only did over three quarters of respondents say it should be an EU priority, but the percentage of affirmative answers rose with each survey — except in the United Kingdom. The respondents' favourable answers to this specific question were probably determined by the conviction that "protecting consumers" was a good thing, no matter who engages in the activity, rather than by particular trust in the EU.

Another question, administered in April–May 1998 (Eurobarometer 49), produced results that suggest that only about one third of Europeans felt that the EU's publicly expressed commitment to consumer protection had had a positive impact. As can be seen in Table 5.24, respondents at European level were

Table 5.23. Role of the EU

Response distributions to the question: "Should protecting consumers and guaranteeing the quality of products be a priority action of the European Union?"

Response category	EU			United Kingdom			Germany			Italy			Finland		
	Late 1998	Early 1999	Late 1999	Late 1998	Early 1999	Late 1999	Late 1998	Early 1999	Late 1999	Late 1998	Early 1999	Late 1999	Late 1998	Early 1999	Late 1999
Priority	76.9	79.2	79.9	76.6	75.3	73.0	68.8	71.5	72.0	76.2	80.2	83.0	77.1	79.5	80.4
Not a priority	17.5	14.0	13.9	15.6	16.2	14.9	24.5	19.7	20.6	18.4	12.4	12.4	20.1	16.3	17.3
Don't know	5.6	6.8	6.2	7.8	8.5	12.1	6.7	8.8	7.4	5.4	7.4	4.6	2.8	4.2	2.3
Total	100	100	100	100	100	100	100	100	100	100	100	100	100	100	100

(Eurobarometers 50.1: November–December 1998, 51.0: March–April 1999 and 52.0: October–November 1999; percentage values)

Sample surveys of

equally split on whether EU policies have had an impact or not, while a quarter reported not knowing what kind of impact those policies might have had. A further weakening of the call for greater EU involvement is mirrored in findings from Eurobarometer 47 (early 1997) relating to preferences for local, national and EU authorities in consumer education. In each country, respondents preferred local authorities over European ones, and national bodies assumed an intermediate status (except in Italy, where European authorities were preferred over national).

▼ Conclusions
• Key findings
According to Eurobarometer results, frequency of meat-product purchase did not change all that much between late 1995 and 1998 at the European level. Within individual countries, purchase frequency declined in Finland, whereas in Germany it increased. In the QPCB study (spring 1997), about half of all respondents said that there had been no significant change in their consumption of various meats over a five-year period. Consumption of beef and pork products declined over the five years for a sizeable minority of respondents, whereas chicken consumption increased. As mentioned above, these consumption data are likely to be related to long-term trends rather than to specific incidents within the BSE crisis. Eurobarometer data from early 1997 indicate that food and medicines were the only product categories causing concern among a general majority of Europeans. The populations of Germany and Italy

Table 5.24. Impact of EU commitment to consumer protection, selected countries

Response distributions to the question: "The European Union has taken actions to improve the level of consumer protection. Overall, do you think that these actions have tended to improve the level of consumer protection, have tended to reduce the level of consumer protection, or haven't they had any impact?"

Impact of EU actions on consumer protection	EU	United Kingdom	Germany	Italy	Finland
Tended to improve level of protection	34.5	30.2	25.9	38.9	31.3
Tended to reduce level of protection	7.8	6.8	12.1	6.9	7.9
No impact	34.6	41.7	31.1	29.9	45.3
Don't know	23.0	21.3	30.9	24.3	15.4
Total	100	100	100	100	100

(Eurobarometer 49.0: April–May 1998, percentage values)

public perceptions and opinion

expressed more concern than those of Finland and the United Kingdom. In general, there was no strong consensus concerning the evolution of food quality: substantial portions of the population felt that food quality was improving, or getting worse, or remaining the same. Nevertheless, perceptions were more negative in Germany and Italy than in Finland and the United Kingdom. National profiles changed somewhat when the questions turned to meat safety (April–May 1998): meat was held to be relatively safe in Finland and Italy, whereas Germans believed the opposite.

In Finland and Germany, perceptions of food quality and safety were more or less consistent across population subgroups, whereas in Italy and the United Kingdom different subgroups seemed to reflect quite different outlooks. However, these outlooks do not seem to have had any deep-rooted, structural features.

According to Eurobarometer data, the relative importance of factors determining the perception of food quality remained unchanged, at the European level, from late 1995 to 1998. The most important factors influencing this perception were: the conditions of hygiene in which a food product is made or produced; "tastiness"; "appetising" appearance; and "natural taste". The importance of hygienic conditions appears to have declined over time. As regards factors affecting meat and poultry purchases, the "look of the product" was by far the most important factor. Low prices, the area/country of production, sale

through a retail outlet and the presence of quality labels were also relatively important. There were some important differences in national profiles.

In Eurobarometer data, no clear consensus emerged among respondents concerning factors that affected the safety of food products. In the QPCB study, the chief concerns relating to the safety of beef were the use of hormones and antibiotics and the risk of contracting salmonella. BSE was also perceived as an important source of risk.

Among the available sources of information about food safety, Eurobarometer studies suggest that consumer organizations were far more trusted than other sources. Finns placed more trust in producers, small grocers, stall-holders and public authorities; this may help explain why Finns were generally less concerned about food safety than other Europeans. In response to Eurobarometer questions concerning food quality information sources, almost 30% of Europeans said that they did not trust any source of information nor did they know whom to trust. Teachers and lecturers, as well as scientists (although sometimes viewed as being pro-industry), were believed to be most truthful. In the QPCB study, the most trusted information sources about meat were meat retailers.

Most people did not feel a compelling need for the EU to be involved in guaranteeing product safety. Respondents preferred local authorities to European ones as guarantors of consumer safety. National authorities were ranked between the two, except in Italy where the EU was preferred to national authorities.

• Implications for communications policy

The results described in the preceding section offer some important lessons for communication, health and risk policy. For example, the fact that foodstuffs were, along with medicines, the product categories that caused most concern among consumers is illuminating, as is the fact that concerns about meat safety appeared to be relatively marginal compared to other food categories. Such simple findings can help to inform policy decisions concerning product safety and related communication strategies, in that they help to identify where consumers have fears that need to be allayed. They can also help to identify critical product types and subtypes that entail risks, and about which the public appears to be unaware. They can suggest whether efforts should be made to counter widespread but in part groundless beliefs (e.g. regarding people's ability to judge quality based on "the look of the product", or assumptions about the competence of butchers to detect BSE risks). The secondary analysis suggests that consumer associations represent an excellent ally for food safety and risk communication campaigns, in that they tend to have a high level of trust among consumers and enjoy an image of impartiality.

The findings described in this chapter show that certain beliefs are more widespread in some countries (or subnational areas) and in some social subgroups (determined by age, educational level, gender, occupational status, household type, etc.) than others. This provides an opportunity for segmentation, i.e. the identification of social sub-groups that have distinctive attitudes, concerns, consumption patterns or trust dispositions, on the basis of which different communication strategies may be shaped. Such segmentation is not available using "qualitative" approaches, which tend to involve research on a small number of subjects. Also, when surveys are based on relatively large samples and sampling has been carried out on probabilistic bases, the researcher may also use inferential statistics to calculate confidence intervals, estimate the size of sampling errors and generalize findings to the population. Qualitative approaches entail greater risks when users of research assume that findings based on a small number of individuals are equally valid for the larger population.

Questionnaire-based survey findings can help to identify more precise and feasible goals for food safety communication strategies: surveys can help to determine in which areas the public should be more or less concerned; whether the public holds incorrect beliefs or has insufficient knowledge, and where such shortcomings lie; and whether consumers adopt risky behaviour. In addition, surveys can help identify the most appropriate methods for implementing those strategies; which population segments should be targeted; which specific media, types of

public perceptions and opinion

retailers, etc., to use for conveying information; what kinds of style and tone to adopt; and so on.

Enthusiasm about such potential benefits needs to be tempered, however, by understanding the weaknesses of the method. The first of these is that sample surveys record stated rather than observed behaviour or actual thought. In other words, even in optimal circumstances, surveys only allow researchers to know what people are willing to say, not necessarily what they really think or what they really do. In contrast, "qualitative" approaches stand a greater chance of unveiling "true" attitudes and behaviour, as well as revealing the underlying social interactions and structures through which they come into being and adapt to changing circumstances. Surveys are also subject to various challenges such as the sampling and questionnaire issues described earlier in the section on conceptual considerations. For all of these reasons, policy-makers who intend to use empirical research must ensure that they are supported by people skilled in social research methods.

Along with these drawbacks, surveys also present many advantages. Since they are relatively straightforward in logistical terms (not least in the fact that there is a thriving market in research firms who can take such work on) and allow a great number of concepts to be operationalized comparatively cheaply, surveys are an excellent way to control hypotheses that otherwise would have no "reality check". They also provide an inferential basis that is more robust than that supplied by other research techniques. Even though there are valid questions that can be raised about the degree to which surveys accurately reflect public opinion, empirically grounded representations of public opinion such as surveys are undoubtedly useful counterfoils to the intuitive interpretations that mass media and policy-makers sometimes feel entitled to make about "what the people think". This is no less true for public perceptions of food safety than for other topics.

References

Becker T, ed. (2000) *Quality policy and consumer behaviour in the European Union*. Kiel, Wissenschaftsverlag Vauk.

Becker T, Benner E, Glitsch K (1998) *Summary report on consumer behaviour towards meat in Germany, Ireland, Italy, Spain, Sweden and the United Kingdom* (http:europa.eu.int/comm/research/biosociety/pdf/bio4_ct98_055_finalreport.pdf.)

Blumer H (1948) Public opinion and public opinion polling. *American Sociological Review*, 13:543–554.

Bourdieu P (1973) L'opinion publique n'existe pas (Public opinion does not exist). *Les Temps Modernes*, 318:1282–1309.

Goyder J (1987) *The silent majority: nonrespondents in sample surveys*. Cambridge, Polity Press.

Hyman H (1972) *Secondary analysis of sample surveys: principles, procedures, and potentialities*. New York, NY, Wiley and Sons.

Kiecolt K, Nathan LE (1985) *Secondary analysis of survey data*. Beverly Hills, CA, Sage.

Payne S (1951) *The art of asking questions*. Princeton, NJ, Princeton University Press.

Price V (1992) *Public opinion*. Newbury Park, CA, Sage.

Schuman H, Presser S (1981) *Questions and answers in attitude surveys*. New York, NY, Academic Press.

Sudman S, Bradburn N (1974) *Response effects in surveys: a review and synthesis*. Hawthorne, NY, Aldine.

Chapter 6

The BSE and CJD crisis in the press

The BSE and CJD crisis in the press

Martin W Bauer, Susan Howard, Vera Hagenhoff, Giancarlo Gasperoni, Maria Rusanen

To what extent can the mass media be used as an index of public perception by policy-makers? This seemingly straightforward question is immediately complicated when the mass media's double character is considered, as an instrument of social influence on the one hand, and as a mirror of public opinion on the other.

Interested social actors such as governments, businesses or nongovernmental organizations (NGOs) use the mass media as a tool to enhance their position in society. The illusion of control over the mass media (or at least the ability to influence it) is an essential part of those actors' confidence, both for their own communication activities and in their polemic against other actors. Similarly, belief in the power of the mass media is implicit both in the public relations activities of societal actors and in the attitudes of those who denounce the mass media as a biased or illegitimate influence on public opinion.

For a disinterested observer, it is more evident that the interplay of many actors, each simultaneously trying to use the mass media for its own particular cause, in fact creates a degree of autonomy for the mass media. By playing those divergent interests against each other, the mass media contribute both a mirror of and a factor of public opinion in society. Thus, although not free of interests, the mass media are not entirely bound to particular interests.

Miller & Reilly (1995) have shown that, from early on in the British BSE experience, the mass media successfully preserved a degree of freedom that enabled them to define events in terms of a social problem ("food safety") despite the communication strategies of key actors. If the working assumption is of the relative autonomy of the mass media, it seems plausible that monitoring — specifically of the salience and the framing of an issue in the mass media — may provide an index of public opinion that is independent of any one actor's dominant voice.

This chapter aims to:

• explore the structures and functions of mass media coverage of issues such as BSE/CJD;

• present results of empirical analysis of mass media coverage of the BSE/CJD issue in four countries;

• demonstrate the use of media analysis methodology to assess public perceptions of issues related to health risks, through investigation of "social representations" of risk; and

• propose ways in which monitoring of the mass media can be used to alert and inform the policy-making process in dealing with risks to health.

The Phillips Inquiry into the Government's handling of BSE/CJD in the United Kingdom (Phillips et al., 2000) did not scrutinize the role of the mass media in the crisis (such an investigation was not part of its remit). This study may contribute to an eventual evaluation of the role of the mass media in the crisis as it unfolded in the United Kingdom by mapping the reporting of BSE and CJD in that country.

• Conceptual considerations

On a conceptual level, this study looks beyond BSE, CJD and surveillance systems in general to explore the idea of a parallel epidemiology. The term "parallel" is used to suggest that, in addition to surveillance of BSE in the animal population and CJD in humans, there is a need to monitor social representations of the problem.

"Social representation" is the generic term for images, beliefs, perceptions, attitudes, concerns and considerations that circulate in the public discussion related to an issue or event. It generally refers to the way a society or a specific milieu in society thinks about an issue at a particular time. Whether or not these images, beliefs, etc., are consistent with or contrary to the latest scientific evidence, they constitute the symbolic environment in which various public actors operate, urging or constraining certain courses of action. They may also reflect particular points of view, such as vested interests, at any moment in time, and some of them may become entrenched as dominant concerns and images.

The monitoring of the mass media allows decision-makers to identify social representations and to consider them in terms of action strategies, either as constraints on what needs to be done or as targets of strategic messages. There are two major approaches to "issue monitoring", as it is technically known. One approach is to monitor continuously the whole output of a mass medium, for example the country's newspapers, and periodically publish a report on the comparative salience of different issues. This information can provide an early warning system for coming issues and a reputation index for societal actors. A second approach is issue-focused, selecting one particular issue and monitoring its coverage in the mass media comparatively and over time. This study follows the second approach.

Such a study of the symbolic content of a public crisis constitutes a practical application of what Sperber (1990) termed the "epidemiology of representations". Symbolic representations of a traumatic event — as a crisis in the first place, and as a particular kind of crisis in the second — help the public to familiarize themselves with uncertainties. They make concrete what otherwise would remain an abstract issue beyond the concerns of everyday life. The two main functions of social representations in public life are: to create familiarity for the purpose of orientation and to enable action (Farr & Moscovici, 1984; Bauer & Gaskell, 1999). The present study compares the prevalence of different definitions of the BSE situation (e.g. defining it as an issue of national identity, of trust in private or public actors, of public accountability, of national interests, of industrial food production, of cost–benefit analysis or of crisis management). Representations of this kind are social facts and part of the public sphere within which government, farmers, meat distributors, food activists and consumers go about their business.

Indeed, BSE and CJD have triggered many such associations and objectifications over the years. Of concern here is the comparison of these meanings (signifiers) both over time and across four different countries: the United Kingdom, Germany, Italy and Finland.

A final conceptual consideration is that symbolic representations form part of the public opinion process in modern societies. In order to study that process, its basic constituencies must be identified. The present study was based on a notion of the public sphere as constituted by government on the one hand and public opinion on the other (Bauer, 2002; Bauer & Gaskell, 2002). Governance is frequently entrusted to the elected government and its administrative departments, legislatures and the judiciary, whose mutual relations and responsibilities are defined by a national constitution. Public opinion emerges from everyday conversations and is reflected and cultivated in the mass media, the latter being for most people the main source of information on most news items. Public opinion is both a source of inspiration and a watchdog for governance. The relationship between government and public opinion, and that between everyday conver-

sations and the mass media, are both complex and subject to normative expectations (e.g. Habermas, 1989). In the short history of empirical research on public opinion, mainly after the Second World War, there has been a trend to equate public opinion with the results obtained by a public opinion poll, i.e. public opinion is no more and no less than whatever the polls can measure. This reduction was diagnosed by Habermas (1989) as the "social psychological liquidation of public opinion", which we want to avoid in our study.

Public opinion is complex and ongoing — it is a process in motion. Any simple, one-time measurement of public opinion necessarily provides only a partial reading of that process and does not capture the process itself. Techniques such as sample surveys, focus groups or mass media monitoring (the focus of this chapter) contribute to understanding the public opinion process; none can be taken as a "true index" of public opinion. Taking mass media coverage into account as an integral part of public opinion goes one step beyond this reductionism of opinion polling.

In this study, therefore, the conceptual distinction between public opinion and social representations is one of elaboration. Opinion refers to a simple evaluative proposition such as "X thinks of the government very favourably" or "X thinks of the government very unfavourably". With representations, the analysis focuses on the discourse elements that

The BSE and CJD crisis in the press

support either favourable or unfavourable judgements. The importance of this distinction can be illustrated by the fact that two newspapers or two persons can favour or condemn a public actor to the same degree but for totally different reasons — as became very clear in the media treatment of government over BSE/CJD.

• The dimensions of mass media coverage

To help understand the symbolic representations used in the mass media, this section considers two basic dimensions of an issue: its salience and its framing.

Salience

Salience is an indicator of the degree of public attention devoted to an issue. Attention is a scarce resource, with many issues competing for the limited attention of the mass media, of government decision-makers, and — finally — of the mind of every member of the public.

Salience is usually measured by the absolute or relative number of press articles or news items on television or radio devoted to an issue, thus "mapping" the development of attention by measuring the amount of coverage given to a topic. It is assumed that the mass media has a limited carrier capacity. If one topic is given a great deal of attention, other topics must be given less. Thus, a count of references to BSE and CJD/vCJD over a period of time will reflect filter activity in newsrooms, itself related to the degree of public interest attributed by journalists or editors to an issue in the wider public. In other words, the more important an issue is assumed to be, the more attention it is given in the newsrooms of media outlets, the more articles are printed on this topic, and the more salient the topic is in the media analysis. It is also assumed that a feedback cycle operates between newsroom attention, news selection and public perception.

Framing

Framing concerns the way the issue is represented in the mass media. It includes such factors as: the actors that become associated with the issue; the aspects of events that are covered; the consequences that are explored; the causes and responsibilities that are attributed; and the conclusions that are drawn. At its most basic, a frame is one way in which an issue is written or talked about; other frames are always possible. In fact, two kinds of conflict frequently develop over an issue or social problem: first, within a frame (e.g. for or against a diagnosis and a solution); and second, between frames (e.g. which frame is the most adequate to discuss the issue and to bring about a solution).

A picture's frame defines its boundaries, and at the same time influences the appearance of the content by managing the inclusion and exclusion of information and thus defining its bias. Changing the frame changes the contextual environment and the meaning of the picture.

In media analysis, framing refers to the problem of selection: the selection of a frame implies definition of a problem, diagnosis of causes, making of moral judgements and suggestion of remedies (Entman, 1993). A media frame suggests a dimension of disagreement (i.e. it is a suggestion of how to disagree) and often offers a key metaphor or image that summarizes its biases. It is likely to be sponsored and endorsed by some actors, and avoided or rejected by others (Gamson & Modigliani, 1989). Frames put some actors in a favourable position and others in an unfavourable one. For this reason, public actors struggle over which frames prevail.

Empirical assessment of public opinion via the mass media raises two methodological issues about framing: how to characterize frames, and how to measure the prevalence or dominance of certain frames in particular contexts.

• Functions of the mass media

The mass media provide a mirror of society, but it is not a faithful reflection. Their main function is to synchronize attention across different fields of societal activity, and thus to provide a sense of actuality; a sense that something and not something else requires urgent action (Luhmann, 1996). Attention is traded in a market (i.e. for media space) that increasingly follows the logic of supply and demand.

Actuality must be distinguished from reality (in German, *Wirklichkeit* as opposed to *Realität*).

Reality is the global horizon or background of all possible topics, which actuality refers to the selection of topics, which then leads to a widespread sense that some topic urgently requires public action. The contributions of the mass media in public opinion partially reflect the current concerns but can also set the public agenda. Empirically these functions are studied by comparing, over time, the salience and the framing of issues in public perceptions, in the mass media and in government. The relative independence of these arenas of the public sphere leaves open who is leading on what topic at what phase of the crisis. Much research goes into specifying the constraints under which it can be predicted when public perceptions lead the mass media, or when the mass media will lead public perceptions and the government, or when government will fuel both the mass media and public conversations.

Mirroring public concern

Many actors in the public sphere see the mass media as key indicators of public opinion. This view is based both on the way the media operate and on their status as a social fact that can be empirically assessed.

First, the mass media operate in a free market of information.[1] Various media outlets will pick up issues that are likely to attract public attention, and which will guarantee sales of copies and advertising. The audience will give their scarce attention to the

The BSE and CJD crisis in the press

mass media only when the latter cover those issues that are important for the audience. In this sense, these media may mirror major concerns of their audience, although exactly how the audience relates to the wider public needs to be assessed in each case. Mass media analysis may therefore provide useful indicators of public perceptions under certain conditions.

Secondly, independently of whether or how the mass media actually mirror public concerns, decision-makers in government and business are exposed daily or weekly to newspapers, radio or television. They do this in order to stay informed about the concerns of the public, or to assess their public standing. Analysis of the mass media thus may provide indicators of "perceived public opinion" — i.e. media coverage is perceived by relevant actors to be equivalent to, or an insight into, public opinion. In this case, media analysis can provide important insights about the constraints on public actors.

Setting the public agenda

Mass media are likely to contribute to the public

agenda on particular issues, such as BSE and CJD. They may or may not prescribe how to think about an issue, but they can tell the public to think about it *now* (McCombs, 1994). The selection of an issue may cause other outlets to follow, thereby amplifying the issue. By amplifying, the mass media attract attention to what hitherto only a few people knew. They may spot issues well in advance of the majority of the population. Over time the critical mass of attention may force governments to respond. But the mass media may also ignore an issue in the continuous flow of events, and thereby deflect its potential for public attention. The media may even lag behind the awareness of sectors of the public.

By amplifying and deflecting, the mass media can perform a watchdog function as the "fourth estate" in the constitution of the modern state, monitoring and stimulating the attention paid by governments, parliament or the judiciary to various issues. Obviously, most mass media are in the business of achieving profits by selling audiences to advertisers, and may perform a social function only as an unintended consequence. However, the social ethos of the mass media should not be ruled out, not least as motivation for those who work there.

Much research has attempted to test empirically the conditions under which the mass media exert control over public perceptions or even policy-making. It is beyond the scope of this study to review all of these conditions (e.g. Bryant & Zillmann, 1994), but a

---

[1] Of course, press freedom must not be taken for granted, and vigilance is necessary. The international organization Reporters sans frontières (RSF) monitors press freedom around the world, ranking countries on a scale of 0 (complete press freedom) to 100 (no press freedom). In 2002, the countries in this study registered on the scale as follows: United Kingdom (6.00), Germany (1.50), Italy (11.00) and Finland (0.50). In contrast, China registered 97 on the RSF scale. See Worldwide Press Freedom Index at http://www.rsf.fr.

few examples can be used to justify the monitoring of mass media as early indicators of public opinion.[2]

• **The quantity of coverage hypothesis** stipulates that, given a controversial issue, a mere increase in news intensity will shift public perceptions towards the negative end of the spectrum (Mazur, 1981). Evidence for this hypothesis is scarce, and little is known about the particular conditions of the effect.

• **The knowledge gap hypothesis** suggests that, under conditions of public controversy, information is likely to circulate more widely than in the absence of controversy (Tichenor, Donohue & Olien, 1970). Controversy over an issue in the mass media therefore contributes to the distribution of information about the issue, and thereby to public education by other means (Bauer & Bonfadelli, 2002).

• **The cultivation hypothesis** suggests that stereotypical framing of an issue that dominates over longer time periods in the mass media is likely to cultivate a matching "world view" among those who are more exposed to that message (Morgan & Shanahan, 1996). Despite an initial context of various opinions, this effect may lead to mainstreaming of opinions towards those offered by the mass media (Bauer, 2002).

• **The "CNN effect"** is a hypothesis about the conditions under which government policy (in this case, foreign policy) is likely to be shaped by 24-hour television coverage of an issue. Research suggests that decision-making can become reactive (to the mass media) in the absence of any strongly held policy or in the presence of known governmental disagreements over policy. Minority opinion in government may mobilize the media with targeted releases of information to gain the ear of the government centre that they would not otherwise obtain (Livingston, 1997).

The evidence for these hypotheses is inconclusive and highly controversial (Livingstone, 1996). However, they give clues as to the conditions under which media analysis is a valid indicator of future public opinion. Because these hypotheses accumulate contradictory evidence, and positive evidence suggests only small effects, the assumption must be that the mass media are in the main resonating current opinion, but that they to some extent also anticipate future opinions that they influence.

▼ Methodology

Content analysis was used to track the salience and framing of BSE issues in the mass media — a method of text analysis highly suitable for comparative and longitudinal research and therefore appropriate to cover mass media across four countries and a 15-year period (Bauer, 2000; more discussion of content analysis as a research tool is provided in Chapter 3).

---

[2] Generally, beliefs about the influence of the mass media on public perceptions oscillate between assuming strong and weak effects. In the last 20 or so years, concepts of and evidence for stronger effects have revived.

The BSE and CJD crisis in the press

• Sampling considerations

The print media in each of the four countries sampled have markedly different characteristics. Readership levels can be discerned by both the newspaper circulation figures (see figures for the relevant British, German, Italian and Finnish publications in Table 6.1) and indirectly through the distribution of advertising investments (Table 6.2). In 1999, the

Table 6.1. Newspaper circulation in the United Kingdom, Germany, Italy and Finland

United Kingdom
(Guardian Media Guide, 1998 survey)

• Daily Mirror	2 478 593
• Daily Mail	2 104 216
• Daily Telegraph	1 073 016
• The Guardian	385 496

Finland
(Levikintarkastus, 2001 survey)

• Helsingin Sanomat	436 099
• Savon Sanomat	67 212
• Turun Sanomat	115 142
• Kauppalehti	85 292

Germany

• Frankfurter Allgemeine Zeitung[a]	407 097
• Frankfurter Rundschau[a]	190 400
• Berliner Zeitung[b]	198 973
• General-Anzeiger Bonn[a]	89 553
• Der Spiegel[c] (weekly)	1.6 million (readership)
• Focus[d] (weekly)	810 931

Italy
(Audipress 1999 survey)

• Corriere della Sera	2 739 000
• Il Sole - 24 Ore	1 421 000
• L'Espresso (weekly)	2 139 000
• Panorama (weekly)	3 610 000
• Venerdi di Repubblica (weekly)	3 382 000
• Oggi (weekly)	4 476 000

[a]H.Meyn for 1999 [b]Medien Markt Berlin for 2000 [c]Die Spiegel-Gruppe for 1999 [d]Medialine for 2000

number (452) of Finnish newspapers sold per 1000 inhabitants was the highest of the study's four countries. The United Kingdom and Germany followed (321 and 300 newspapers sold per 1000 inhabitants, respectively) while the Italian circulation index was much lower (102 newspapers sold per 1000 inhabitants). A comparison between German and Italian advertising distribution reveals a similar picture, with German daily newspapers receiving 45.4% of advertising investments, in contrast to Italian dailies, which received 22.3% of advertising investments.

For the purposes of an international comparative content analysis, it would be ideal to employ the same sampling rationale for each country. However, with four very different media environments this is an unrealistic proposition. Each country's sampling strategy is briefly described below.

United Kingdom. Content analysis was performed over a subsample, as the intensity measure revealed more material than was manageable. In order to represent the British national press coverage of the debate, broadsheets and tabloids, left and right, daily and Sunday editions were all included. The *Telegraph* and the *Guardian* are the two leading broadsheets in terms of circulation according to the *Media Guide* figures for 1998 and they were

Table 6.2. Distribution of advertising investments among selected media in the United Kingdom, Germany and Italy (1999, percentage values) and Finland (1997, percentage values)

Medium	United Kingdom	Germany	Italy	Finland
Television	33.2	23.1	52.9	21.8
Radio	4	3.3	5.2	3.5
News dailies	34.5	45.4	22.3	56.2
Periodicals	23	23	15.2	17.2
Cinema	0.8	0.8	0.5	0.1
Outdoors	4.5	4.5	3.9	3.3
Total	100	100	100	100

Source for United Kingdom, Germany and Italy: Zenith Media, cited in *Media Key*, June 1999
Source for Finland: Gallup Mainostieto, cited in *World Press Trends*, 2002, World Association of Newspapers

The BSE and CJD crisis in the press

available almost from the beginning of the debate (the *Guardian* since 1985, the *Telegraph* since 1987). The *Sun* (by far the highest circulation) was not available on-line, so the tabloids with the next two largest circulations were analysed: the *Mirror* and the *Mail*. Articles were available for the *Mail* from 1993 and for the *Mirror* from September 1994. Because of the systematic random procedure used, each newspaper's weight in the final sample is proportional to the total article count.

Finland. The Finnish papers chosen were *Helsingin Sanomat* (one of the largest national circulation newspapers), *Savon Sanomat* and *Turun Sanomat* (regional papers) and *Kauppelehti* (specializing in finance and economics). All are quality daily papers; popular newspapers were not used in the study. They provide a relatively low intensity of articles in the period from 1990 to 1999, and none before that. All relevant articles were included.

Germany. As the intensity measure revealed more material than manageable, content analysis was performed over a subsample. To represent the German national press coverage of the debate, six publications were included — four newspapers and two news magazines — all of which were considered to be opinion leaders. Among the dailies, *Frankfurter Allgemeine Zeitung* and *Frankfurter Rundschau* represent right-wing and left-wing quality press, respectively, *Berliner Zeitung* is a high-circulation Berlin daily, while *General-Anzeiger*

Bonn is an apolitical Bonn paper. They have been chosen to contrast with each other. *Der Spiegel* and *Focus* provide examples of weekly coverage said to present "permanent themes in contrast to daily news" (Hagenhoff, 2000, German national report).

Italy. Two daily newspapers were selected, partly on the basis of their nationwide readership and partly because there were electronic archives available from 1996. The decision to focus on two newspapers also stemmed from the relatively marginal nature of newspaper reading in Italy. The *Corriere della Sera* is Italy's most "institutional" newspaper. It has a reputation for having no specific political orientation other than being generally "progovernment" no matter which parties or politicians comprise the majority coalition government. *Il Sole-24 Ore* is one of Europe's most widely read economic and financial newspapers, and has a reputation for backing business interests. Both are based in Milan. Four national weeklies are also included: *L'Espresso* and *Panorama* are the two leading news weeklies; *Oggi* is a weekly magazine with a more popular appeal and orientation; *Venerdì* is a weekly magazine supplement to the daily newspaper *La Repubblica*. Media coverage of BSE was practically non-existent before March 1996. For this reason (and reflecting the study's parameters of 1985–1999), content analysis was performed only from 1996 to 1999 (missing the peak of coverage in 2000).

• **The coding frame**

The conceptualization of the coding frame followed the idea of news as a "narrative". Newspaper writing about BSE/CJD takes the form of storytelling involving storytellers, actors, events, consequences, backgrounds of events and morals. Each of these elements of narration was measured and assessed as a variable in the press material (Table 6.3). The key variable for the results of the content analysis is the "frame", which defines the context and "flavour" of the narrative in terms of its main argument. The same events and themes can be reported within different frames. A description of the frames used in the study is given later in this chapter.

In order for the data to be comparable across the four countries, the coding process was the subject of intense discussion between the four teams during its development. Coder training was undertaken, and the reliability of the process was formally tested. The data are saved as an SPSS data file and are available for future secondary analysis.

▼ **The changing salience of BSE**

The number of newspaper articles written on BSE and/or

Table 6.3. The narrative of BSE /CJD in the media

Aspect of narrative	Corresponding variables
Storyteller	Newspaper, author
Actors	Actors, primary and secondary
Plot, events	Themes, location, time horizon, types of risk/benefit
Context, background	Frame
Consequences, moral	Demands and evaluations of actors

The BSE and CJD crisis in the press

vCJD is an indicator of the salience of the topic among competing issues. Figure 6.1 compares the monthly numbers of articles in each of the four countries. For simplicity of presentation, the graphic shows the intensity of coverage on the basis of two newspapers in each country (left scale, logarithmic), and charts these against the number of BSE cases detected in the United Kingdom per year (right scale).

Before 1996, the number of newspaper articles ranged from none to one a day or one a week. This changed significantly after March 1996 in all four countries. The change is readily explained by the March 1996 announcement in the United Kingdom

Figure 6.1. Monthly coverage in two daily newspapers in the United Kingdom, Germany, Italy and Finland, and British BSE cases, 1995–2001

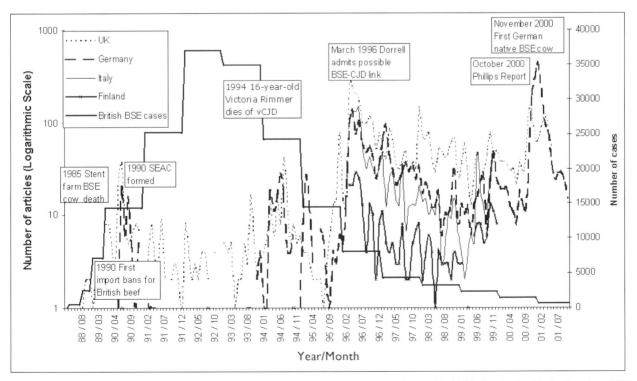

Source for United Kingdom, Germany and Italy: Zenith Media, cited in Media Key, June 1999

of the possible link between BSE and vCJD. Although cases of BSE in the United Kingdom had been steadily decreasing since 1993, the Government's admission of there being a risk to human health triggered media attention to the issue as never before. In general, the level of coverage was highest in the United Kingdom, where the issue originated. The second highest coverage was in Germany, where significant interest in the topic had already been evident before 1996. Following the British announcement in 1996, the Italian press matched the degree of attention given to the topic by the German press, and in certain periods even exceeded it. Finnish media coverage was the lowest of the four before and after 1996. There are few or no data for Italy and Finland before 1996, and Italian and Finnish colleagues confirm that very little attention was paid to BSE before that turning point.

The overall picture of intensity of coverage shows some convergence across the four countries. While BSE was defined as an animal health crisis, the events did not constitute a major media issue before 1996. It only became an issue once BSE was also defined as a human health issue, as vCJD, in March 1996. Although BSE prevalence in animals was at its peak in 1992 and 1993, this did not constitute a topic for much press coverage; it seemed to fall outside the criteria that guided the selection of news.

However, there are two periods when press coverage may have performed a sort of early warning function.

First, between 1988 and mid-1990, press coverage captured the rising number of incidents in Germany and the United Kingdom, with a peak in published articles in April–June 1990. The peak declined after a number of European governments declared a ban on British beef and SEAC was set up in the United Kingdom in April 1990. Secondly, there was increased press activity on the BSE issue between the end of 1993 and mid-1994, suggesting a build-up of pressure on governments to clarify unanswered questions about BSE raised by the death of Victoria Rimmer in 1994. The pressure to acknowledge the public health issue increased during that period, not least with Germany's ban on imports of British beef.

Following the simultaneous explosion of coverage in all four countries in March 1996, attention stayed consistently higher than before, but receded to a low point at the end of 1998 (Finland and Germany) and mid-1999 (Italy and the United Kingdom). After 1999, attention reached an unprecedented peak in Germany at the end of 2000 and beginning of 2001, when the first cases of domestic BSE were confirmed. Similar events were reported in Finland and Italy during 2001, although this study did not document that increase. In summary, after the initial synchronization of mass media coverage of BSE/CJD in March 1996, national media tended to respond primarily to the detection of domestic BSE and vCJD cases, but did so with particularly high salience once local public opinion was primed after 1996. A more detailed examination of daily news shows

The BSE and CJD crisis in the press

Table 6.4. Peaks of coverage in the United Kingdom, Germany, Italy and Finland, 1990–2001[a]

United Kingdom	Germany	Italy	Finland
April 1990	June 1990		
September 1993			
July 1994	March 1994 July 1994		
	February 1995		
December 1995			
March 1996	April 1996	June 1996	May 1996 September 1996
	February 1997	January 1997 July 1997 December 1997	January 1997 July 1997
December 1997			
	November 1998		
		June 1999	October 1999
	November 1999	November 1999	
		(no data for 2000)	(no data for 2000)
October 2000			
	January 2001		
		(no data for 2001)	(no data for 2001)

[a]Boxed dates are the highest peaks of coverage.

little correlation between the four countries. The BSE crisis runs to a different clock in the four contexts. Table 6.4 shows the timing of relative peaks in the coverage of BSE for the four countries. In the United Kingdom the story culminated in 1996 with a kind of "media quake", which had clear repercussions in the other countries. In Germany, Italy and Finland this wave of attention became only the pre-history of the local "media quakes" that erupted during 2000 and 2001.

• The British "media quake"

More detailed analysis of British media coverage of BSE/CJD reveals a phase structure that might be characterized as follows, using the analogy of an earthquake in the public sphere.

1985–1993: sporadic warnings (one article or fewer a week)

On 11 February 1985, cow 133 on Peter Stent's farm in Kent, United Kingdom, died. Its remains were investigated in November 1986, and BSE was identified. The oldest CJD reference in the study's sample is in the *Guardian* of 2 August 1985.

Noticeable coverage occurred only three years later during 1988, when the Southwood Working Party was constituted to investigate BSE, its causes and implications. They concluded in February 1989 that there was minimal risk to humans, while admitting that, if estimates were wrong, the

implications would be very serious. In this period, the *Guardian* took the lead among national newspapers, running more than half of all articles published on BSE until the end of 1988. *Guardian* headlines included "Brain disease in food" (4 June 1988) and "Butchers selling diseased meat" (29 June 1988).

In February 1989 beef was banned from use in baby foods, and in May from use in pies. In 1989 other countries and the European Commission started to ban beef imports from the United Kingdom. These domestic and international measures were reported in the press. The *Guardian*'s story "Mad, bad and dangerous" (10 November 1989, by Nigel Williams) reviewed the literature on the health risk to humans and challenged the official version according to which British beef was safe.

Press coverage on BSE and CJD rose to its first noticeable peak in April-June 1990 (which the study team termed "the year of media hype"). A number of events accumulated in this period and were reported. The Government formed the Spongiform Encephalopathy Advisory Committee in April 1990. In May 1990, the first case of feline spongiform encephalopathy (FSE) was diagnosed following the death of a cat named Max who had eaten cat food made from British beef, suggesting that BSE crosses the species boundary. On 10 May, Professor Richard Lacey gave a radio inter-

The BSE and CJD crisis in the press

view calling for 6 million cows to be slaughtered as a precautionary measure. Professor Lacey established himself as a dissident voice in the national BSE and CJD debate. The *Sunday Times* covered this under the headline "Leading food scientist calls for slaughter of 6m cows".

In the aftermath of these events, the Minister for Agriculture, John Gummer, tried to calm the public by feeding a hamburger to his daughter in front of the cameras, providing a picture that travelled the world. There were 79 press articles on BSE and/or vCJD in 1989 but seven times more (570) were published in 1990, with the press led by the *Times* and the recently founded *Independent*. After 1990, coverage of the issue declined again to previous levels until the end of 1992. The report of the Lamming Committee on animal foodstuffs in that year (Expert Group on Animal Feedingstuffs, 1992) received little media attention. Yet 1992 was also the year in which TSE emerged in zoo animals, and the authoritative *British Medical Journal* wrote in an editorial that further information was necessary if BSE beef were to be declared safe for humans.

Mid-1993–1995: pressure building (two articles per week)

Although the BSE epidemic reached its climax in 1993 with over 35 000 diagnosed cases, media coverage was low, although there was visibly an increased interest in CJD. From the beginning of 1994 until mid-1995, coverage gained new momentum with two articles on BSE and/or vCJD published per newspaper per week. Events that received coverage in 1994 included the death of a 16-year-old girl, Victoria Rimmer, from vCJD, the revelation that the computer system used for BSE surveillance was ineffective, and further EU restrictions on British beef. The following year brought evidence of maternal transmission of BSE (from cow to calf) and the death of two dairy farmers from vCJD. The fact that all these deaths were in relatively young people, rather than among the aged as expected for CJD, was remarkable – and was remarked upon.

A linkage between BSE and CJD emerged in the print media's focus during 1994 and 1995. Until 1993, less than 5% of press articles had linked BSE and CJD in terms of a possible transmission from infected cattle to humans via the consumption of beef. This changed in 1993–1994, rising to 15%, and in 1995 fully 35% of all articles associated BSE and CJD – the highest proportion in the whole period of observation.

As the coverage of BSE and/or vCJD increased, so the public suspicions increased. The decline in beef consumption is an indication of this, albeit other factors were involved. For the early period of the BSE crisis, Tilston et al. (1992) convincingly show with econometric time-series analysis that media coverage of BSE negatively influenced beef consumption in the United Kingdom. Although the

National Food Survey shows a long-term decline in British beef consumption since the late 1950s, a closer look at the data shows that this long-term trend was accentuated between 1987 and 1996, levelling off only after 1997.[3]

March 1996: the quake (daily articles)

The "earthquake" struck on 20 March 1996. SEAC had already reviewed the accumulating evidence over vCJD and informed the Secretary of Agriculture (Hogg) and Secretary of Health (Dorrell). On the afternoon of 20 March, Dorrell informed Parliament of new disease control measures, the implicit meaning of which was summarized in the *Mirror* under the headline "Official — mad cow can kill you". This framing of the message was reported around the world. In the same issue of the *Mirror*, Professor Lacey alleged an official cover-up of vital evidence and an orchestrated attempt to silence dissident voices like himself since 1989.

The earthquake struck at the moment when the BSE epidemic in British cattle seemed well under control. BSE cases were down to a quarter

of 1992–1993 levels, although they were still very much above reported levels in any other country.

The year saw a flurry of national and international measures to contain the crisis. In June 1996, at its Florence summit meeting, the EU agreed on a framework ultimately to lift the ban on British beef exports. The following month, the European Parliament set up an inquiry into the handling of BSE by the European Commission and the British Government.

1997–1999: "aftershocks preceding the beef war"

During the first aftermath period, which featured considerable media interest peaks in the second half of 1997 and in mid-1998, coverage focused on issues related to government activities such as the management of external blame (e.g. BSE is an EU problem) and damage containment, public information campaigns stressing national interests and British beef as a matter of identity, evaluation of government processes for policy-making about food, and other issues. The issue of national identity was exemplified in the *International Herald Tribune*, albeit on an ironic note, with an earlier article characterizing the BSE crisis as the ultimate demise of the British Empire: "The virile beefeaters are poisoning themselves" (March 1996).

▼ The narrative framing of BSE/CJD

In addition to salience, the study team analysed the print media's framing of the BSE/CJD crisis. Each

---

[3] Average consumption declined from 300 to 200 grams weekly per person between 1958 and 1987; and from 200 to 100 grams between 1989 and 1996 — a clear acceleration of decline.

The BSE and CJD crisis in the press

Table 6.5. Frames used in analysis of press coverage of BSE

Frame names	Examples		
	Sponsor	Polarity within frame	Key metaphor
National interest	British Conservative party, sectors of the press, farmers	Actions in or against national interests	Beef war
National/regional identity	Just about anybody	Actions that highlight national differences and place domestic practices in a favourable light	"Us" versus "them" Domestic versus foreign Domestic versus Europe or globalization
Industrial production of food	Vegetarian, organic farmers, food industry	BSE as a necessary outcome versus a temporary deviation	Transgressing the natural boundaries Messing with nature
Costs/benefits of the crisis	Farmers, victims, corporations, government	How much does it cost, is it worth the cost, what are the benefits of crisis Unnecessary crisis	Waste of money Financial disasters
Public accountability	Media, parliament, NGOs	Who is responsible, denial of responsibility	Scapegoating Image: cow bigger than the Minister
Food or product safety/ public health	Retailers, consumers, industry, medical profession	Is food related to cows safe or unsafe	Image: agriculture minister feeds himself/his daughter a hamburger
Trust	Media, NGOs, government	Mistrust in institutions or procedures Independent vs dependent institutions Is the institution or the process trustworthy or not	Image: MAFF "in bed" with the industry/farming
Scientific expertise	Scientific community, government, NGOs	Is scientific expertise sufficient/conclusive, other forms of expertise Certain or uncertain knowledge Quantified risks	Image: scientist in laboratories Quarrel between scientists
Food ethics	NGOs, religious groups	Ethical, unethical practice	Adulteration, messing with nature

NGOs = nongovernmental organizations.

article was coded according to whether BSE was presented predominantly as being "about" one of the frames shown in Table 6.5. The table also gives examples of the narrative or descriptive elements that were considered in coding an article as representing one or another frame.

Coding for each frame took into account a variety of elements. For example, the frame of "costs" included references to the collapse of beef prices, the future viability of farming under changed conditions, and the costs of containing and controlling the epidemic, like the cull of affected herds. Each article was also coded according to the main theme and the main public actors that were associated with the events of the crisis. Analysing the data along these variables allowed comparison of the trajectory of the BSE crisis in the four countries over time.

"National interest", "food safety and public health" and "cost of the crisis" were the frames that most frequently defined the BSE situation in all four countries. "Food safety and public health" dominated the representation of the BSE crisis in the United Kingdom followed by "costs" and the "national interest". In the British case, "national interest" mainly meant lifting the bans on British beef. Finland and Italy were mainly concerned with the "costs" followed by "food safety" and issues of "national interest". Here, as in the case of Germany, "national interest" meant banning

British beef as long as it was unsafe. In Germany, this was the main concern followed by "food safety" and "scientific expertise" (i.e. in the controversy over the safety of British beef). The Germans alone read more articles referring to "scientific expertise" than to "costs of the crisis".

The most frequent themes of BSE coverage in all four countries were: banning or lifting the ban on British beef; the viability of farming under changing conditions; the implementation and enforcement of control measures; beef prices and beef consumption; and the sporadic discovery of single indigenous BSE cases outside the United Kingdom.

A final point of analysis was the question of location. In the United Kingdom the focus of media attention was on domestic events, with a small proportion of articles on the EU (often referred to simply as "Brussels"). The other countries divided their attention between the national context, the United Kingdom and the EU.

In the case of Finland, more attention was paid to the EU than to national events. In terms of national news, BSE was a non-event until 2001. This reflected the United Kingdom as being the origin of the BSE events, and Brussels as the source of expected solutions to the crisis, at least as it related to the emerging European common market and its institutions.

The BSE and CJD crisis in the press

• Crisis management and the meaning of the crisis
The study team also carried out an analysis of the framing press coverage before and after the key national BSE events in the United Kingdom and Germany, respectively. In the United Kingdom, this key event was the 20 March 1996 announcement, while in Germany it was the detection of indigenous BSE at the end of the year 2000. Figure 6.2 shows how, after the key event in the United Kingdom, the coverage shifted away from food safety to the costs

of the crisis and a discourse of national identity: "British beef is best". Figure 6.3 reveals that, in Germany, the discourse shifted away from scientific expertise and national interests (justifying the banning of British beef) to a discourse of the costs of crisis containment. It also reflected concerns over industrial food production, which was characterized as a root cause of the problem.

These shifts show the diversification of the media

Figure 6.2. British framing, 1988 to February 1996 and March 1996 to 1999

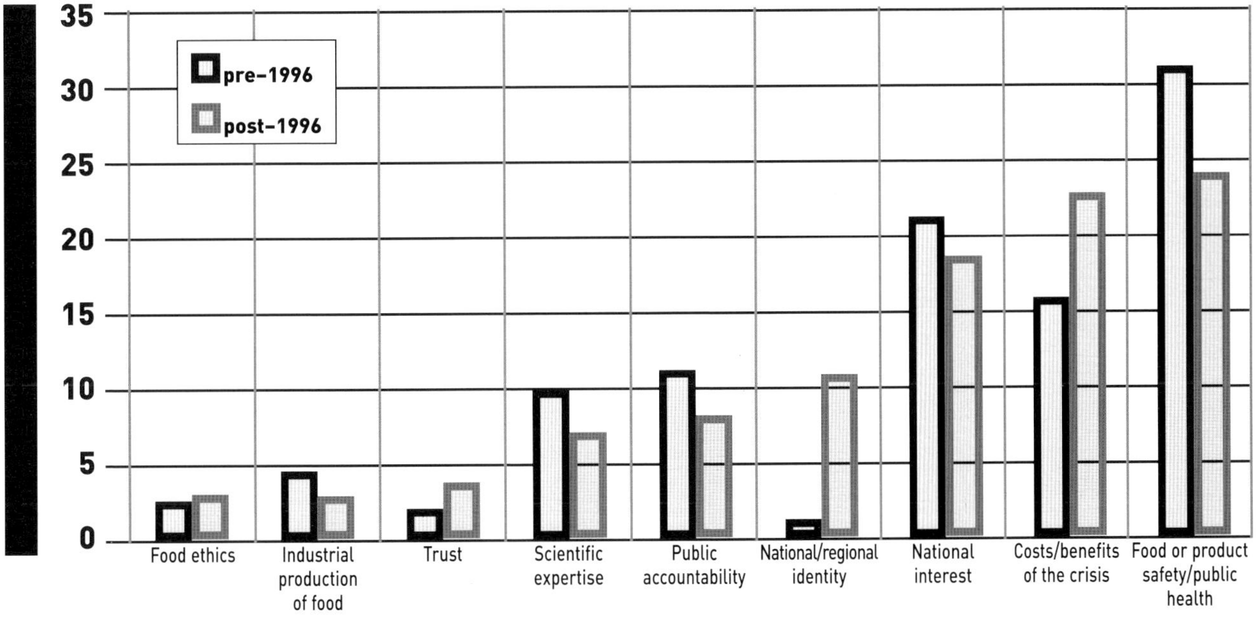

coverage in response to significant national events, and at the same time how this discourse reflected crisis management concerns, on the one hand, and the symbolic nature of the crisis on the other. The crisis meant different things in different countries, or at least in their respective newspapers: a threat to national pride in the United Kingdom, a crisis of industrial food production in Germany. In the British case, raising the national flag reflected the temporary success of the Government in deflecting responsibility for the crisis away from

itself and towards appeals to patriotism and criticism of "Eurocratic procedures". In contrast, the study team's research shows that the symbolic element of the crisis in Germany resonated with environmental and consumer concerns in the wider population.

• **National interest and national identity**

The BSE crisis was often framed as a matter of measurable (mainly economic) national interests, mainly related to the benefits of banning British beef from the national food markets, or the lifting

Figure 6.3. German framing, 1990–1999 and 2000 to June 2001

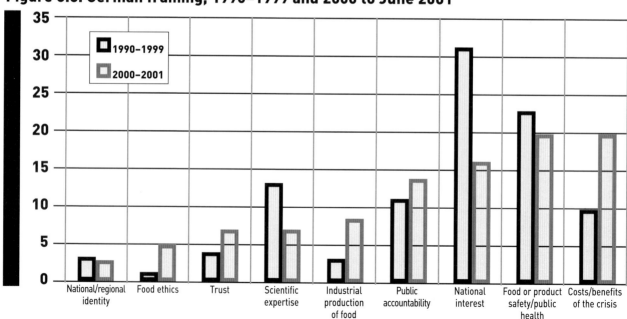

The BSE and CJD crisis in the press

of such bans. It was also framed as a matter of symbolic national identity; less a question of economic rationale than of appeal to patriotic feelings, as well as to the national food culture and the need to preserve it as an expression of national virtues and achievements. In the United Kingdom, this culminated in the repeated call to eat British beef despite all the controversy, because "British is best". Such national feelings can only be invoked in response to some polluting force that comes from "outside".

Figure 6.4 shows the overall trends of the frames of national interest and identity in all four countries, and indicates that national identity followed national interests. While "national interests" was clearly the more important discourse frame, the two fluctuated jointly. The curves show that 1990, 1994 and 1999 were the years when the discourse of "national interest" was at its highest. This reflected anticipation of and reaction to the unilateral banning of British beef, and served to establish legitimacy for these measures within the context of European institutions.

Figure 6.4. Articles framed by national interest or national/regional identity in the United Kingdom, Germany, Italy and Finland, 1988–1999

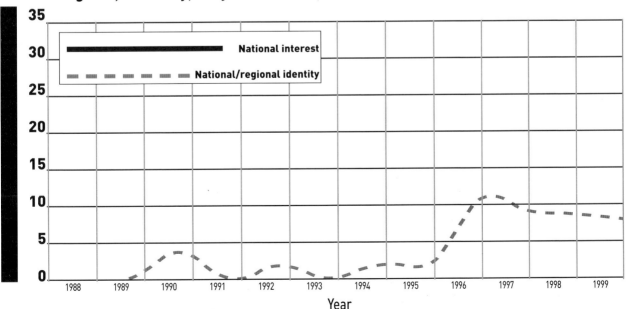

"National identity" became an issue after 1996, signalling desperation over lost beef markets in public discourse particularly in the United Kingdom.

Figure 6.5 shows how the "national interest" discourse fluctuated over time in each of the four countries, and clearly indicates that different "rhythms" were involved. Germany seemed to lead this concern in the middle and at the end of the 1990s. In Finland national interest was the big issue in 1994. In the United Kingdom it was the focus of public concern in 1990, in 1994, and again in 1999. References to public concerns were also prominent in Finland and Italy by the end of the 1990s.

• Public health and industrial food production

The frame "food safety and public health" has always been prominent in the BSE press coverage, and remains so today. Before March 1996, however, BSE was officially defined in the United Kingdom as an animal health problem and not as a public health problem; that framing was widely reflected in the coverage by the British print media. Prior to that

Figure 6.5. Articles framed by national interest by individual countries, 1985–2001

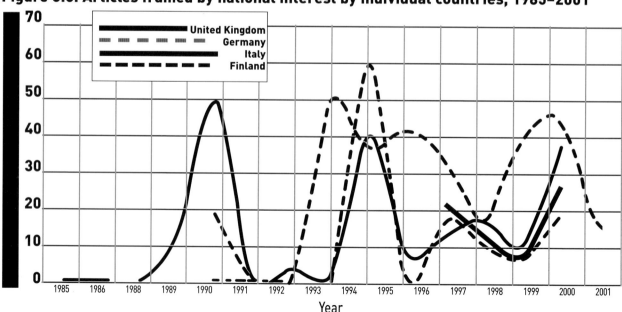

The BSE and CJD crisis in the press

date, BSE was seen in several continental countries as a potential risk to human health, but also as a problem confined to the United Kingdom. Such a framing of the issue propagated a view that BSE was an alien disease that needed to be kept out. Figure 6.6 shows how, prior to March 1996, the press across all four countries invoked the "food safety and public health" frame on average in one third of its coverage. This rose strongly during 1994

and 1995 when the suspicions of a link with CJD began to circulate following the unusual cases of CJD. Once the link was acknowledged in March 1996, that prevalence declined and the coverage changed.

The frame of "industrial food production" (which places agro-industrial techniques in opposition to small and organic farming) had some prominence in the years before March 1996, although these were

Figure 6.6. Overall view, through press coverage analysis, of the changing discourse (frames relating to industry and the consumer) across the United Kingdom, Germany, Italy and Finland, 1988–1999

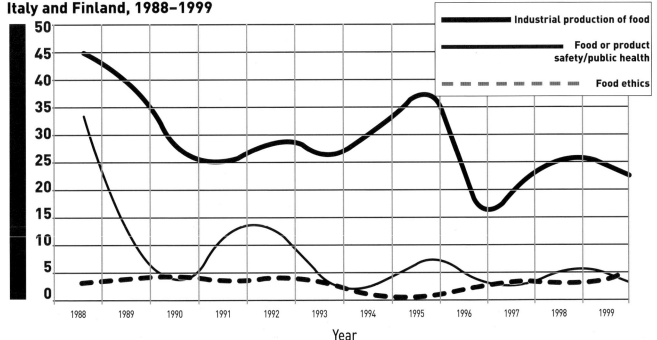

Year

years of relatively little overall coverage. The frame lost much of its currency over the years and flattened out at around 5% of coverage in 1993.

Figure 6.7 shows changes in the distribution of the "cost of the crisis" frame in the four countries. This appeared to have registered as a significant focus twice in the United Kingdom, first in 1990–1991 and then again in 1995–1996, both times appearing in over one third of all articles. This concern was shared by the press of other countries: in 1995 by Finland (half of all articles) by Italy

in 1996 (one third of all articles) and by Germany in 1996 (15% of all articles). Germany became aware of the "cost" issue when domestic BSE cases were detected.

• **Actor prominence and the trust paradox**
The study team tracked press coverage of actors in the BSE/CJD story as an indicator both of the focus of public attention and of how those actors were evaluated. In the United Kingdom, overall press coverage was clearly dominated by references to government (23% of all actors) and to parliament (13%), although the food industry and

Figure 6.7. Overall view, through press coverage analysis, of the changing discourse (costs and benefits of the crisis), by individual country, 1985–2001

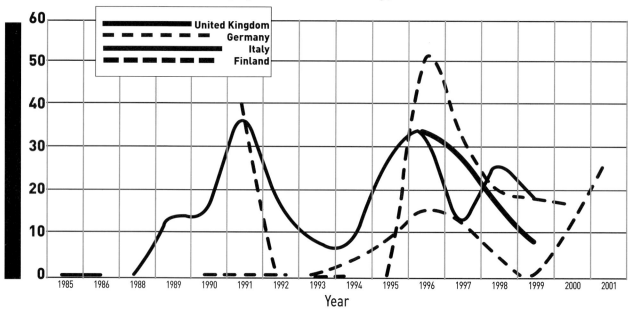

The BSE and CJD crisis in the press

farmers got some attention as well. This was rather different in the other countries. In Germany, Italy and Finland, the EU (the European Commission and European MPs) was the focus of attention. Additionally, food producers and farmers got attention in Finland and Italy, while in Germany more attention was focused on the national Government.

"Trust" is generally another important frame with which to define the BSE situation, i.e. a crisis of trust in the institutions and actors involved in producing and regulating a country's food production. In social relations, trust is characterized by a number of paradoxes. When trust becomes a topic of conversation (e.g. in the form of a question: "can we trust each other?" or in form of a request: "trust me!") it already signals a problem, as the interaction process cannot take trust for granted any longer. Trust often needs to remain implicit, meaning that explicit discussion of trust reveals a lack of trust in the process. The study used this paradox as a basis to construct an indicator of public trust. Actors that appeared in stories on "trust" may have a trust problem, otherwise they would not appear under this topic. The more an actor is mentioned in relation to trust, the more likely it is that this actor has a trust problem. However, this is not to conclude the inverse: that those actors who were not mentioned were seen as trustworthy.

In general, "trust" registered as a frame relatively rarely, with an average of around 5% of the coverage. This is considerably lower than the other frames already discussed (see Figures 6.2 and 6.3 above). The trajectory of the "trust" frame is shown in Figure 6.8, and provides more evidence that the definition of the BSE crisis in the press changed over time, with the issue of trust moving into and out of coverage. In the United Kingdom, "trust" became an issue for the press early in the crisis, and again in 1997, when the Labour Government was taking over from the Conservatives. The year 1997 was also the one of prominence for the "trust" question in Finland and Italy, while in Germany this occurred a year later and has continued to have some prominence. In Finland, "trust" returned as an issue in 1999.

The majority of articles reflecting the "trust" frame mentioned international actors, mainly the EU; about one quarter mentioned public sector actors such as national government and politicians, while one fifth referred to private sector actors such as the food industry and farmers.

Stories linking trust and BSE/CJD were often about distrust of the figures of power engaged in risk management and the dissemination of information. Coverage of BSE risk management activities provided a chance for the press to scrutinize figures of responsibility, an opportunity the press clearly relished. The data suggest that, when "trust" was the frame in such stories, the British press was most likely to refer to the national Government, while in Germany and Italy the press tended to mention international actors, mainly the EU. Finland was most concerned by this issue, with 10.4% of articles published there being framed by "trust". Unlike in other countries, the actors most often scrutinized by Finnish newspapers were private sector food producers and farmers, along with the EU. However, in all four countries, when the media suspected outright duplicity, it was governments and administrators to whom they turned first. Even this had important nuances: the "Eurosceptic" United Kingdom was mainly preoccupied with the activities of its own Government, with the EU showing up only as a marginal issue in the "trust" frame.

Another feature of "trust" in actors was the positive

Figure 6.8. Overall view, through press coverage analysis, of the changing discourse (trust), by individual country, 1985–2001

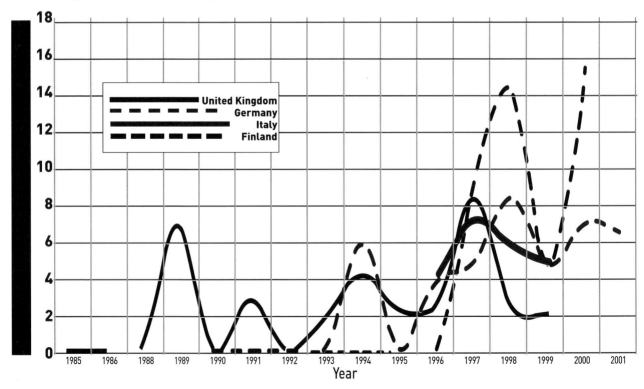

The BSE and CJD crisis in the press

or negative evaluation these received in press coverage. Overall, actors that were mentioned in articles were mostly evaluated negatively: in this the press seemed to apply the rule of "only negative news is news". Among these actors, the EU and the national governments received predominantly negative evaluation. Actors were not always evaluated in the same article but, if evaluated, EU and national governments made up 84% of all evaluated actors. Of all four countries, the British press coverage was the most negative. The national Government was judged very negatively in the United Kingdom compared to the others. In both Germany and the United Kingdom, the press was more critical of their national governments than of the EU, while Italian articles rated both negatively in equal measure. The Finnish press was positive about its own Government's handling of the BSE situation. In 2000–2001, the German press turned strongly against both the EU and the German Government, indicating that the domestic BSE cases had brought the story definitely "back home". Since then, the German Government has been presented as less reliable, open, competent, responsible and powerful than it was before, but also as increasingly self-critical. The EU, while being attributed an increase in competence, obtained a similarly unfavourable judgement for its handling of the situation.

▼ Focus on the British press

Further examination of the British articles' evaluation of the national Government and civil service

yields a more detailed picture. The first article in the British sample with a very negative evaluation, written by the *Guardian*'s consumer correspondent James Erlichman ("A cow disease to beef about", 11 July 1988), identified the Ministry of Agriculture as "penny pinching" and suggested it was incompetent. It is at this point that the public image of the Ministry of Agriculture began a long journey downhill, at least as regards the BSE issue.

A less negative report by David Brown appeared in the Conservative *Sunday Telegraph* the following November ("Cattle disease 'no risk to milk'", 13 November 1988), describing the occurrence of the disease. The Government came under attack in this article for paying farmers too little in compensation for incinerated BSE-infected cattle. Where the *Guardian* championed the consumer, the *Telegraph* took up the banner of livestock farmers. In both cases, the Government was evaluated negatively. Thus, from very early on in the debate, doubts about BSE crisis management were found across the national print media's political spectrum. Some articles criticized the Government for being overly focused on the interests of beef farmers, while others criticized it for taking insufficient care of those interests (see also Miller & Reilly, 1995).

By 1996, inflamed commentary on the Government's handling of BSE and CJD had given way to a resigned scepticism. Simon Heffer in the *Daily Mail* reflected with cynicism when he wrote:

> I am bored with calling for Mr Hogg to be sacked, and replaced by someone who can convince a justifiably anxious public and a devastated beef industry that he knows what is going on ... if you didn't believe me at the time of the Florence summit, when I said it was a lie for Mr Major to suggest he had won the beef war, perhaps you will believe it now (Add weight to the argument, 3 August 1996).

Early in 1999, the *Sunday Mirror* was drawing conclusions from the Government's handling of BSE, making a warning analogy for the new public issue of genetically modified (GM) crops and food. The Labour cabinet were warned, after news of Dr Arpad Pusztai's research on GM potatoes: "That is exactly what happened with BSE. Warnings ignored, research dismissed — until people started dying and British beef was banned all over the world. If this Government makes the same mistake, they will never be forgiven" ("We must not have another BSE debacle", 14 February 1999). Government, regardless of party politics, was represented as blundering or, worse still, callous. The repercussions of BSE policy failures included a relentless battering of government on behalf of the "victims" (consumers and industry) in relation to other food or health risks. (This will seem familiar to those who read the British press coverage of the "foot and mouth" crisis in 2002.)

• The special role of the *Guardian* newspaper

The *Guardian*'s BSE/CJD coverage followed a different pattern from the other national newspapers in the period prior to 1996. The *Guardian* was the first paper to raise the BSE and CJD issue in public in 1985. In 1988 it ran more than twice as many articles on BSE than any other quality paper in the United Kingdom, and in 1994 it was far more attentive to the emerging BSE/CJD issue than the other quality papers. The *Guardian*'s consumer affairs correspondent, James Erlichman, covered issues of food safety early on: his newspaper was therefore already on the alert about BSE and looking for public health news angles. In some ways the *Guardian* took on the role of watchdog, which it shared with outspoken commentators such as food scientist Richard Lacey. The commentary was often met by other journalists with the suspicion that the media were exaggerating or propelling public hysteria. An example can be seen in Christopher Booker's article for the *Sunday Telegraph* ("Twenty-four words that will cost us billions", 24 March 1996), in which he gave implicit support to many of the objectives of government policy while criticizing ministers for their shortcomings in the attainment of those objectives.

Analysis of article salience confirms the special role of the *Guardian*. Newspapers tend to watch closely what competing papers write about, in order not to miss an interesting story. This leads to a high correlation in the distribution of stories over time.

The BSE and CJD crisis in the press

However, analysis of the two periods before and after March 1996 shows that while the *Mail*, the *Mirror* and the *Telegraph* correlate very highly with each other ($r > 0.80$), the *Guardian* has its own rhythm ($r < 0.58$). This is due to its writing about BSE when the others were still ignoring the topic. The situation changed after 1996, when all the papers joined in the dance around BSE with the same rhythm, albeit to a slightly different tune.

• Self-reflexivity in the British press

BSE was news, but "news of BSE" also became news occasionally too. It is a feature of the modern mass media that, in the course of a crisis, they become aware of their functions in society. When this happens, their focus tends to be one either of self-congratulation or of critical examination of the coverage by competitors. In practice, this means that newspapers audit their own contributions to public opinion as opinion leaders or as mirrors of public concerns, and make this contribution a matter of commentary. Some newspapers even publish a weekly or monthly count of their news stories, often comparing themselves to other newspapers and claiming the role of opinion leaders, with or without evidence, on particular issues. Examining the coverage of the competition may involve attributing irresponsibility, misinformation or deliberate bias — which in itself intensifies the coverage of an issue. Self-reflexivity adds to the level of reportage, increases the flexibility of the framing, and thus may usher in a change in the dominant framing of an issue. In media monitoring such as that done in this study, it is therefore important to identify when and how self-reflexivity of the mass media reportage comes into play.

The Phillips Inquiry was a large-scale investigation into the management of BSE and vCJD in the United Kingdom. Its remit, focusing on the conduct of public administration (rather than the functioning of societal institutions in general), did not include an assessment of the role of the mass media in the BSE and CJD process. However, comments hinting at the role of the mass media can be found scattered in the Inquiry reports. The study team found 15 such references, for example to a television programme and to the coverage by (mainly broadsheet) newspapers:

> To an extent the Government's response to BSE was driven not by its own, and its advisers', assessment of risk, but by the public's perception of risk. The introduction of the human SBO ban is the most notable example. At times media response to BSE was exaggerated, but often media critique was pertinent and well informed. <u>The media played a valuable role in reflecting, and stimulating, public concerns which proved well founded and which had a beneficial influence on government policy</u> (Phillips et al., 2000, Vol.1,13: 1190) [underlining added].

On the basis of this judgement of the official Phillips Inquiry, the British media had reasons to be self-congratulatory. However, the basis of this conclusion is unknown and no evidence to warrant this judgement is provided anywhere in the text.

Although tabloid and broadsheet papers normally differ considerably in style and content, a crisis (in the best known example, a war) can bring them closer together. Nonetheless, the division between left and right political affiliation remained marked in the treatment of the BSE/CJD crisis. Over many years of the BSE story, the Conservative Government was loyally supported by the *Telegraph* until March 1996. On the other side of the political divide, the *Guardian* and the *Mirror* were consistently unabashedly critical and cynical of government actions and intentions.

In view of this the study team looked at the articles in which the British newspapers commented on their own role in the BSE crisis. This was done to demonstrate the reflexive element in press coverage of BSE/CJD; it was not intended to evaluate the role of newspapers in the BSE crisis or to ascertain the basis for any of their claims. Some of the highlights include the following.

• **1989: self congratulation.** "In the last year [The Food Programme] reacted brilliantly to the never-ending food crisis and they infuriated many assorted bodies, the animal feed manufacturers, the government when Cooper investigated "the mad cow disease" (BSE) and salmonella in eggs and the British Nutrition Foundation when he looked at commercially sponsored teaching materials..." (Tearing at the bone: a look back ... and into the future for The Food Programme, Colin Spencer in the *Guardian*, 2 September 1989, page 13).

• **1993: personalization of the controversy.** "Every year, without fail, Professor Richard Lacey of Leeds University blazes across our screens and, like an Old Testament prophet ... alerts us to some deadly poison lurking in our food. Listeria, salmonella, BSE ... his battle honours are impressive and, if he tends to overstate his case, his scaremongering has the not unwelcome effect of forcing the Department of Health to take food poisoning seriously. The food industry regards him as the Devil in human form, but the media adore him. The fact that other experts have examined the same topics and come to less sexy conclusions is generally overlooked" (The essential ingredient — Television, Max Davidson in the *Daily Telegraph*, 11 February 1993).

• **1996: disassociation from other media.** This occurs where journalists refer to "the media", excluding themselves whilst attacking the other writer. This is particularly relevant in the case of BSE, where the media set themselves up as "judges" over government, science and the farming industry; newspaper journalists, it seems, are also in judgement of their peers in the press. " ... But of that, of

The BSE and CJD crisis in the press

course, we hear very little from the media. It would never do to admit what havoc their self-righteous hysteria can help to create. This time they have created a real beauty ..." (Twenty-four words that will cost us billions, Christopher Booker in the *Sunday Telegraph*, 24 March 1996).[4]

• **1997: self defence.** "Cabinet minister Roger Freeman launched an astonishing attack on the *Mirror* during the BSE debate. [He] accused us of 'sheer irresponsibility' for breaking the BSE story last March. But Labour Chief Whip Donald Dewar blasted: 'It was childish stuff from Roger Freeman. The Tories have been reduced to abusing the press for doing its job. It's very sad.' " ('Childish' Tory attacks Mirror: Roger Freeman launched an attack on the *Mirror* during the BSE debate, the *Mirror*, 18 February 1997).

One of the most visible dichotomies in the print media's self-reflexivity is that of self-congratulation and self-denigration. In covering their peers, journalists can provide praise (for example the 1989 *Guardian* article cited above) and blame (the 1996 *Sunday Mirror*). The importance of the media is assumed (rightly so, according to the BSE Inquiry); articles appear to take for granted that the media have a powerful role in stimulating public opinion and defining government policy. Where the media references itself, praise and blame are also attached to those who oppose journalistic "excess". In doing so, the media both protects itself and attacks its critics. This type of commentary is closely connected to party-political affiliations. The lines were clearly drawn in the *Mirror* article above: Conservative Roger Freeman accuses the (left wing) *Mirror* of irresponsibility and Labour Whip Donald Dewar retaliates; the *Mirror* claims "astonishment" while reporting the spat with uncontained glee.

The attribution of blame spreads far and wide. The *Sunday Telegraph* article above undermines what it calls "rogue scientist" Richard Lacey by depicting him as an Old Testament prophet (imposing but hardly scientific) and sensationalist, and dismissing his warnings as "sexy". Again, party politics are at work. The right-wing *Telegraph*'s alarm about the health risks described by Lacey is tempered by a relatively gentle treatment of the Conservative cabinet, much assailed by crises of food safety.

▼ Monitoring of the press by policy-makers

Chapter 8 of this study investigates the means used by governments in the four countries to gather information on public opinion, perceptions and attitudes to BSE/CJD, including the opinions and information available in the mass media. It is useful to summarize some of the findings about how (if at all) the press was monitored in such efforts, and the

---

[4] The "24 words" refer to those uttered by Steven Dorrell on that momentous day, 20 March 1996.

extent to which this changed over time.

• Press monitoring in the four countries

As can be seen in more detail in Chapters 8 and 9, there was no formal monitoring of public opinion or attitudes in the United Kingdom during the early years of the BSE crisis. The main concern was with formulating messages to the public rather than with monitoring public opinion. That the latter might be used to inform and shape the former appears not to have been considered. An audit report of 1993 concluded that knowledge was lacking in MAFF about how to monitor public opinion, and that there was a notable absence of two-way communication. While officials seem to have had access to press cuttings, there is no evidence that these were analysed in any systematic manner or that they influenced policy significantly. While such cuttings served as windows onto "public opinion", they were mainly used to explain negative images of the ministry as "media misrepresentation". Similarly, occasional surveys of public opinion focused on the perception of MAFF. In general, the administration took the view that public opinion was not an input but a target, although there was some admission that it might have been useful to know about public attitudes earlier on.

The establishment of the FSA in 2000 has apparently changed the situation in the United Kingdom. The agency makes a "commitment to listen carefully".

This includes some monitoring of attitudes and public beliefs in the food safety area on the basis of large-scale surveys and stakeholder consultations in the process of risk assessments. However, the results of the monitoring of public attitudes seem not to be widely known within the FSA. A prevailing view among the experts seems to be that knowledge of public opinion is important, though, not to influence policy but to make it look appealing (in the United Kingdom known as "spin").

In Germany, neither the national nor the *Länder* governments seem to have carried out any monitoring of public opinion on BSE/CJD at all before 2000, when the local crisis broke out. Finnish government officials seem to have considered a small range of sources — statistics on meat consumption, some media reports and parliamentary debates — to be adequate indicators of public attitudes to BSE/CJD. They also had some direct contacts with consumers over the phone and via e-mail. The prevailing view among officials seems to have been that public opinion was essentially "irrational worries".

Italian policy-makers appear to have had no systematic means of assessing public opinion or perceptions about BSE/CJD, and no communications specialists appear to have been available or consulted to remedy this. In general, policy-makers felt the media (particularly television) were prima-

The BSE and CJD crisis in the press

rily interested in bad news, were not interested in science, and were more intent on boosting their viewing audience or newspaper circulation by sensationalism rather than serious reporting.

This overview suggests that none of the four countries made the continuous and systematic monitoring of the media an integral part of the management of the BSE crisis, beyond the unsystematic perusal of press cuttings. The limited media monitoring that was carried out was not used to learn about public concerns in order to consider them as part of policy-making. It can be concluded that such data are currently not part of health and food intelligence systems in the four countries, and that those systems have not considered the potential use of media information as a source of insight into public perceptions. This may be a missed opportunity with considerable costs.

▾ Discussion: the potential value of press monitoring

To return to the question posed at the beginning of this chapter: Can the mass media be used as an index of public perception by policy-makers? The answer is necessarily qualified: carefully designed media analysis can provide useful indicators of public opinion and how it evolves over time. This is complementary to other ways of gathering public opinions, such as focus group discussions or opinion polls. The latter provide information about how such opinions are formed, and what are the factors influencing them. The various ways of understanding different aspects of public opinion are discussed in the concluding chapter of this book.

As noted earlier, the mass media carry out concurrent functions of (a) mirroring public perceptions and (b) setting the public agenda (i.e. forming public perceptions). These functions are not constant: one or the other function may be more important at any given time on any given issue. Therefore, systematic analysis — empirical study of salience and framing — that understands and investigates these two functions can indeed provide useful information to policy-makers without claiming to represent a complete or authoritative indicator of public opinion.

The study findings suggest that systematic media monitoring using both quantitative and qualitative methods (in fact, the two are complementary) could aid policy-makers in the following ways.

• **Provide an index of trust**. Occasional and selec-tive use of some press cuttings for the purpose of evaluating the image of the government was made in the countries studied (e.g. MAFF in the United Kingdom). This narrow use of press monitoring can be useful if done systematically and when care is taken not to reinforce existing prejudices about the press and contribute to a "bunker mentality", especially when a government finds itself dealing with a crisis.

• **Summarize information and avoid overload**.
The use of complete press cuttings as a form of data collection may serve some purposes, but only as long as the articles are few and infrequent. However, once a story breaks, the number of articles is likely to exceed the capacity of any single reader. Without systematic analysis, civil servants and politicians are likely to be overloaded with information and unable to reach a considered judgement about public opinion as expressed in the media, its trends and variations.

• **Avoid or prevent stereotypical assessment of public opinion.** The study findings (most visibly in the British and Italian cases) suggest that a narrow or unsystematic reading of the media is likely to lead to stereotypical interpretations and simplistic dismissal of the press coverage as "misrepresentation" of the issues.
This attribution is only self-serving and does not provide any information to evaluate and direct current crisis management. Systematic coding of press materials can provide policy-makers with a clearer understanding of how an issue is being shaped in the press, in particular by alerting them to changes in framing and thematic focus.

• **Provide early warning as to the likely future public opinion**. Continuous monitoring of the trends in press coverage as they happen can draw attention to changes in the press coverage early on. In view of the influence of press coverage over public opinion, this monitoring may also anticipate themes and ways of framing an issue that may become important in the mind of the public.

• **Strengthen understanding of public opinion as measured by other methods**. Media monitoring can be carried out relatively cheaply and can provide continuous indicators that lead other types of data. The results can be used in conjunction with parallel data on public attitudes such as focus groups and survey methods. Because media monitoring is continuous, it may be particularly useful in spotting trends relatively early on. This contrasts with data collected by the other methods that are generally spot observations (unless they are repeated at short intervals — an expensive activity).

• **Facilitate consideration of public concerns as part of policy-making on issues involving health risks**. The proposed use of media analysis can make it feasible to include information on public perceptions as a regular input to health intelligence systems, along with information on diseases. Having indicators of media perception as part of the usual information handled by health intelligence systems would underscore the need to take people's perceptions into account, and could facilitate a more

The BSE and CJD crisis in the press

systematic feeding of public perspectives into the policy-making process.

The use of media analysis (particularly of the press, as in this study) as a proxy for public opinion in between waves of other types of data collection is likely to be context-dependent, i.e. to depend on the issue itself and on a variety of other conditions occurring at a given moment. Other media such as television and radio may also be worth exploring as early "sensors" of opinion among particular parts of society. Whatever happens, new ways of using media analysis to integrate people's perspectives into health intelligence systems will need to be pilot tested and evaluated to determine their feasibility and cost benefits. How those analyses might be used will depend on whether public opinion is seen by policy-makers merely as a target or as an input.

▾ Conclusions

This study confirmed that the amount of press coverage and the actual number of BSE/CJD incidents were not directly related, reinforcing the notion that the mass media constructed an "artificial horizon" (Kepplinger, 1989), which, however, took intermittent clues from the disease process. For some observers this dissociation provides grounds for a normative critique of the media system (Adam, 1998; Kepplinger, 1989); for others it is just an operational characteristic of the mass media. It does not mirror events in real time but modulates public opinion

about such events. It is our view that the mass media system has to be assessed by its contributions to public opinion rather than by its correspondence with the real-time events. Key findings across the four countries include the following.

• Throughout the period examined in this study, there were both similarities and dissimilarities in the way the BSE situation was reported in the four countries. In all countries, March 1996 clearly marked a synchronization of international public attention. It was the peak year in all four countries in the period until 1999 (coverage of 2000 exceeded this peak in Germany). Before 1996, Germany and the United Kingdom had a similar cycle of attention, with peaks in the summers of 1990 and 1994.

• After 1996, an emerging disjunction in salience could be observed. In the United Kingdom, salience was highest, in Germany, medium, and in Italy, low. From the end of 1997 to the beginning of 1999 the development of the German and Italian salience was parallel, but in complete contrast to the United Kingdom where the 1998 commissioning of the Phillips Inquiry began a time for evaluation of crisis management.

• There were both similarities and significant differences in the framing of articles about the crisis. Overall, "cost/benefits of the crisis", "food safety and public health" and "national interest" were the three dominant frames in the United Kingdom, Finland and Italy, while in Germany the "cost/benefits of the crisis" frame was eventually replaced by "scientific expertise". In the United Kingdom, the most frequent frame was "food safety and public health"; in Germany the most frequent frame was "national interest", while in Italy and Finland it was "cost/benefits of the crisis". However, the most marked differences between the countries were in the actors reported and the thematic content of the articles. In the British case the most frequent main actor was "national government", while Germany and Italy focused most on the EU, and Finland on its farmers and producers.

• Protecting the national (agricultural) interest from the threat of BSE infection in Germany, Italy and Finland, or in the United Kingdom from other countries or EU limits and bans, was clearly a dominant frame. "National interest" was a significant frame in all countries, exceeding articles framed by "national identity" The three main peaks of framing by "national interest" were echoed by somewhat smaller peaks of "national identity", which reached its apogee in 1996.

• Speculation about the safety of British beef may have driven the increase in articles framed by "food safety and public health", which

reached a peak in 1995 and declined thereafter. The "cost/benefits of the crisis" frame appeared more frequently than the "food safety and public health" frame in 1996; this may reflect the way that the March 1996 announcement permitted speculation to cease and assessment to begin. The "industrial production of food" theme echoed the "cost/benefits" frame.

• Thematically, Finland and Germany were similar, most frequently discussing lifting the ban on British beef and implementing controls. In contrast, the Italian press found beef prices and expenditure implications to be more pressing. In both the United Kingdom and Finland, the viability of farming was also important.

• An overall observation can be made, that the framing of the BSE issue did not remain con-stant over time, most noticeably regarding "national identity" or in terms of "industrial food production". Such fluctuations in framing illustrate the fluidity of media discourse. While the overwhelming majority of coverage in the United Kingdom concerned national events, in the three other countries, concern for their own national situation was balanced by interest in the EU and the United Kingdom. This was particularly true for Finland. The United Kingdom evaluated its "national government"

The BSE and CJD crisis in the press

negatively compared to the EU, while the other countries were more positive about their own governments.

• Around 10% of articles dealt with the trustworthiness of actors in the crisis. Over 50% of articles framed by "trust" took international institutions as their main actors (specifically the EU). This tends to confirm that the media constructed or reflected the international conflict hinted at by the frequent framing by "national interest". Moreover, international actors (along with the public sector) were given the most negative evaluations.

As to whether the mass media be used as an index of public perception by policy-makers, this study's findings suggest that systematic media monitoring could aid policy-makers in the following ways:
• provide an index of public trust for those concerned about public trust;
• summarize information and avoid overload;
• avoid or prevent stereotypical assessment of public opinion;
• identify themes that may grow in importance in the mind of the public;
• strengthen understanding of public opinion as measured by other methods; and
• facilitate consideration of public concerns as part of policy-making on issues involving health risks.

A more general implication of this research is the potential value of media monitoring and analysis as a contribution to health intelligence systems. Continuous monitoring of the trends in press coverage as they happen can draw attention to changes in press coverage early on. In view of the interaction between press coverage and public opinion, this monitoring may also anticipate themes and ways of framing an issue that may become important in the mind of the public. The validity and reliability of such development would need further investigation; its feasibility and cost benefit would also need to be tested.The potential value of media monitoring in the policy process is discussed further in Chapter 10.

References
Adam B (1998) *Timescapes of modernity, the environment and invisible hazards.* New York, NY, Routledge.

Bauer MW (2000) Classical content analysis: a review. In: Bauer MW, Gaskell G, eds. *Qualitative researching with text, image and sound.* London, Sage: 131–151.

Bauer MW (2002) Controversial medical and agri-food biotechnology: a cultivation analysis. *Public Understanding of Science*, 11:93–111.

Bauer MW, Bonfadelli H (2002) Controversy, media coverage and public knowledge. In: Bauer MW, Gaskell G, eds. *Biotechnology –the making of a global controversy.* Cambridge, Cambridge University Press: 149–177.

Bauer MW, Gaskell G (1999) Towards a paradigm for research on social representations. *Journal for the Theory of Social Behaviour*, 29:163–186.

Bauer MW, Gaskell G (2002) The biotechnology movement. In: Bauer MW, Gaskell G, eds. *Biotechnology –the making of a global controversy.* Cambridge, Cambridge University Press: 379–404.

Bryant J, Zillmann D, eds (1994) *Media effects. Advances in theory and research.* Hillsdale, NJ, LEA.

Entman RM (1993) Framing: forwards clarification of a fractured paradigm. *Journal of Communication,* 43:51–58.

Farr R, Moscovici S, eds (1984) *Social representations.* Cambridge, Cambridge University Press.

Gamson WA, Modigliani A (1989) Media discourse and public opinion on nuclear power. *American Journal of Sociology,* 95:1–37.

Habermas J (1989) *The structural transformation of the public sphere.* Cambridge, Polity Press [German original 1961].

Hagenhoff V (2000) *Media coverage of BSE/CJD crisis in the press – 1985-1999. National report of Germany, WHO project 'public perception of BSE and CJD risk – media module'.* Kiel, University of Kiel, Agricultural Economics.

Kepplinger M (1989) *Künstliche Horizonte, Folgen, Darstellung und Akzeptanz von Technik in der Bundesrepublik. [Artificial horizons, consequences, representation and acceptance of technology in the Federal Republic of Germany].* Frankfurt, Campus.

Lamming E (1992) *The Report of the Expert Group on Animal Feedingstuffs to the Minister of Agriculture, Fisheries and Food, The State Secretary for Health, and the Secretaries of State for Wales, Scotland and Northern Ireland.* London, Her Majesty's Stationery Office. (http://www.bseinquiry.gov.uk/report/volume9). (See also:http://www.bseinquiry.gov.uk/files/ws/s012.pdf).

Levikintarkastus (2003) "*Sanomalehtien Levikit 1992-2002*" *[The circulation of the newspaper 1992-2002].* (http://www.levikintarka-stus.fi/Levikintarkastus/tilastot/periodicals10years.pdf.)

Livingston S (1997) *Clarifying the CNN effect: an examination of media effects according to type of military intervention.* Harvard University, The Joan Shorenstein Center (Research Paper R-18).

Livingstone S (1996) On the continuing problem of media effects. In: Curran J, Gurevitch M, eds. *Mass media and society,* 2nd ed. London, Arnold: Ch. 15.

Luhmann N (1996) *Die Realität der Massenmedien. [The reality of the mass media].* Opladen, Westdeutscher Verlag.

McCombs M (1994) News influence on our pictures of the world. In: Bryant J, Zillmann D, eds. *Media effects. Advances in theory and research.* Hillsdale, NJ, LEA.

Mazur A (1981) Media coverage and public opinion on scientific controversies. *Journal of Communication,* 31:106–115.

Miller D, Reilly J (1995) Making an issue of food safety: The media, pressure groups and the public sphere. In: Maurer D, Sobal J, eds. *Eating agendas: food and nutrition as social problems.* New York, NY, Greuyter: 305–336.

Morgan M, Shanahan J (1996) Two decades of cultivation analysis: an appraisal and meta-analysis. *Communication Yearbook,* 20:1–45.

Peak S, Fisher P, eds (1998) *The media guide.* London, Fourth Estate.

Phillips N, Bridgeman J, Ferguson-Smith M (2000) *The BSE Inquiry: Report: Evidence and supporting papers of the inquiry into the emergence and identification of Bovine Spongiform Encephalopathy (BSE) and variant Creutzfeldt-Jakob Disease (vCJD) and the action taken in response to it up to 20 March 1996.* London, The Stationery Office. (http://www.bseinquiry.gov.uk/index.htm.)

Sperber D (1990) The epidemiology of beliefs. In: Fraser C, Gaskell G, eds. *The social psychology of widespread beliefs.* Oxford, Clarendon Press: 25–43.

Tichenor PJ, Donohue GA, Olien GN (1970) *Community conflict and the press.* Beverly Hills, CA, Sage.

Tilston CH, Sear R, Neale RJ, Gregson K (1992) The effect of BSE: consumer perceptions and beef purchasing behaviour. *British Food Journal,* 94:23–26.

World Press Trends (2002) Paris, World Association of Newspapers.

Risk communication strategies in public policy-making

Risk communication strategies in public policy-making

Patrick van Zwanenberg, Erik Millstone

The purpose of this brief chapter is to provide an analytical context for the subsequent description and analysis of BSE risk communication strategies in the four countries in this study.

The chapter begins with an historical and theoretical account of some of the main developments in thinking about risk communication in modern industrialized countries. It identifies three analytically distinct ways in which risk communication has been conceptualized and practised, and how these are in turn connected to more general ideas about the relationship between science and policy-making. In the following chapters, based on this theoretical framework, the study team explores such questions as: how well informed official bodies were concerning the beliefs, wants and behaviour of their publics; how they could become better informed; and what the conditions for, and consequences of, improved dialogue might be.

▾ Evolution of thought and practice in risk communication

The official and scholarly literature on risk communication can be characterized in several different ways. These include characterization by disciplinary perspective (e.g. Turner & Wynne, 1992), by broadly chronological phases (Powell & Leiss, 1997) or in terms of competing conceptual approaches (Pidgeon et al., 1992).

One of the difficulties in providing an historical characterization of risk communication is that there has not

necessarily been a convergence between the scholarly literature, official guides and actual practices within policy institutions. Furthermore, particular risk communication practices may not constitute a coherent strategy as such. What is clear, however, is that shifts in both scholarly and official thinking about risk communication, as well as actual practices, can usefully be thought of as an ongoing retreat from naive positivism, i.e., the progression is away from the view that communication is essentially about displacing false public beliefs about risk by substituting assertions about probabilities of harm.

Fischhoff (1995) described such a shift when he characterized the history of risk communication in seven discrete developmental stages, each of which, he argued, can be identified by a focal communication strategy. Fischhoff suggests that practitioners initially thought that "All we have to do is to get the numbers right". He suggests that practitioners have had to learn that such an approach is not sufficient, and that "All we have to do is tell them the numbers", is also insufficient. Eventually, policy-makers had to work their way through more assumptions: "All we have to do is explain what we mean by the numbers" was followed by "All we have to do is show them they've accepted similar risks in the past", followed by "All we have to do is show them that it's a good deal for them", and "All we have to do is treat them nice [sic]". Fischhoff's final stage in the development trajectory is to suggest that practitioners have had to learn that "All we have to do is make them partners". While elements of Fischoff's scheme are reflected in the discussion below, the study team has instead identified three different ways in which the purposes and nature of risk communication have been conceptualized and, at least to some extent, practised. These three approaches are termed the "technocratic approach", the "decisionist approach" and the "deliberative approach".

It is important to note that the three approaches are analytical and explanatory ideals, and in actual practice elements of more than one may be reflected in any one jurisdiction or policy arena. Each of the three approaches (actually sets of conceptual modes and practices) concerning risk communication is, however, tied to a broader set of consistent ideas and assumptions through which analysts and practitioners have understood the nature of science-based policy-making. The discussion in this chapter therefore relates risk communication ideas to those more generalized models of the nature of science-based policy-making.

• The technocratic approach

Explicit and sustained attention to the communication of risk as a topic of public policy dates from the 1970s, in particular as a response to public controversies about the risks and social acceptability of nuclear power. The dominant assumption on the part of industry, officials and many experts was that public fears and scepticism about safety claims concerning nuclear power and other controversial technologies reflected public misunderstanding, media misinformation, scientific illiteracy and plain ignorance (MacGill, 1989; Otway & Wynne, 1989; Stern, 1991; Shrader-Frechette, 1998).

According to this approach, the public's understanding of issues of science and risk was conceived as a "deficit", and it was problematic to the extent that it failed to coincide with the views of officials and ministers — or at any rate failed to coincide with the views that ministers and officials wanted the public to accept. Scientists were presumed to be in possession of "the truth", or at least reliable knowledge about risk (defined as an objective probability of harm), whereas the general public was understood or represented as being at best ignorant, and at worst possessed of false and unscientific beliefs. From that perspective, risk communication was seen as the attempt to provide science-based representations of risk that were sufficiently simplified to be readily transferable into the minds of the general public in order to diminish their ignorance or to displace alternative representations of risk.

To the extent that the media might disseminate representations of risk that were at variance with those officially approved, they too needed to become "better informed". From this point of view, the media were seen as being irresponsible if they saw their role as providing representations of the public's views to the policy-makers rather than the other way round. Bottom-up communication had no place within the technocratic model.

Early and historically dominant models of risk communication thus conceived of it as a tertiary consideration (i.e. subsequent to, first, the assessment of risk and, second, the identification of policy responses). Risk

Risk communication

communication was thus a one-way, top-down process running from the experts to the government and thence to industrial stakeholders and the general public. It involved the provision of predominantly technical, and often quantitative, information about risk (Nelkin, 1989; Powell & Leiss, 1997). The challenge was to provide information that was sufficiently clear so that public views would comply with official expectations of reasonable belief and behaviour.

Such models of risk communication were typically articulated by those who assumed (or at least asserted) that risk policy-making could be based solely on scientific considerations, i.e. that science provided not just a necessary but also a sufficient basis for policy decision-making. They also assumed or asserted that science functions in complete independence of social, political, cultural and economic conditions.

During the 1970s and early 1980s, much of the academic work on risk perception was motivated by a wish to understand why people's perceptions deviated from what was sometimes assumed to be a proper rational understanding of risk. Psychometric research suggested that a number of "risk attributes", in addition to the normal scientific dimensions of risk, affected public risk perceptions and that such attributes meant that people placed different weights on different risks even where the numerical magnitude of the frequency of death from those risks was the same (Fischhoff et al., 1978; Slovic, 1987).

Risk attributes included, for example, the relative voluntariness of risk, the potential for catastrophic or chronic harm, and the degrees of familiarity and uncontrollability of the risks. Risks that were involuntary, potentially catastrophic and unfamiliar, such as nuclear power generation, were typically interpreted by different social groups as far less tolerable than voluntary and familiar risks, such as the consumption of alcohol. Interpretation of the psychometric work on risk depends crucially on whether such "risk attributes" are assumed to be legitimate or whether they are seen as external to properly rational definitions of risk (Turner & Wynne, 1992).

Even if policy practitioners assumed that "risk attributes" were ultimately irrational (in other words, that the objective/subjective distinction between experts and the public was maintained), an important lesson drawn from this work was that a more careful tailoring of communication messages to the antecedent perceptions of the audience might be required. To do otherwise, it was recognized, would devalue the perspectives of those bearing the risks. As well as various strands of research into risk perceptions, the experience of commercial advertising also indicated to some practitioners a need to take into account the characteristics of the audience and their perceptions in order to maintain credibility. One research technique designed to support risk communication that was developed in response to such concerns was known as the "mental models" approach. It sought first to identify lay publics' beliefs about a hazard and then to develop the content of subsequent communication by strengthening correct

strategies in public policy-making

beliefs, adding missing concepts, correcting mistakes and de-emphasizing peripheral beliefs (Jungerman et al., 1988; Pidgeon et al., 1992).

In contrast to the psychometric focus on various properties of risk as relevant factors in explaining public perceptions, sociological research into risk perception in the 1980s placed far more empirical and explanatory emphasis on the social and institutional structures of risk-generating processes. Factors that were taken by those in the psychometric field to be properties of risk, such as controllability, were interpreted by some as being reflections of the social institutions responsible for controlling risks (rather than, or as well as, properties of the technical risks themselves). This body of work suggested that people's experiences of risk are socially framed and are not purely about attributes of physical harm, but rather primarily stem from the perceived threat to social relationships and identities (Turner & Wynne, 1992).

Social theorists of risk argued that the extent to which lay publics find particular decisions about risk acceptable is connected with their perceptions of the credibility of the institutions responsible for managing and controlling risk. It was noted, for example, that if regulatory bodies had a history of incompetence or secrecy then lay publics would judge the risks that those bodies were responsible for controlling as greater than would otherwise be the case. Empirical work seemed to suggest that trust, or rather lack of trust, was one factor responsible for the gulf between official technical

assessments of risk and public perceptions. One lesson widely drawn by risk communication analysts and practitioners was that if lay publics do not trust the source they will not trust the message (Covello, 1993).

Technocratic approaches have by no means disappeared in practice. Nevertheless, the fact that those approaches had failed to prevent or reduce social conflict over new technologies, together with evidence that the institutions engaged in orthodox forms of risk communication lacked credibility, began to prompt changes in both thinking and practices, especially from about the mid-1980s, in both Europe and North America. Risk communicators, it was argued, should understand the bases of public risk perceptions and the social context within which regulatory activities took place, and then proceed on that basis with a tailored process of targeted information dissemination (Covello & Allen, 1988; Powell & Leiss, 1997: 36). In other words, risk communication should not be thought of as merely information transfer but rather as a type of political discourse (Stern, 1991).

Crucially, however, much of this new thinking still embraced the deficit model of the public understanding of science; representations of technical risk, provided by the officially selected scientific experts, were deemed to be unproblematically correct and adequate. Furthermore, risk communication practices still sought not only to achieve unconditional acceptance of assessments of risk but also of official risk management decisions. The only difference was that the new risk communication strategies were based on some intelligence about

Risk communication

how people construct their assumed misperceptions of risk. Those strategies could then be tailored to the misunderstandings and concerns of the target audience.

• The decisionist approach

The decisionist approach shares an important similarity with the technocratic approach: both assume that the representations of technical risk provided by officially selected expert scientists are unproblematically correct. However, the decisionist approach typically recognizes that public views about what is a fair trade-off between the physical or social risks and the advantages of the technology or process generating those risks should be considered a legitimate source of information for risk managers. In other words the decisionist approach takes public attitudes (and perforce the media) into account, but their relevance is confined to informing evaluative judgements — for example, about the acceptability of the risks — once experts have delivered their authoritative conclusions.

Under the decisionist approach, risk communication is understood as a two-way rather than a one-way process. On the one hand, technical attributes of risk are communicated in one direction, from the experts to the government and thence to the general public. On the other hand, the media and other mechanisms have a legitimate role to play in helping policy-makers to understand the conflicting concerns and interests of different social groups and their varying willingness to tolerate different kinds of risks in exchange for different kinds of benefits. From the point of view of policy-

makers, the public need to be persuaded that risk management decisions are prudent and fair, but that can only be accomplished if policy-makers understand how the public view issues such as prudence and fairness as they apply to the issues at stake. Contemporary official risk communication guidelines typically stress the importance of both understanding the attitudes to risk of affected and interested citizens and of incorporating those views and preferences into policy (e.g. Inter-Departmental Liaison Group on Risk Assessment, 1998).

Many regulatory bodies, whilst recognizing that what counts as an acceptable level of risk is partly a matter of social values, nevertheless have not necessarily sought actively to solicit public views about what is fair, preferring instead to rely on rules-of-thumb or official judgement. For example, in 1983, the British Royal Society (1983:179) suggested that an annual risk of death of 1:1000 population might not be totally unacceptable provided that countervailing benefits existed, that everything reasonable had been done to reduce the risk and that the individual at risk was aware of the situation. It also suggested that an annual risk of death of 1:1 million population was the point at which an imposed risk could be treated as trivial by policy-makers. In 1988, the British Health and Safety Executive subsequently based its own guidelines on acceptable levels of risk on the Royal Society report (Royal Commission on Environmental Pollution, 1998: 53).

Some regulatory organizations have not, however, relied entirely on official judgements about fairness and accepta-

strategies in public policy-making

bility and have commissioned research on public attitudes to risk, for example by using questionnaires to derive data on people's willingness to pay to avoid certain risks (Wynne, 1989: 120). Many regulatory institutions also routinely rely on standard public consultation processes to solicit views on whether regulations are viewed as fair, reasonable and practicable. In most cases, however, those consultation processes are not aimed at lay citizens.

Policy-makers who acknowledge that risk communication, under the decisionist approach, is a two-way process typically conceive of the relationship between science and policy as one in which science is necessary but not sufficient for policy decision-making. Once scientific judgements have been made, and once advice has been provided by scientific experts, a number of social, economic, cultural and evaluative considerations necessarily have a downstream contribution to make to policy decision-making. Those downstream evaluations might be concerned, for example, with the economic costs of risk reduction, or the civil liberties implications of imposing restrictions on the actions of individuals or corporations, or the relative suitability of different policy instruments. A representation of the structural assumptions of what can be termed the "decisionist model of science in policy-making" is provided in Figure 7.1. The model assumes in effect a clear, straightforward and strict division of labour between (a) the scientific community

Figure 7.1. A decisionist model of science in policy-making

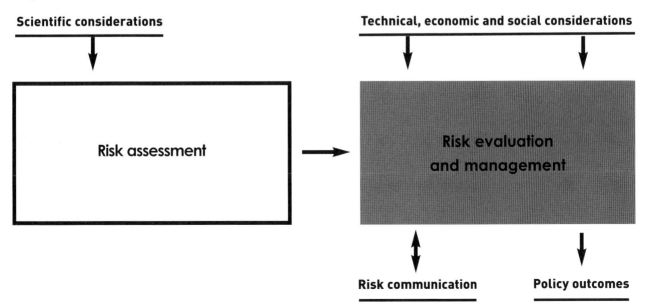

Risk communication

which can and should assess risks in a socially and ethically neutral way, and (b) policy-makers who subsequently and legitimately take into account the possible risks, costs and benefits of accepting or diminishing those risks, as well as the distribution of those costs and benefits.

• The deliberative approach

A key assumption underlying most risk communication practices is that scientific knowledge is essentially neutral and objective and that the key problems are both the public's inability to understand the "correct", expert-defined messages about risk and the failure of governments, media and scientists to communicate that message effectively to the public (Stern, 1991; Pidgeon et al., 1992).

Several problems have been raised with that assumption and consequently with the dominant interpretation of the key problems faced by risk communicators. Firstly, many commentators have argued that risks can never be assessed in a value-neutral way because value judgements, often referred to as "framing judgements", are involved in defining a regulatory problem and specifying the scope and limits of any subsequent risk assessment. These refer, for example, to often tacit decisions about which risks are deemed to be significantly adverse, how different dimensions of risk should be ordered and aggregated, and which benchmarks should be used against which to measure risk (Levidow et al., 1997; Stirling, 1999). These are not in themselves questions that scientific experts can decide, although

they do shape the conduct of subsequent scientific deliberations and risk assessments. Framing judgements also help to shape research agendas within regulatory programmes and thus the kinds of evidence available and unavailable for subsequent risk assessments (Stern, 1991).

Wynne (1995) has argued that expert risk assessments are also typically framed by assumptions about the behaviour of social institutions and practices. One example provided by Wynne concerns expert assessments of nuclear reactor safety that are predicated on the assumption that the quality of manufacture, maintenance, operation and regulation will persist long into the future. While that kind of commitment might turn out to be justified, it is nevertheless a conditional social commitment rather than a purely scientific claim. Wynne also notes that different views between experts and lay citizens about the long-term stability of such social institutions often underpin controversies about nuclear safety.

A second reason why critics have argued that scientific knowledge about risk cannot be socially or politically neutral is because there are often scientific uncertainties involved in assessing risk issues, and because scientists interpret shared bodies of evidence in differing and conflicting ways (Pidgeon et al., 1992; Wynne, 1992). Indeed, scientists have also disagreed about which bodies of evidence are relevant when conducting risk assessments (van Zwanenberg & Millstone, 2000). Decisions about how to manage uncertainties and con-

strategies in public policy-making

flicting approaches to analysis within risk assessments are partly non-scientific in nature, and this point is often obvious, especially when disputes arise or risk assessments are subsequently demonstrated to be misconceived in the light of new data or events (Shrader-Frechette, 1998).

Many analysts have consequently argued that, since framing commitments and the kinds of judgements involved in assessing incomplete and equivocal bodies of knowledge are not solely dictated by scientific reasoning or evidence, the values and knowledge of non-experts have a valid role to play in risk assessment (Fiorino, 1990; Royal Commission on Environmental Pollution, 1998). This implies a more thorough two-way and deliberative process of communication than envisaged in decisionist approaches to risk communication.

A key feature of a deliberative approach is that risk communication is not treated entirely as an object of policy — it is not an exercise "bolted on" at the end of a conventional, specialist-led process (Stirling, 2003). Nor is it restricted to dialogue about the appropriate trade-offs between the costs and benefits of particular forms of regulatory intervention, as in the decisionist model. Instead, risk communication needs to involve dialogue about the definition and analysis, as well as the evaluation, of any particular risk issue.

Several contemporary official sources recognize at least some elements of a deliberative approach. For example, the British Government suggests that regula-

tors find out how much risks matter to whom and why, prior to a regulatory response (Inter-Departmental Liaison Group on Risk Assessment, 1998) and that departments involve the public in framing key issues and discussing possible policy solutions (Cabinet Office, 2002: 86). Similarly, the Royal Commission on Environmental Pollution in the United Kingdom (1998: 105) argues that the public should be involved in the formulation of regulatory strategies, rather than being merely consulted on draft proposals. The National Research Council in the United States of America (1996) goes further, suggesting that deliberative processes — involving all interested and affected parties — are necessary when deciding which types of harm to analyse, deciding how to describe scientific uncertainty and disagreement, analysing evidence, generating policy options, and deciding on policy outcomes.

Recent years have seen the development of a wide range of deliberative forms of communication through which public input into processes of framing, analysing and evaluating risk issues might be achieved. Public consultation and participation on risk policy-making has been attempted using techniques such as surveys, focus groups, consensus conferences, citizens' juries, deliberative polls, multi-criteria mapping and representative commissions (Parliamentary Office of Science and Technology, 2001; National Research Council, 1996: Appendix B). Thus far, however, the actual experiences of using these new forms of deliberative and participative communication have been subject to little critical analysis (Holmes & Scoones, 2000).

Risk communication

As with the technocratic and decisionist approaches to risk communication, the deliberative approach presupposes a particular model of the relationship between science and policy decision-making. This model emphasizes that science-based risk assessments always involve a prior set of non-scientific framing assumptions within which selected scientific information is analysed. The model also acknowledges that, even after a set of decisions and commitments have been made defining the scope and nature of risk assessments, the risk assessments themselves will involve evidential assumptions and decisions about issues such as how uncertain and incomplete evidence should be interpreted and represented. The model assumes,

furthermore, that once expert risk assessors have (a) reached conclusions about the existence of a risk, its probability and severity, and (b) acknowledged some of the scientific uncertainties with which they have had to grapple, it is then up to policy-makers to make a further set of specific downstream evaluative judgements to decide how the conclusions of the risk assessment will influence policy decisions. A representation of the structural assumptions of this alternative "co-evolutionary model of policy-making" is provided in Figure 7.2.

▾ Dimensions of analysis

The study team's research has sought to explore the

Figure 7.2. A co-evolutionary model of science in policy-making

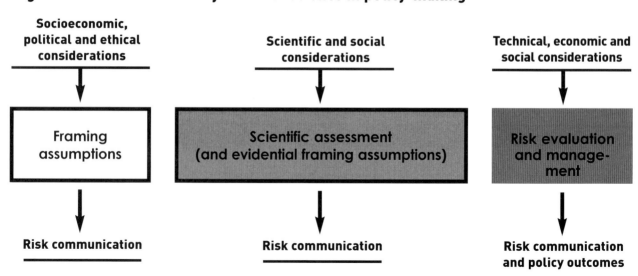

strategies in public policy-making

extent to which risk communication did and could play a key role in BSE policy-making. The fullest account thus far of the potential function of risk communication is the "deliberative" one that corresponds to a "co-evolutionary" model of the interaction between science and policy-making, as indicated in Figure 7.2. Accordingly, the study team approached the task of examining and analysing risk communication strategies on the basis of certain ideas about which dimensions of analysis might be particularly important.

- **Explicit or implicit.** It would not have been realistic to assume that all risk communication strategies were fully and explicitly articulated, nor that explicit accounts were always fully accurate, and therefore the team approached this study by assuming that risk communication strategies could be implicit as well as explicit.
- **Unidirectional and top-down or part of a dialogue.** Some (indeed many) approaches to risk communication by BSE policy-makers might have been conceptualized as a matter of sending messages out, typically to stakeholders, citizens and consumers. Others can be thought of as bilateral or multidirectional in that policy-makers are also concerned with listening, receiving and digesting signals as well as with sending messages out.
- **Science-based or driven primarily by non-scientific factors or a combination of the two.** Some approaches to risk communication may have assumed that what needs to be communicated is essentially scientific information and scientific

accounts of what the risks might be (or might have been) and about what is being done to control and manage, diminish or eradicate them. A contrasting approach to risk communication might assume that it is not only about scientific information but also about a range of non-scientific factors such as the competence, legitimacy and trustworthiness of institutions and their decisions.

- **Acknowledge or deny uncertainties.** Some approaches to BSE risk communication may have been characterized by an assumption or assertion that, while there may be some uncertainties about the science of BSE, policy measures were based on sound and secure science. A contrasting approach would be to emphasize the uncertainties, and the difficulties in anticipating the risks or the future epidemics of BSE and/or vCJD.
- **Acknowledge or deny "evidential framing assumptions".** Some approaches to BSE risk communication might be predicated on the assumption that scientists can and do assess the risks of BSE without presupposing any policy considerations. A contrasting approach would be to assume that scientific deliberations about, and assessments of, the risks from BSE depend on what has been termed "evidential framing assumptions" about which there can also be communicative exchanges.
- **Acknowledge or deny wider framing assumptions.** Some approaches to BSE risk communication could acknowledge that BSE policy can depend, for example, on broad issues such as the accept-

Risk communication

ability of recycling animal waste (especially from slaughterhouses) into the animal feed-chain. A contrasting approach, however, would be one that addressed relatively narrow technical issues about risks of exposure to the BSE pathogen, without acknowledging or questioning those broader choices.

- **Acknowledge or deny risk–cost–benefit trade-offs.** Some approaches to BSE risk communication might assume that policy-making decisions typically need to juxtapose, for example, the costs of reducing or eradicating the hazards posed by the BSE pathogen against the benefits of adopting a range of alternative courses of action. A contrasting approach, however, would be to presume that issues of risk and safety can or should be addressed without reference to countervailing costs or benefits.

- **Communicating about what?** Key features of the risk communication strategies of official policy-makers, and other key stakeholders, may also depend on the assumptions being made about the topics on which risk communication may be necessary, appropriate or desirable. Is there a need only to communicate the outcome of scientific and/or policy deliberations? Should it also address the assumptions about the objectives of policy, or just the means by which policy goals are achieved?

- **Assumptions about recipients.** Official risk communication strategies can also depend crucially on the assumptions that are being made about the publics to whom the communications are

directed, in particular about the publics' beliefs, wants and behaviour. One assumption underlying this entire research project, and the European Commission's funding of it, was that public policy-makers could be, and should be, far better informed about public beliefs, attitudes and wants.

In the two chapters that follow, the study team draws on many of these dimensions of risk communication in order to describe the kinds of information gathered and disseminated by surveillance institutions, and to characterize the risk communication strategies adopted by the governments of the United Kingdom, Germany, Italy and Finland. The team also explores how well informed official bodies were concerning the beliefs, wants and behaviour of their publics, how they could become better informed, what the conditions for improved dialogue might be and their consequences, and how considerations of risk communication can most effectively contribute to overall policy-making about risk.

References

Cabinet Office (2002) *Risk: improving the Government's capability to handle risk and uncertainty.* London, Cabinet Office Strategy Unit.

Covello V (1993) Risk communication, trust and credibility. *Journal of Occupational Medicine*, 35:18–19.

Covello V, Allen F (1988) *Seven cardinal rules of risk communication.* Washington, DC, Office of Policy Analysis, United States Environmental Protection Agency.

strategies in public policy-making

Fiorino DJ (1990) Citizen participation and environmental risk: a survey of institutional mechanisms. *Science, Technology and Human Values*, 15:226–243.

Fischhoff B (1995) Risk perception and communication unplugged: twenty years of process. A critical review. *Risk Analysis*, 15:10–14.

Fischhoff B et al. (1978) How safe is safe enough? *Policy Sciences*, 8:127–152.

Holmes T, Scoones I (2000) *Participatory environmental policy processes: experiences from north and south*. Brighton, Institute for Development Studies (IDS Working Paper 113).

Inter-Departmental Liaison Group on Risk Assessment (1998) *Risk communication: a guide to regulatory practice*. London, Risk Assessment Policy Unit, Health and Safety Executive.

Jungerman H, Schutz H, Thuring M (1988) Mental models in risk assessment: informing people about drugs. *Risk analysis*, 8:147–155.

Levidow L, Carr S, Wield D, von Schomberg R (1997) European biotechnology regulation: framing the risk assessment of a herbicide-tolerant crop. *Science, Technology and Human Values*, 22: 472–505.

MacGill S (1989) Risk perception and the public: insights from research around Sellafield. In: Brown J, ed. *Environmental threats: perception, analysis and management*. London, Belhaven Press.

National Research Council (1996) *Understanding risk: informing decisions in a democratic society*. Washington, DC, National Academy Press.

Nelkin D (1989) Communicating technological risk: the social construction of risk perception. *Annual Review of Public Health*, 10:95–113.

Otway HJ, Wynne B (1989) Risk communication: paradigm and paradox. *Risk Analysis*, 9:141–145.

Parliamentary Office of Science and Technology (2001) *Open channels: public dialogue in science and technology*. London, Parliamentary Office of Science and Technology (Report No.153, POST).

Pidgeon N et al. (1992) Risk perception. In: *Risk: analysis, perception and management. Report of a Royal Society Study Group*. London, Royal Society: 89–134.

Powell D, Leiss W (1997) *Mad cows and mother's milk. The perils of poor risk communication*. Montreal and Kingston, McGill-Queen's University Press.

Royal Commission on Environmental Pollution (1998) *Setting environmental standards*. London, The Stationery Office (21st Report, Cm 4053).

Royal Society (1983) *The assessment of risk. A study group report*. London, Royal Society.

Shrader-Frechette K (1998) Scientific method, anti-foundationalism and public decision-making. In: Lofstedt RE, Frewer L, eds. *Risk and modern society*. London, Earthscan.

Slovic P (1987) Perception of risk. *Science*, 236:280–285.

Stern PC (1991) Learning through conflict: a realistic strategy for risk communication. *Policy Sciences*, 24:99–119.

Stirling A (1999) *On science and precaution in the management of technological risk. An ESTO project report*. Seville, Institute for Prospective Technological Studies (Report No. 19056 EN).

Stirling A (2003) Risk, uncertainty and precaution: some instrumental implications from the social sciences. In: Berkhout F, Leach M, Scoones I, eds. *Negotiating environmental change*. London, Elgar.

Turner B, Wynne B (1992) Risk communication. In: Durrant J, ed. *Biotechnology in public: a review of recent research*. London, Science Museum.

van Zwanenberg P, Millstone E (2000) Beyond sceptical relativism: evaluating the social constructions of expert risk assessments. *Science, Technology and Human Values*, 25: 259–282.

Wynne B (1989) Building public concern into risk management. In: Brown J, ed. *Environmental threats: perception, analysis and management*. London, Belhaven Press.

Wynne B (1992) Uncertainty and environmental learning. Reconceiving science and policy in the preventive paradigm. *Global Environmental Change*, 2:111–127.

Wynne B (1995) Technology assessment and reflexive social learning. Observations from the risk field. In: Rip A, Misa TJ, Schot J, eds. *Managing technology in society: the approach of constructive technology assessment*. London, Pinter.

8

Surveillance systems: their information and communication practices

Surveillance systems: their information and communication practices

Patrick van Zwanenberg, Kerstin Dressel, Maria Grazia Giannichedda, Meri Koivusalo, Eeva Ollila

All the countries in this study have been engaged in veterinary, food and human health surveillance activities related to BSE. This chapter describes the surveillance activities of the EU and the national regulatory regimes in the four study countries, and outlines the types of information gathered and disseminated by surveillance institutions. The discussion covers why certain types of information were and are gathered and disseminated and to whom (as well as why some types of information are not gathered or disseminated), and some of the impacts of those choices on policy-making. In the following chapter, that discussion will contribute to an analysis of the more general risk communication activities undertaken by regulatory regimes.

The term "surveillance" is normally understood in a rather narrow technical sense as applying only to diseases or pathogens responsible for disease, and this was certainly the case for the study countries. As will be seen, none of them made any systematic efforts to obtain non-veterinary data about BSE, such as public perceptions of the BSE-related events. They did not see that aspect as being part of surveillance or as relevant to policy-making. Not only was there no systematic surveying or monitoring of such information, but also such data were not thought to be worth gathering or taking into account even where they were available.

The veterinary surveillance methods most commonly used through most of the 1990s to identify suspect BSE cases were passive rather than active. Farmers and veterinary surgeons were expected to report cases of cattle displaying clinical signs compatible with BSE, after which the animals would be tested. This meant that the success of the surveillance depended to a great extent on (a) the willingness of farmers and veterinarians to report cases and (b) their awareness of symptoms. Even where these conditions were satisfied, the technology of testing presented additional difficulties. Since BSE does not produce an immune response in the host animal, diagnosis could only be undertaken once clinical symptoms of the disease were manifest. Clinical diagnosis required testing of brain tissue, which is expensive and time consuming and needs specialist expertise. More active forms of surveillance required either a survey (using histopathological, immunohistochemical and/or scrapie-associated fibrils (SAF) immunoblotting methods) of cattle brains or, more accurate but also more complicated, experiments in which brain tissue was taken from a sample of cows and injected into rodents known to be susceptible to BSE. Indications of the scale of infection would then be provided by the numbers of rodents that subsequently contracted a TSE.

The introduction of rapid postmortem tests in 2000 made it much easier to perform active surveillance. Such tests can be conducted on random or targeted subpopulations of national cattle herds. These rapid tests, however, are not used to confirm the presence of infection in clinically suspect animals.

EU surveillance policy?
BSE surveillance
A common, EU-wide surveillance policy for BSE has

been in place only since April 1998. From that date, all Member States were required to ensure training of people working with cattle so that they could identify signs of BSE. EU Member States are also required to implement a monitoring system and test, by histopathological examination, the brains of all animals older than 20 months that are displaying behavioural or neurological symptoms.

In 1997, the Office for Veterinary and Phytosanitary Inspection and Control was moved from the European Commission's Directorate-General for Agriculture to the Directorate-General for Consumer Policy and Consumer Health Protection, and in the process was renamed the Food and Veterinary Office (FVO). The FVO is now responsible for conducting audits on food safety controls in the Member States and in countries exporting to the EU. A key part of the FVO's responsibilities is to inform all stakeholders of the outcome of evaluations. Thus, information supplied to the FVO from Member States concerning surveillance strategies is made publicly available, as are the FVO's findings and recommendations.

Since January 2001, the European Commission has required Member States actively to monitor for BSE using the new tests. Such testing must be carried out on:
• all cattle aged over 30 months slaughtered due to an emergency or showing signs of any kind of illness at the antemortem inspection in the slaughterhouse;
• a random sample of cattle that have died on the farm;
• a targeted sample of animals; and
• all healthy animals over 30 months destined for human consumption (this requirement does not apply in the

United Kingdom, since domestic regulations permit only animals under 30 months of age to enter the human food-chain).

Some countries discovered that, once an active surveillance regime had been established under EU requirements, cases of BSE were found in their domestic herds although previously they had believed themselves to be disease-free.

Rapid tests can only detect subclinically infected animals (i.e. infected but not showing clinical symptoms) a few months before the onset of symptoms. Given that the average incubation period of BSE in cattle is five years, the rapid tests currently available (2003) cannot reliably differentiate between uninfected animals and subclinically infected cattle.

• **CJD surveillance**
In view of growing concern about the potential transmission of BSE to humans through the food-chain, a number of measures were implemented in Europe during the 1990s to enable the identification of changes in human spongiform encephalopathies. This started in 1990 with the establishment of the British CJD surveillance unit in Edinburgh. Since then, two important projects have been initiated with funding from the European Commission. The first is the European and Allied Countries Collaborative Study Group of CJD (EUROCJD), set up in 1993 to compare data from national registries in Australia, Austria, Canada, France, Germany, Italy, the Netherlands, Slovakia, Spain, Switzerland and the United

Surveillance systems:

Kingdom. In 1998, the Extended European Collaborative Study Group of CJD (NEUROCJD) started up after the European Council recommended that epidemiological surveillance of CJD be extended to all Member States. Both projects are coordinated by the CJD surveillance unit in Edinburgh (National CJD Surveillance Unit, undated). WHO works closely with EUROCJD and NEUROCJD in European countries, including the countries of eastern Europe and the Russian Federation.

The European Research Action Plan on TSE Diseases was started in 1996 by the European Commission's Directorate-General Research, to strengthen surveillance, understanding, prevention and treatment of TSEs. A regularly updated inventory of TSE research in Europe was created in 2000, along with a TSE research expert group to reinforce coordination of national activities in this field (European Commission, 2002). On a global level, WHO is working directly with countries to help create or improve vCJD surveillance systems, and to conduct risk analysis for BSE (WHO, undated).

▾ The United Kingdom

The study's information on surveillance activities in the United Kingdom was gathered from a variety of sources. These include the evidence made available by the Phillips Inquiry, government publications and web sites, and interviews with senior officials and scientists in the Department for Environment, Food and Rural Affairs (DEFRA) (formerly the Ministry of Agriculture, Fisheries and Food, MAFF), the Food Standards Agency (FSA) and the Spongiform Encephalopathy Advisory Committee

(SEAC). Until 1999, national surveillance of animal diseases in England and Wales was undertaken by the State Veterinary Service (SVS), which was part of MAFF. National surveillance of food, on the other hand, was the responsibility of a wider set of organizations including MAFF, the Department of Health, the Public Health Laboratory Service and local government.

The SVS comprised: (a) the Veterinary Field Service, which dealt with abattoir inspections among other tasks; (b) the Veterinary Investigation Service, a network of laboratories providing a regional diagnostic and surveillance service; and (c) the Central Veterinary Laboratory, which was the research base of the SVS. In 1995 the Veterinary Investigation Service merged with the Central Veterinary Laboratory to form an executive agency known as the Veterinary Laboratories Agency. The majority of veterinary surveillance in England and Wales, including surveillance for BSE, is now carried out by the Veterinary Laboratories Agency with the assistance of the Veterinary Field Service in collecting samples. The Agency produces data on diagnosis of BSE in suspect animals, ad hoc surveys of cattle (since 1999), surveillance of BSE in exotic species, and epidemiological analysis of BSE. It is also responsible for the development and validation of tests for BSE and the testing of animal feed for mammalian protein. Since the demise of MAFF in 2001, the Agency has operated under the aegis of DEFRA.

Surveillance and inspection of cattle at slaughterhouses, as opposed to on-farm surveillance, was conducted by meat inspectors working for around 300 local authorities

their information and communication practices

until 1995. Meat inspectors were responsible for ante-mortem inspection of animals entering slaughterhouses and postmortem inspection of carcasses. This also involved ensuring compliance with the specified bovine offal ban in animal and human food-chains (see Chapter 2). Responsibility for monitoring oversight of local authorities rested with MAFF's Veterinary Field Service. In 1995, a new Meat Hygiene Service was established within MAFF, which took over meat inspection duties at slaughterhouses from the local authorities. In 2000, the Meat Hygiene Service was transferred to the new FSA.

• BSE surveillance policy

Before 1999, BSE surveillance in the United Kingdom was entirely passive. Notification was dependent on farmers and their private veterinary surgeons informing the Ministry of Agriculture of suspected BSE cases. Historically, the accuracy of BSE surveillance in the United Kingdom has been hampered by a number of factors. First, it was not compulsory to notify the Government about cases of BSE until two years after the epidemic was first recognized. Following the introduction of a legal requirement for notification in 1988, compensation was set at just 50% of the market value of the animal. Farmers had no incentive to report the incidence of the disease, until 1990 when compensation was increased to 100% of the market value of the animal.

Secondly, when the BSE epidemic was first recognized, and for many years thereafter, British surveillance was hampered by inadequate record-keeping. Investigation of

the possibility that BSE might be maternally transmissible required complete and accurate identification of the offspring of BSE-affected animals. British farmers were required to tag animals and to keep documentary movement records of cattle on and off the farm for three years. However, there was no legal requirement for farmers to keep breeding records that might enable the offspring of the mother to be established. In 1990, MAFF imposed a more stringent regime of identification and record-keeping. The new legislation required farmers to keep their records for 10 years. At about the same time, the House of Commons Agricultural Select Committee recommended that the Government should establish a central computerized system for identifying and tracking animals.

MAFF officials did not, however, agree that it might ever be necessary to slaughter offspring of BSE cases, even if maternal transmission was shown to exist. The Agricultural Select Committee's recommendation for a computerized central scheme was rejected, largely on the grounds of cost.

A computerized system for identifying and tracking animals was only established in the United Kingdom in September 1998, two years after the Florence Summit of the European Council had agreed on a framework of action to permit lifting the worldwide export ban on British beef. The actions required of the United Kingdom before the ban could be lifted included the introduction of a passport system for all cattle and the establishment of a computerized cattle-tracking system.

Surveillance systems:

Prior to the availability of rapid postmortem tests in 1999, it would have been possible to estimate the numbers of subclinically infected animals close to clinical onset by conducting histopathological diagnosis or transmission experiments on a sample of animals. However, such surveys or experiments were never undertaken in the United Kingdom. Furthermore, the Government did not even use routine statistical methods to estimate numbers of subclinical infections in British cattle (or if it did, such estimates were never publicly disclosed).

When the specified bovine offal ban was introduced in 1989, the Institute for Environmental Health Officers (responsible for enforcing regulations in slaughter-houses) warned about the impracticality of implementing and enforcing the requirements of the legislation (Phillips et al., 2000, Vol. 6, paras 4.120–4.124). Over the next five or six years, however, the Veterinary Field Service failed to detect what were later found to be quite significant failures in complying with, and enforcement of, the specified offal ban. It was not until April 1995, when the Meat Hygiene Service was launched as an executive agency of MAFF, that the extent of compliance failures became apparent. A major benchmarking exercise was undertaken by the Meat Hygiene Service. This discovered that more than 40% of all plants showed some degree of non-compliance with the ban's regulations (Swann, 1998, para 14).

Active surveillance of BSE in the United Kingdom only started in 1999 when a survey was conducted in 3950 cattle brains from animals that had been slaughtered under the Over-Thirty-Month Scheme (OTMS). Under EU legislation, the United Kingdom also began a survey in January 2001 of fallen stock, testing for BSE in the brains of at least 6500 cattle over 30 months of age that had died on farms or in transit, or that had been killed on farms but were not eligible for the OTMS. The United Kingdom was also required, by the EU, to test all casualties over 24 months of age, all cattle slaughtered under the OTMS that had been born between August 1996 and July 1997, and a sample of 50 000 other OTMS cattle (MAFF, 2001). It remains the case, however, that no neuropathological or experimental survey of animals destined for the human food supply has yet taken place. In the summer of 2001, the European Commission's Food and Veterinary Office noted that since "active surveillance is practically not performed [in the United Kingdom], it has to be assumed that the BSE incidence for GB has to be seen with a considerable degree of uncertainty" (FVO, 2001).

At present, the Veterinary Laboratories Agency produces surveillance information on diagnosis of suspect cattle, ad hoc surveys and testing of animal feed, and also performs epidemiological analysis of BSE. In 2000, veterinary officials acknowledged that there were gaps in the current surveillance strategy, at least in so far as MAFF's risk management activities were concerned, and that a more effective strategy ought to involve making available information to help form an integrated view of the entire food-chain: from farm inputs, production and slaughter to processing, retail and finally to the consumer. This might include topics such as control processes on farms, the prevalence of pathogens in "high-risk" foods, contamination during

their information and communication practices

processing and transport, control processes in processing and retail, and human epidemiology. Obtaining such integrated information would require
better coordination of existing research and surveillance activities between different institutions, rather than something that the Agency itself would necessarily provide (MAFF, 2000a). Information on public attitudes and media coverage was not viewed as relevant to overall risk management.

• Dissemination of BSE surveillance data
Until the FSA was established in 2000, the communication of surveillance information on BSE was the responsibility of MAFF rather than the surveillance services themselves. As far as these services were concerned, the purpose of producing surveillance information was to inform MAFF's disease control policies and to provide information to other countries on the health status of British livestock (MAFF, 2000a).

During the first eight months following the official discovery of BSE, the policy adopted by senior MAFF officials was to restrict the dissemination of any information about BSE, even within the SVS. That policy was based primarily on an anxiety on the part of senior veterinary officials that reports of the emergence of BSE would damage cattle exports. One consequence was that the regional SVS, private veterinarians and farmers were initially unaware of the new disease, and that inevitably hindered identification and accurate reporting of possible cases of BSE. As the chair of the British Cattle Veterinary Association stated:

Throughout most of 1986 and 1987 most veterinary surgeons in practice, who were in the front line of disease diagnosis and control, were ignorant of the presence of this disease, and were not informed of its clinical signs or its significance as a potential national disease problem.

(Phillips et al., 2000, Vol. 3, para. 2.171).

After late 1987, surveillance data and other information about BSE were made available to the public domain. For the next nine years of the British BSE epidemic, however, those surveillance data were only communicated publicly in summary form, either in press releases from the Ministry of Agriculture or, after 1992, within six-monthly progress reports. Scientific papers about BSE epidemiology were also occasionally written by Ministry of Agriculture scientists for publication in the academic literature. MAFF also received numerous individual requests for surveillance information and data, and provided some (but not all) data to selected members of the scientific community and to other government departments.

A number of independent academic scientists and medical professionals have claimed that the data released by MAFF did not always contain those types of information that would have been most useful, in terms of public policy concerns (Phillips et al., 2000, Vol. 11, ch. 5). For example, it might have been useful to know how many subclinically infected animals were entering the human food-chain. A senior epidemiologist within MAFF has acknowledged, however, that there was a policy of not

Surveillance systems:

releasing figures on estimated rates of subclinical infection (Phillips et al., 2000, Vol. 11, para. 5.150). Many people were therefore unaware that many thousands of infected animals had been, and were being, consumed.

Many of the scientists and officials who requested surveillance data from MAFF have also claimed that agriculture officials were reluctant to release raw data or data in a form that enabled independent analysis of the epidemic. For example, a Department of Health official who was part of the secretariat of the Government's early advisory committees on BSE claimed that a "continual concern was over the restricted use made of the wealth of data available within the Central Veterinary Laboratory (CVL) on the animal epidemic. ... I was frustrated at the lack of analysis at CVL and the reluctance to share raw data with me or anyone else" (Pickles, 1999).

Constraints on dissemination of surveillance data had unfortunate consequences. For example, a group of epidemiologists from Oxford University had, in the late 1980s, made a series of unsuccessful attempts to gain access to raw epidemiological data from the Ministry of Agriculture. Access to the data was only granted in June 1996 and even then only after pressure had been exerted on ministers by the Chief Scientist, the Director of the Wellcome Trust and the President of the Royal Society of London. The research group in question has claimed that, had appropriate mathematical and statistical methods been employed in 1989 to analyse MAFF's BSE database (as they say they were then able to do), that analysis would have shown that there was a more serious epidemic

than officially predicted and that controls on the animal feed-chain were ineffective (Anderson, 2000). The research group has also claimed that improved advice on how best to limit the size of the epidemic could have been provided, and that, if that advice (to slaughter affected herds) had been followed at the end of 1989, approximately 330 000 animals infected with the BSE agent would have been prevented from entering the human food supply.

Surveillance of the extent to which regulations were being followed in slaughterhouses was undertaken by the Ministry of Agriculture, but the information was not publicly released. On some occasions, particularly where the information was anecdotal in nature, data on compliance were not even released to SEAC, the main scientific committee advising the British Government on BSE. That meant that it was not only consumers who were uninformed about the extent of non-compliance but also the government expert advisers — who for several years were not even told privately about the Government's concerns about shortfalls in following regulations. SEAC's advice was therefore given to ministers who did not have the benefit of vital information.

Since March 1996, and especially since the establishment of the FSA in 2000, the British Government's risk communication policy regarding surveillance data has undergone a marked shift. Veterinary surveillance data continue to be disseminated in a summary form as before, but in addition a monthly *BSE Enforcement Bulletin* and a monthly report on BSE to the Commission (a requirement under EU legislation — Decision 98/256) are made publicly

their information and communication practices

available. Publicly available information now includes: details of suspected and confirmed BSE cases; information on the progress of the BSE epidemic; information from surveys of fallen stock and OTMS cattle; the results of audits of the specified risk material controls and the feed sampling programme; details of cattle passports issued and movements recorded; details of the selective cull; details of the offspring cull; and details of inspection of plants exporting bovine products and of exported meat. It also includes details of enforcement action and prosecutions.[1]

The Ministry of Agriculture has also now allowed at least some members of the broader scientific community access to raw surveillance data. Nevertheless, several respondents to a consultation on veterinary surveillance, published in 2000, argued that MAFF's (now DEFRA's) surveillance system should provide epidemiological data in a form that allowed a proactive approach to risk assessment to be taken by interested parties. This would include, for example, the dissemination of data on the animal population surveyed and on the methodological techniques used (MAFF, 2000b).

An internal review of veterinary surveillance, conducted by MAFF in 2000, concluded that greater efforts needed to be made to generate awareness of the Ministry's surveillance programme and for overall risk appraisal and management

activities to include the dissemination of surveillance information (MAFF, 2000a: 36). The review reported that veterinary officials believed surveillance information to be of value to external stakeholder groups such as primary producers, veterinarians and consumer groups — not least in order to demonstrate the value of surveillance, given the substantial costs of producing the information. The review noted that it was not clear if and how surveillance information was actually used by external stakeholders.

Since the FSA was established in 2000, it has demonstrated a greater willingness than MAFF to release potentially sensitive surveillance information. On such issues as surveillance of regulatory compliance, enforcement and fraud, the FSA has taken a relatively open approach. For example, it has publicly commented on breaches in BSE controls on both domestically produced beef and imported beef, naming the firms and abattoirs involved. The FSA's web site also provides detailed information on seizures of specified risk material in imported meat, listing the date of discovery, the location from which the meat was imported and the number of beef quarters found to contain specified risk material.[2]

The FSA does not possess a communication strategy in terms of formal guidelines, but it does have overall goals, for example to be as open as possible (FSA, 2000c). FSA officials interviewed in this study were of the view that being open with information was important to engender trust. The point was made, however, that trust was required both from the people to whom information is disseminated and in the people who provide information.

---

[1] See, for example, the information provided on the DEFRA web site at http://www.defra.gov.uk/animalh/bse/index. html.
[2] See "BSE Controls Review" at http://www.food.gov.uk/bse/what/about.

For example, it was important to reassure the industry that the FSA was not going to release "everything" to the media in an irresponsible way.

• Surveillance of public attitudes

During the late 1980s and early 1990s, risk communication by MAFF was essentially a one-way activity (Breakwell & Purkhardt, 1993). There were virtually no communication channels or mechanisms by which to monitor public opinions and attitudes to BSE.

In the late 1980s, following crises concerning the microbiological safety of foods, MAFF had established a Risk Assessment and Risk Management Strategy Branch in its Food Science Division, which was responsible for some work on risk communication. As one official involved commented, however:

> In this initial period [1988–1991] the main work was concerned with developing the thinking on priority setting, the role of consumer perceptions in policy development, and in considering risk communication issues, particularly in relation to food scares. The importance of effective communication was already recognized, though at that time the concern was mainly about formulating messages effectively for outside consumption and the importance of taking outside views into account in policy-making was not yet fully understood.
>
> (Fisher, undated).

An unpublished audit of MAFF's risk communication strategy, conducted by independent academic consultants in 1993, reported that there was a significant degree of ignorance within MAFF about what the British public understood about foodborne risks and how it reacted to a range of signals. It also said that there was no effective mechanism by which the public's concerns, misunderstandings or interests could have entered into the policy-making process. The audit reported that understanding the public's risk evaluations was widely viewed, amongst a sample of MAFF officials, as an essential part of risk management (although not risk assessment) but that the problem lay in knowing how to monitor such evaluations. In the absence of two-way communication channels and mechanisms by which to monitor public opinions and attitudes to food risks, officials used the interpretation of media coverage as the major means for monitoring public reactions to MAFF activities and statements. Interestingly, those officials also viewed the media as misrepresenting MAFF to the public. It is thus not clear why officials consequently expected the media to reflect public opinion accurately.

Following that audit, a "tool kit" was designed in collaboration with the University of East Anglia for assessing the views of consumers on different types of food risk. The tool kit was based on the assumption that risk communication should be two-way and that public participation should be included at all stages of the risk management process, not just at the risk prioritization stage. It recommended the development of a software program that could be used by members of the public to record the

their information and communication practices

values they placed on the risks and benefits of different food-related hazards. Although the software program was commissioned and tested within several focus groups and with professionals in the food safety field, participants felt that the program was too time consuming. MAFF therefore decided to drop the idea on the grounds that it was an impractical tool. Further expenditure to make the tool kit more user-friendly was not considered to be cost-effective. No detailed basis for that decision was, however, provided (MAFF, 1999).

In the wake of the acute BSE crisis of March 1996, and other high-profile issues such as the management of agricultural biotechnology commercialization, the British Government has been reviewing its approach to risk appraisal. As far as risk communication is concerned, DEFRA and other government departments recognize that it should be interactive and facilitate participation. For example, the Government's response to the Phillips Inquiry, which was written by DEFRA, stated that: "Good risk communication is a two-way process, starting with consultation and continuing throughout the risk analysis" (DEFRA, 2001).

Despite these policy ambitions, DEFRA's Animal Health Group still views risk communication as being predominantly a one-way exercise (interview, DEFRA official). There are still no mechanisms either to involve the public in policy processes, beyond routine consultation exercises, or to monitor the attitudes and beliefs of the public about BSE. A DEFRA official noted that, in the past, MAFF's Communication Department had occasionally

conducted public surveys in which a question was asked about "trust in MAFF". Officials in the BSE division take the view that in general they do not need to know about public attitudes in order to form policy, and that with BSE in decline, the need to know is past (interview, DEFRA official).

MAFF did (and DEFRA continues to) monitor the media, but only by using a cuttings service. There is also some proactive work with the media through meeting journalists and developing relationships with the key correspondents. Thus, in 2001, agricultural policy officials continued to assume that media coverage provided a reasonable proxy representation of what the public think (interview, DEFRA official).

In the process of formulating policy, DEFRA officials did not (and do not) actively take media coverage — or indeed public beliefs and attitudes — into account when setting policy goals or deciding what kinds of risks are acceptable. Officials asserted that the issues were too subtle and complex. They also felt that the general public would always take the most risk-averse approach since they were not themselves responsible for bearing the cost-regulatory measures (interview, DEFRA official).

The assumption that media coverage provides an adequate proxy for public attitudes is problematic. An example can be found in the comments of one official, who asserted that public reaction to a policy decision in 1997 to ban "beef on the bone" indicated the policy as being actually more precautionary than the public wanted (interview,

Surveillance systems:

DEFRA official). The official did not differentiate between the media reaction to the ban (which was highly sceptical) and public perceptions. In this particular case, it is impossible to know whether media coverage reflected or coincided with more general public concerns.

Although MAFF/DEFRA policy-makers may not have shifted their risk communication strategy since March 1996, the approach adopted by the FSA is substantially different. When the FSA was first established, it outlined three core values that would guide its work: to put the consumer first, to be open and accessible, and to be an independent voice. That ambition was no doubt a reaction to what was perceived to be one of the principal faults in the approach to policy-making taken by MAFF. On the issue of risk communication the FSA has stated that:

> We will be open in all our decision making ... We will also listen carefully to what people tell us. Except in an emergency, we will discuss the risks and the options for handling them with those who may be affected, and we will be open about doing this. We value the input that we can get from everyone who may be affected by our decisions — such as the public, consumer representatives, enforcement authorities and industry.
>
> (FSA, 2000a).

By comparison, DEFRA does not have a similar formal commitment to deliberative forms of communication (apart from adhering to the British Government's re-

sponse to the BSE Inquiry, as all British Government departments are expected to do). One DEFRA official has characterized the department's approach to risk communication as "information in and communication out" (interview, DEFRA official). However, since the FSA was established, DEFRA officials have taken the view that responsibility for the communication of food risks belongs to the FSA. In practice, it is indeed the FSA that takes the lead in risk communication on all food safety issues.

The FSA has been conducting at least some monitoring of the attitudes and beliefs of the public about BSE. There has been one externally commissioned survey on public attitudes to food safety in general. Apart from such general surveys, the FSA publishes information and consults on risk assessments and the proposed range of policy responses to those assessments. One FSA official has claimed that feedback from those risk assessment consultations provides relevant information to policy-makers (interview, FSA official).

An FSA review of BSE controls on the food-chain, conducted in 2000, was the first example of a wider consultation process within the FSA on food safety policy-making. A series of meetings was held before and during the review process with stakeholders, including representatives of the British Health and Agriculture Departments, consumer organizations and industry experts. Initial meetings were concerned with the framing of the review process, including the types of questions and issues to be addressed. An interactive FSA web

their information and communication practices

site was also established, and both official and public comments were listed on the site. The review raised a number of sensitive issues that were made public despite concerns expressed by the industry. For example, the review was explicit about the fact that no one knew whether BSE was present in the national sheep flock, and that if that were indeed the case, the current offal controls on sheep would not be sufficient to protect public health (FSA, 2000b).

One senior member of the FSA has claimed that, among other benefits of the BSE review, stakeholders from other government departments had to make and perhaps defend their arguments in public (interview, FSA official). Another benefit was that reaction to the report was gathered in the course of the various drafts, i.e. during the review process. This had the effect of rendering less controversial certain pieces of information, such as the public acknowledgement that, if BSE were found to be present in sheep, existing controls would not be sufficient to deal with the situation. Finally, in response to input from broader stakeholders, the review process managed to reframe some of the issues in a constructive way. For example, such input led to the inclusion of a section on imports, and the final review dealt with the issue of risks from "private kills" (animals slaughtered by the farmer, ostensibly for private consumption), which had previously been overlooked by the FSA.

FSA officials did not view public perceptions and media coverage of BSE as problematic for policy-making, except in so far as the public was not generally aware of the legal constraints on policy-makers, such as the rules governing the operation of the single European market (interview, FSA official). Nor did they feel that the public necessarily had all the information required to make informed judgements about policy. Despite the greater degree of openness on the part of the FSA, the officials interviewed were not very clear about how the results of monitoring and surveillance of public attitudes and media coverage could be, or had been, incorporated into policy decision-making. One suggested that the FSA was aware of public concern about imported meat and that, for example, when making risk management judgements, interaction within policy processes with the families of people who had suffered from vCJD provided an important reminder of the severity of the possible risks that need to be weighed up against the costs of any restrictions (interview, FSA official). In this case, therefore, it is not the formal input of the public through a specific mechanism that the official believes is helping to influence risk management decisions, but rather the mere presence in the policy process (for example, at public meetings) of those who have to bear the risks.

One member of the principal expert advisory committee, SEAC, argued that information on public attitudes would be "extremely relevant" to that committee's deliberations (interview, SEAC member). He conceded that he did not know about public perceptions of BSE and stated that such information would not make a significant difference to SEAC's recommendations, although it might influence the ways in which risks were represented in SEAC's public statements, interviews and press releases. More

Surveillance systems:

generally, the SEAC advisers thought that information on public perceptions should affect the way governments deal with risks.

▾ Germany

Germany played an important role inside the European Community after BSE emerged in the British cattle herd. Germany was the first Member State to insist that the previously unknown cattle disease might constitute a risk to public health. In 1989, Germany placed unilateral restrictions on imports of British beef, a measure that led to the first EU-wide precautionary controls. Several years later, in 1994, Germany was once again insisting on further Community measures to protect public health (Dressel, 1999, 2002).

Despite these concerns and actions, German policy-makers were confident that the risks from BSE were confined to British cattle and beef, and that there was no domestic problem with the disease. German surveillance efforts were, as a consequence, very weak prior to the introduction of European legislation on BSE surveillance. The small German TSE research community, however, took a more sophisticated view than public policy- makers. While these researchers supported the policy of excluding the BSE agent from Germany, they also took the view that the potential risk of BSE in the German cattle herd — although probably low — should not be neglected by policy-makers. There is also evidence that the two German fede-ral ministries involved in the regulation of BSE did not always share the same ideas about the most appropriate policy on BSE and the protection of public health.

At the time the research for this book began, German policy-makers still believed that the country was free of BSE. That assumption was based on the fact that, apart from six BSE cases, all of which had occurred in cattle imported from Switzerland or the United Kingdom, there had been no cases detected in the domestic herd. During the course of the study team's research, the situation changed dramatically: the first domestic German BSE case was reported, followed by many more cases once the country's surveillance methodology was changed from passive to active. Furthermore, public pressure triggered by the detection of the German BSE cases resulted in the restructuring of surveillance systems (e.g. the foundation of a new ministry in Bavaria and a complete reorientation inside the former Federal Ministry of Agriculture towards an emphasis on consumer protec-tion). Subsequent interviews reflected changes in atti-tudes about the relevance of public perception issues (the interviews were also harder to obtain).

• BSE surveillance policy

BSE surveillance is currently undertaken largely at state level by the regional State Veterinary Laboratories. There is also a single federal public sector research institution, the Federal Research Department for Animal Virus Diseases (BfAV, now located on the Island of Riems), which is the country's reference centre for BSE.

BSE surveillance is carried out under two separate pro-grammes, which spring from two different legislative Acts: (a) the Animal Disease Act (*Tierseuchenrecht*), in force since 1999, and (b) the Meat Hygiene Act and Food

their information and communication practices

Act (*Fleischhygienerecht und Lebensmittelrecht*), in force since December 2000. Under the first of these Acts, monitoring is carried out on a specified range of animals (fallen stock, emergency-slaughtered animals or animals displaying BSE-like symptoms), in accordance with EU requirements. The second Act, originally supervised by the Department of Health, makes testing obligatory for every bovine animal older than 24 months (30 months according to EU legislation, with the higher standard coming into force in Germany on 25 January 2001). The two Acts were originally supervised by different bodies (the Ministry of Agriculture and the Ministry of Health, respectively) but are now under the single responsibility of the Federal Ministry of Consumer Protection, Food and Agriculture. The Federal Ministry of Health retains responsibility for animal health vaccines.

In principle, procedures for dealing with suspected cases of BSE are the same whether the case comes under one programme or the other. An animal suspected of having BSE as defined in the Animal Disease Act should be reported by the farmer or a vet to the district veterinary officer. The veterinary officer should then initiate histolo-pathological and/or immunohistochemical examinations and is also responsible for initial etiological and epi-demiological investigations. If suspicions of BSE persist, the district veterinary officer should contact the state's veterinary examination office, which would carry out further tests. If that office could not exclude the possibi-lity of BSE infection, the sample would be forwarded to the national reference centre for animal diseases, the BfAV, which is responsible for the final analysis (as requi-red by the Office International des Épizooties) and certifi-cation of the animal. The BfAV reports all cases of BSE to the respective state ministry and to the Ministry of Food, Agriculture, and Forestry (BML).[3]

Under the Meat Hygiene Act and Food Act, every slaugh-tered bovine animal older than 24 months is subjected to a rapid postmortem test (*fleischhygiene-rechtliche Untersuchung*) in a state or private laboratory. The labora-tories receive material to be tested straight from the slaughterhouses, which are required to await the final results before they are allowed to process the slaugh-tered carcass. If laboratories at the district level find inconclusive or positive samples, the procedure is the same as described above.

• A historical perspective
BSE surveillance policy started in 1990 when BSE was made a notifiable disease inside the EU. In the same year, BSE was added to the German list of infectious diseases that were notifiable (i.e. compulsory reporting) under the German Animal Disease Act (*Tierseuchengesetz*). Surveillance activity increased in 1992 after the first case of BSE was found in an imported

---

[3] European Commission decision 2000/374 required Member States "to list the national reference laboratories for TSEs". In March 1999, Germany had already announced that the BfAV would be the national reference laboratory for BSE. Since the introduction of the Meat Hygiene Act and Food Act, the BfAV is contacted only as the final authority, e.g. if a definitive diagnosis cannot be achieved at the state level or if the sample tests positive in the state-level laboratory.

Surveillance systems:

animal from the United Kingdom. The same event led to an emergency session in the BML, which concluded that the Federal Research Institute for Animal Virus Diseases should set up a BSE surveillance unit to act as the national reference centre. This was done.[4] Nonetheless, until Germany implemented a nationwide monitoring programme for BSE in 1999, as directed by European Commission Decision 98/272/EC, surveillance was voluntary, unsystematic, and poorly funded and staffed. In addition, the *Länder* had responsibility for BSE monitoring. Between 1991 and 1999, only about 1500 brains of neurologically suspect cattle were examined in all of Germany for BSE (interview, scientist).[5]

Surveillance activities prior to 1999 focused primarily on the monitoring and control of the import of, and trade in, live cattle and bovine meat products. The aim was to prevent the BSE agent from crossing German borders. A more active domestic surveillance programme was per-

ceived by German policy-makers as unnecessary. Germany was believed to be — and represented as — a country free of BSE, especially by the agriculture ministry. In the words of a German scientist: "The result was, of course (...) not enough was done on the issue (...). It [the BSE surveillance] was not a priority".

Even in 1999, the federal Ministry of Agriculture only required the *Länder* to test cattle on a voluntary basis, in order to meet the new EU requirements. The *Länder* were generally reluctant to establish their own surveillance programmes (with the exception of North Rhine-Westphalia, see below). In their view, the EU decision was unnecessary and too expensive in a country assumed not to have BSE in its domestic herd. In 1999, a proposed trial of the new rapid postmortem tests in North Rhine-Westphalia was opposed by the federal agriculture ministry and by several other *Länder*. The Bavarian Health Ministry, for example, labelled the tests "a waste of money in a country with no BSE". According to one official, the possibility was also raised that systematic surveillance might threaten Germany's BSE-free status.

Germany's assumption that it was free of BSE was challenged in June 2000 when the European Commission released a geographical risk assessment that concluded, "it is likely that domestic cattle are (clinically or preclinically) infected with the BSE agent but it is not confirmed" (European Commission, 2000a: 30). The EU's assessment was based on the assumption that "the current surveillance system is passive and therefore not able to detect all clinical BSE cases". In November 2000, the first

---

[4] Until the BSE surveillance unit was fully established at the BfAV, another German institute, the State Veterinary Laboratory of North Bavaria (*Landesuntersuchungsamt Nord*) acted as a kind of unofficial national reference. The laboratory had already begun BSE testing, having sent a pathologist to Weybridge, United Kingdom, to learn the necessary methodology.

[5] It was suggested in the interview with a German scientist that it might well be the case that more tests were carried out, but that numbers were not officially provided by the state governments to the Federal Government. It is hence not surprising that other numbers are circulating. For example, according to a letter of a civil servant of the responsible federal ministry (BML) to a citizen asking for those numbers in 2001, a total of 3725 out of 18 994 cattle with neurodegenerative behaviour were examined for BSE between 1991 and 1999.

their information and communication practices

unambiguously German case of BSE was detected in Schleswig-Holstein using a rapid postmortem test, at that time a voluntary measure. Following the introduction of the active surveillance programme (under EU rules) many more cases of BSE in the domestic herd were discovered (189 cases by August 2002, about half of which were reported in Bavaria). Not surprisingly, this led to a major crisis in consumer confidence.

• A tale of two *Länder*

As has been discussed in Chapter 2, Germany consists of 16 states (*Länder*). Legislation on surveillance of BSE and CJD is made by the Federal Government, usually in response to EU legislation, but the *Länder* are responsible for implementation of that legislation. The different political cultures of the German states and current policies result in quite distinct surveillance programmes, at least for BSE. CJD surveillance is somewhat different, in that it is more centrally organized at the federal level.

Nineteen interviews were conducted during the course of this study's research with both senior and mid-level civil servants responsible for the surveillance of BSE and CJD, and with federal and state politicians responsible for public risk policy. Journal articles, leaflets, web sites and media reports were also scrutinized. As it was impossible to examine all 16 *Länder* in detail, two very different ones were chosen: North Rhine-Westphalia and Bavaria.

Bavaria is traditionally a Conservative-led state. In contrast, North Rhine-Westphalia is historically a stronghold of the Social Democrats and is currently led by a cabinet of Social Democrats and members of the Green Party. The agriculture minister and the health minister in Bavaria belong to the Conservative party, whereas the minister responsible for BSE in North Rhine-Westphalia is a member of the Green Party. The two have occasionally clashed, most notably over the North Rhine-Westphalia minister's decision in 1999 to use the then newly available Swiss "Prionics" test on more than 5000 cattle — a decision that was heavily criticized by the Bavarian ministry as a "waste of money".

About one third of the German cattle herd is located in Bavaria, whereas only about one sixth is located in North Rhine-Westphalia. The opposite is true for the human population: North Rhine-Westphalia has the highest density population of the German states, whereas Bavaria is of about medium density. Unlike Bavaria, North Rhine-Westphalia has traditionally had a strong history of consumer protection.

With hindsight, the contrast between the surveillance efforts in the two *Länder* are striking. Whilst North Rhine-Westphalia had voluntarily performed a trial of the rapid diagnostic tests, Bavaria argued that there was no need to take such a measure, particularly since the test applied had not yet been fully validated by the EU. Although Bavaria was the first German state to begin BSE surveillance in 1992 (and thus carried out most of the German BSE tests until 1999) it became obvious in 2000 that surveillance and control of BSE in the Bavarian cattle herd were deeply problematic. For example, in one of the two Bavarian state veterinary laboratories, over 80% of brains from German cattle were assessed as "unsuitable" for BSE testing, whilst all brains originating from animals born in countries with indigenous BSE were tested (European Commission, 2001). According to one interviewee, the Bavarian State Veterinary Service was "afraid" of writing BSE on the form when asked for the examination of neurologically suspicious or moribund cattle. As one Bavarian senior civil servant put it (interview):

> We were absolutely convinced that we have had no BSE. We thought of BSE as a danger, but — mark you — not for us ... But we hadn't taken into account that it might have already arrived here latently by winding paths.
> That didn't occur to us.

Consequently, BSE surveillance was not a top priority in the responsible ministry; moreover, the monitoring programme was seriously understaffed (European Commission, 2001). As a result, Bavaria, with one third of the German cattle population, was faced with rising numbers of BSE cases.

The situation was substantially different in North Rhine-Westphalia. Unlike in Bavaria, BSE had already become an issue of public attention and increased policy awareness in 1994–1995. Whereas only two veterinarians were responsible for all Bavarian BSE surveillance, six were involved by the responsible North Rhine-Westphalia ministry (Ministry for the Environment, Environmental Planning, and Agriculture, MURL) despite a relatively smaller cattle population. Although the actual number of cattle brains examined prior to 1998 was low (in total less than 100 tested cattle brains per annum in those years, according to the annual reports of the State Veterinary Service) BSE monitoring reflected a very different set of priorities, as this testimony suggests:

> Regarding examination, it was clear that no additional jobs were allowed. But it is of course always a question of judgement and assessment of a problem we had to deal with ... On the one hand, I could say, 'I don't have the staff, therefore, I am not able to do something'. That is one position. The other position is, if I don't have enough staff, I need to reassess the situation ... And I could say, 'You don't have time for examination of cattle brain for BSE pathology, but you have the time to examine the excrements of saddle-horses'.
> ... Well, we were never quite sure whether we got it right ... But we said, we need to have new priorities.
> (interview, North Rhine-Westphalia official).

The new priority in this case was testing and monitoring for BSE. This was given extra impetus by the events of November 1998, when the EU Agricultural Council decided to relax the export ban on British beef, and also by the fact that the Prionics company had just developed a BSE test system. The North Rhine-Westphalia agriculture minister, Bärbel Höhn of the

their information and communication practices

Green Party, took the initiative and informed the public that she was determined to apply the Prionics test to 5000 slaughtered cattle:

> The goal is to achieve inside of the European Member States a maximum of consumer protection ... The Swiss test system was approved by scientific accompanying research ... Without such a test, I think the impending loosening of the export ban of British beef is irresponsible.
>
> (MURL, 1998).

This announcement received a negative response from the federal agriculture ministry and several German states, including the Bavarian Health Ministry (interviews, various politicians and civil servants). For example, the initiative was heavily criticized by other German states and by the BML, which had shown no interest in the question of whether such a quick detection test was applicable in daily practice (interview, North Rhine-Westphalia scientist). Nevertheless, between March and June 1999, North Rhine-Westphalia conducted a Prionics test series on 5029 cattle brains, examining them for BSE (MURL, 1999). The testing included 21 different breeds of cattle from various parts of Germany and other European countries. It also took into account age distribution, ranging from cattle under two years to cattle over four years of age. With that initiative, North Rhine-Westphalia made itself Europe's front-runner on BSE surveillance, for in no other EU

Member State were precautionary BSE assays carried out at that time.

No BSE was detected during the experiment. Although the scientists involved in the tests gave many public talks about it, the relevance of the experiment was still not obvious to everybody. For instance, when it was suggested that a paper about the trial should be given at the annual conference of the German Veterinary Association (*Deutsche Veterinärmedizinische Gesellschaft*, a German-language conference involving Austria, Germany and Switzerland), the request was rejected on grounds of the paper's "lack of practical applicability" (interview, North Rhine-Westphalia scientist).

In the course of the events at the end of 2000, the North Rhine-Westphalia trials received enormous attention. What had formerly been described as a waste of taxpayers' money now emerged as a brilliant model for Germany and the EU, showing that BSE testing was possible on a large scale and was applicable to the routine functioning of abattoirs. After the first German BSE cases were detected, the federal and state governments were then quite happy to bask in the glow of North Rhine- Westphalia 's experience. At the time of writing, only two cases of BSE have been detected in North Rhine-Westphalia.

A draft report of a German veterinary mission by EU inspectors, performed in October 2000, focused on the two states (European Commission, 2001). It indicated substantial differences in the monitoring systems between those two *Länder*. The publication of the report contributed to the resignation of the Bavarian Minister of Health.

• CJD surveillance policy

CJD surveillance is more centrally organized than BSE sur-veillance in Germany. Or as one interviewee described the actual situation, "State sovereignty, which played a role in the BSE case, did not play any role for CJD" (interview, German CJD scientist). CJD surveillance formally started in 1994, when CJD became a notifiable disease under the Federal Law of Diseases (*Bundesseuchengesetz*, or *BseuchG*). Under that act, doctors must report any suspec-ted case of CJD to the local public health department, which would then report the case to the state authority. The latter would then report the case both to the Robert Koch Institute (RKI), a public sector research institute reporting to the Federal Ministry of Health, which is the main German institution for infectious diseases, and to the respective state health ministry.

After a judicial modification in January 2001, the Federal Law of Diseases was replaced by a newly implemented Act for Infection Prevention (*Infektionsschutzgesetz*, or *IfSG*), although the RKI is still the institution in charge of formal CJD surveillance. Under the new Act, the RKI is obliged to investigate each CJD case systematically and continuously, and to report regularly (currently, twice a year) on actual numbers of CJD cases in order to make any changes in numbers transparent.

This statutory CJD monitoring system is supplemented by a sophisticated epidemiological research programme undertaken by the Surveillance Centre for CJD (*Surveillance Zentrum für die CJK*, or SZG) at the University of Göttingen and Munich, with funding from the Federal Department of Health (it is also part of the EU's above-mentioned activities on CJD surveillance). Established in 1993, in the wake of the BSE events in the United Kingdom, the centre's research team consists of epidemiologists, neurologists and neuropathologists whose activities include not only epidemiology but also clinical diagnosis, genetics and pathology. Every three months, the team sends a letter to each neurological and psychiatric hospital in Germany (about 1300 in total) both to update them and to increase awareness of the disease — and thus to increase the number of notifications. The team also supplies differential diagnoses to show which other diseases might similarly appear as CJD. Finally, the team will visit any patient in Germany about whom they are notified.[6]

• Dissemination of BSE surveillance data

Both federal and state-level German government depart-ments are responsible for communication of surveillance information on BSE. The research institution responsible

---

[6] Though the RKI is the official national reference centre, the SZG is the de facto CJD reference centre. This was rec-ognized by all interviewees in the various ministries as well as those in the RKI itself, who acknowledged that the SZG team is notified more frequently about cases than the RKI. With the implementation of the Act for Infectious Diseases, increased cooperation between the RKI and SZG was agreed upon by both institutions.

their information and communication practices

for surveillance, the BfAV, has neither the resources nor the authority to engage in communication activities aimed at the public. For example, requests by the media to the BfAV are forwarded to the Ministry of Agriculture.

Since BSE surveillance was not a top priority in Germany until very recently, relatively few surveillance data were available, and even less of this information was distributed. In practice only small amounts of information were made available to the public or to interested researchers or other professionals. When surveillance data were required for the EU's geographical BSE risk assessment, the BML did not have the human resources to contact every single state and investigate available data. That would have been, in any case, a difficult task as every state had until then collected its own sets of data that were sometimes not comparable.

During most of the 1990s, BSE was a topic of public discussion, but only in so far as other countries were affected. Information was given by the BML to farmers and practitioners "upon request" but, as an EU inspection discovered in 1996, "no information was available on specific training programmes for veterinary practitioners, vets in slaughterhouses, etc." (European Commission, 1996). The fact that several animal pathologists were nevertheless trained in BSE diagnosis was due to their own initiative in arranging in-service training rather than to actions of the state or federal governments.

After the discovery of BSE in the domestic herd in 2000, however, the new Ministry of Consumer Protection, Food

and Agriculture appeared to adopt a new communication strategy. Publicly available information was markedly more straightforward and critical than previously.

Again, Bavaria and North Rhine-Westphalia differed significantly as far as the dissemination of surveillance data was concerned. The official "line" that there was no BSE in Bavaria meant that there was no interest in the topic — apart from worrying news from abroad — among professionals, journalists or the general public. A Bavarian senior civil servant put it as follows in an interview:

> It is strange, but I'd like to stress that the interest regarding BSE was always like a wave: If there wasn't Cindy or Maise [the names of imported cattle which developed BSE in Germany in 1997] or whatever, no one was interested. Well, maybe not no one, but certainly not the media.

This situation changed dramatically in the latter part of 2000. When the BSE crisis occurred, officials at the local, district, regional and ministerial level were unprepared and unable to respond. The situation was unexpected and made a mockery of an implicit communication strategy that was based on the assumption that Bavaria, with its putative high standards and control, was not at risk from BSE. There is now considerably more public information available on the Internet, in particular from a self-styled consumer protection information system (*Verbraucherschutzinformationssystem*) introduced in November 2001

Surveillance systems:

(see http://www.stmgev.bayern.de or http://www.vis. bayern.de).

North Rhine-Westphalia has followed a completely different communication strategy, at least since 1995 when the new minister was appointed. In this strategy, BSE was never described as a purely external problem, and it was always stressed that scientific knowledge was still inconclusive and that BSE might well constitute a risk for humans. For example, when the testing of over 5000 slaughtered cattle was carried out in late 1998 without identifying any cases of BSE, the official "line" was not that the state had no BSE but that it was at least possible to state that the incidence of BSE was lower than 1 in 5000 (interview, North Rhine-Westphalia politician).

The MURL undertook a series of campaigns to provide information, including surveillance data, to all those interested in BSE. In particular, a proactive information campaign targeted consumer protection associations, the regional farming associations, associations for organic farming and intensive farming, nature conservation movements, and any other group within the Ministry's mandate (interview, North Rhine-Westphalia politician). Intensive cooperation was pursued between the Ministry and diverse consumer protection organizations.[7]

Another component of the information campaign was the Ministry's web site (see http://www.murl.nrw.de). In contrast to the approach of the federal and Bavarian governments, the web site produced relatively sophisticated information about BSE for the public domain, embracing not only typical consumer questions but also information about the history of the BSE crisis, scientific evidence about the disease, political responses, and a selection of press cuttings (not only in relation to the ministry). The BSE portion of the web site starts with a statement by the Minister about the current and past BSE situation, both in Germany and in North Rhine-Westphalia. According to an interviewee in the Ministry, the BSE web pages logged 6000 daily requests from citizens at peak times. The Ministry also placed advertisements regarding BSE and its risks in newspapers.

The Ministry also employed professional agencies to canvass public opinion on topics like BSE and, if specific individual questions were asked, to refer the questioners to consumer protection associations or related nongovernmental organizations. A substantial part of the agencies' work is to provide feedback to the Ministry about the consumer concerns they find (interview, North Rhine-Westphalia politician).

• Surveillance of public attitudes
German officials dealing with BSE policy at the federal level and in Bavaria did not commission any survey of public attitudes, nor did they see a need for such information. However, two surveys conducted on related issues prior to the German BSE crisis included some questions on the public perception of BSE risk, although

---

[7] Note that in spring 2000, prior to the German BSE crisis, the MURL was re-named the Ministry for Consumer Protection, an aspect that had always been an inherent part of its mandate.

their information and communication practices

they did not focus on it as a matter of its own (Noelle-Neumann & Köcher, 1997). For example, the Allensbach Institute asked in March 1995 whether people considered British beef to be dangerous or whether the danger was exaggerated. The results indicated that 51% of the German population thought of it as a "great danger". Also high were numbers in another poll by Allensbach in November 1995, which asked "what are the most urgent problems to solve for policy-makers in Europe?". Some 63% of respondents stated that BSE was one of the top priorities for policy-makers to tackle (Noelle-Neumann & Köcher, 1997: 369 and 1156). But, as there was no awareness of these surveys in any of the interviewees in the present study, it is very unlikely that they have had any influence on actual policy-making.

As mentioned above, North Rhine-Westphalia has for some years canvassed the public on topics like BSE or genetically modified organisms. However, the principal aim of these efforts has not been to gather public attitudes but to "enlighten" the public about current food risks and to present alternatives, e.g. options for consumers to switch to organic products and organic farming in general. The intense information campaign includes an easily accessible (in terms of language and layout) Internet web site and extensive use of leaflets distributed in areas such as public departments, schools and offices of consumer organizations.

▼ Italy

The following section attempts to reconstruct the adaptation of the Italian surveillance system to BSE risk since 1980. The study team's research included interviews with 17 key persons and analysis of 56 provisions (laws and government decrees, Ministry of Health circulars, directives and orders) that represent the main policy initiatives taken at national level.

The BSE problem arose at a time when relations between the Italian state and the regions were getting more tense and during which the role of the state (in the case of BSE, the Ministry of Health) had weakened. The process of redefining the division of powers and tasks between the state and the regions is still under way, and has influenced both the reactions of the surveillance system to the BSE problem and the ways in which information passes through and leaves that system.

Although not federal in the strict sense, the Italian political system gives the regions a high level of autonomy in many areas, including health, for which they may pass laws, plan spending, and organize and manage the health structures. The Italian state, through the Ministry of Health, has retained the powers and duties required for the guidance and coordination of the regions in all matters regarding health. Likewise, the Ministry of Agriculture is in charge of the animal and agricultural production sectors, except for those involving animal health, the state of hygiene of stock farms, animal food, etc., which come under the control of the health authorities.

The Ministry of Health, with its Department for Food, Nutrition and Public Veterinary Health and the Health Protection Department, is at the top level of the surveil-

Surveillance systems:

lance system. The veterinary services at ports, borders and airports are also part of that Ministry as well as the Superior Institute of Health (SIH), a technical and scientific institution with a remit for research, training and consultancy in the field of human and veterinary health and food hygiene.

Throughout Italy there are 10 experimental animal health institutes (EAHIs), laboratories that diagnose and treat infectious diseases in animals. These institutes are defined by law as technical–scientific instruments of the state and of the regions, and are supposed to work in close collaboration with the veterinary offices of the local health agencies.

Each of the 19 regional governments has a Regional Minister for Health and a Regional Health Office that, in the same way as the Ministry of Health at national level, is the technical organ responsible for all health policy. While the organization and actual name of the regional offices may vary significantly, all the regions have a regional veterinary service which, on the basis of health ministry guidelines, decides on the timing and type of controls that the local health authority veterinary surgeons must carry out, and establishes the minimum number of samples and examinations as well as the frequency and type of reports to be sent to the region. Each region has a public health department that, on the basis of health ministry guidelines, decides on controls that the local health authority Public Hygiene Service must carry out.

Each region is divided into districts, each with local

health authorities of varying size. Each local health authority has a local veterinary service employing a variable number of veterinary officers. The veterinary officers basically carry out administrative work, draw up monitoring plans, and conduct examinations that evaluate the presence or otherwise of disease in each stock farm. Treatment of the animals is left to vets in the private sector. All the local health authorities also run a public hygiene service responsible for the surveillance of health conditions in public places (restaurants, canteens, cafeterias in schools, hospitals, shelters, etc.).

At the most grassroots level, the mayor is the local health authority. The mayor is responsible for informing the regional health authorities about the ongoing situation regarding infectious diseases in animals and humans, and for implementing health measures, from surveillance measures to closure of any public or private place if there is a health risk.

• BSE surveillance policy

The Italian surveillance system first took note of the BSE problem in 1989 when the Ministry of Health banned imports from the United Kingdom of live animals born before 18 July 1988, in accordance with the relevant European Commission decision issued a few weeks earlier. In 1991, again following a European Commission decision, scrapie and BSE were added to the list of animal diseases that must be compulsorily notified. Within the surveillance system, the first operational agency for BSE was established. Two of the 10 experimental animal health institutes — one in Turin (Piedmont) and the

their information and communication practices

other in Teramo (Molise) — were designated national centres of reference and entrusted with special functions regarding the epidemiological surveillance of TSEs.

In 1993 there was a further institutional change within the surveillance system. The Government established a "Permanent Commission on the Emergency to coordinate the measures adopted by the regions to control all infectious diseases in animals". Members came from the regions, the Ministry of Health and the Ministry of Agriculture. This Commission highlighted a problem that was destined to get worse over the years: that of the relationship between the central administration of the state and the regions.

In October 1994, two cases of BSE were discovered in Sicily. The local surveillance system raised the alarm and the SIH was brought in. However, even though it was known that the two infected cows were part of a group of 25 animals imported from the United Kingdom in 1989, no further attempts were made to trace them all. The year 1994 also saw the first Italian provisions banning the use of proteins in feed from mammals, in accordance with measures taken by the European Commission, along with increased controls on imported meat from the United Kingdom. BSE remained "a British problem" and was of little interest to the media until 2001, when the first cases of BSE originating in Italy emerged.

In 1996, following the announcement of a possible link between BSE and CJD, the Italian Ministry of Health immediately confirmed the European Commission ban on imports from the United Kingdom, and followed up with precautionary measures against meat and animals imported from France, Ireland, Portugal and Switzerland. For the first time, the Italian surveillance system raised the alarm and clearly recognized the need to intervene at the base of the system. The Decree No. 429 of 8 August 1996 spoke of the "extreme seriousness" of the BSE epidemic and the "extraordinary urgency with which health controls must be strengthened". Under the same Decree, a "Bovine Meat Guarantee Certificate" system was established. It was, however, left to later provisions to define the procedures and criteria for this certification system. The control of animal feed remained the exclusive responsibility of the Inspectorate for the Repression of Fraud within the Ministry of Agriculture.

In 1997 the Ministry of Health set up a National Surveillance Unit for Animal TSEs at the Reference Centre for Animal Encephalopathies in Turin, and also established local units for animal encephalopathies (LUAEs) at every experimental animal health institute. The epidemiological TSE surveillance system began in this way with various tests on animals displaying symptoms that could be caused by TSEs. These tests all gave negative results in regard to BSE. The ban on the use of animal proteins in feed for ruminants was confirmed. It was established that the carcasses of suspect animals would be destroyed and other possibly contaminated animals would be killed, with compensation in line with market prices.

Decree No. 196 of 22 May 1999 implemented the 1997 Directive obliging all Member States to send a report to the

Surveillance systems:

European Commission on infectious diseases in animals and on disease eradication programmes. This meant that the Ministry of Health, the regions and the local health authorities had to work together to manage a database with full information on every head of cattle in their territory. Such an objective was not easy to achieve in Italy, due to the differences between regions as regards the availability of services and data and the methods used in data collection.

In January 2000, the FVO mission to Italy found epidemiological surveillance to have serious shortcomings, and the mission submitted a very critical report. The Ministry of Health, sent more details and asked for corrections to be made, all of which were accepted. However, the final version of the FVO report confirmed all the criticisms (European Commission, 2000b). The two main points were: serious shortcomings at the base of the surveillance system, above all in controlling slaughtered animals and animal feed; and serious shortcomings at the national level in that there were no standardized written instructions, and significant differences existed from region to region. Nevertheless, the FVO report did not have any important effects either on the inside of the surveillance system or on the outside, since it did not reach the media. And so, up until the summer of 2000, the surveillance system tended to reject or at least to minimize the results of a second Community report — on the assessment of the geographical risk of BSE — which placed Italy in the third risk band, i.e. among countries where BSE was presumed if not actually confirmed (European Commission, 2000b). But at this stage the Italian media were on alert, and therefore the Ministry of Health issued a press release on this

report, stating that it "cannot be considered a cause for alarm since it is only a theoretical analysis of the risk and not an assessment of the Italian health system".

The summer of 2000 marked the beginning of a crucial stage for the BSE question in Italy. Policy initiatives began to be taken that were consistent with those of the European Community and with what was happening in France, Germany and Spain. Various decrees dealt with the problem of specified risk materials, including compulsory testing on all cattle older than 24 months. At the same time, there was a rapid increase in the information released on BSE, much of it contradictory. For the first time, the different roles and agencies at the top of the surveillance system became visible to the general public and certain differences of opinion became evident. This was the case with top-level politics: the Minister of Health, the Deputy Health Minister and the Minister of Agriculture all gave very different assessments of the seriousness of the situation, their own and others' responsibilities and of the measures to be adopted. The endemic tension between the Ministry of Health and the regional health offices also blew up again, each blaming the other for any shortcomings. The experts — SIH and EAHI researchers and various university researchers — were also consulted by the media about BSE risk and they expressed apparently contradictory points of view. In a very short time, a climate of chaotic communication was created that continued until March–April 2001.

In December 2000, the Government appointed Mr Guido Alborghetti as Government Commissioner for BSE.[8] One

their information and communication practices

of his first acts was to call a meeting with the heads of department from the ministries involved in various ways in the BSE problem: environment, health, agriculture, community policy, industry and finance. At this meeting, a commitment was made to prepare, before 15 January 2001, an extraordinary plan for the BSE emergency with the aim, declared in a press release, "of providing a total health guarantee for consumers and protecting the productive activities of the sector". A few days later, Mr Alborghetti met representatives of the associations of animal feed producers and meat distributors and he reported that, "the will of the Government is to define an urgent provision on the collection and management of animal bone meal".

In the meantime, beginning in the second half of November, the volume of meat consumption in Italy began to fall. First in Milan and Rome, school canteens in many districts took bovine meat off the menu. The producers' organization estimated that, between mid-November and mid-December, consumption had fallen by more than 35%. It rose slightly over the Christmas period but then plummeted by 60–70% in relation to the same period the previous year when the first "home-grown" cases of BSE were discovered.

The beginning of 2001 witnessed a promise of transparency, which was in fact kept: on 5 January a monitoring system was started up to verify the progress of the rapid tests carried out by the EAHIs. This system provided for a weekly update of the test results. In the following week, the first official case of an Italian cow with BSE was discovered, cow No. 103 from the Cascina Malpensata herd. Media coverage of this event was massive, and provoked considerable alarm among consumers. Cow No. 103 had been housed in a cowshed with another 189 animals. The terms of the 1998 law made it compulsory to destroy the entire herd. In the face of this possibility, fellow farmers formed a cordon around the farm in their tractors. They in their turn were surrounded by a police cordon. After a few days, a compromise was reached and 26 animals were released for research purposes.

A second case was discovered on 16 February, after 23 000 tests, and a few days later a third case came to light. By the end of 2001, 50 cases had been diagnosed. Of these, two animals had been born in Germany and the other 48 in Italy. Thirty-eight cases of BSE were recorded in 2002.

• CJD surveillance policy

In 1993, within the framework of a European research project, the SIH Virology Laboratory, in collaboration with some Italian universities, started organizing a national register and a surveillance programme for CJD, which was gradually extended to cover the whole of Italy. The SIH appointed a team of experts, launched a campaign to raise awareness in the medical world and contacted all neurological hospitals, health managers and doctors'

---

[8] This was not an unusual step for a government to take. Italian law provides for the appointment of an "extraordinary" commissioner who, in some particularly complex or urgent situations, can be appointed and endowed with powers of initiative and coordination.

Surveillance systems:

organizations, and drew up standard intervention and diagnosis procedures to be applied following a report of a suspected case. In this way the present national register for CJD and correlated syndromes was established and then entrusted to the Department of Degenerative Diseases of the Nervous System and Viral Etiology within the SIH.

Since February 2001, CJD has been on the list of diseases requiring compulsory notification, and is classed among the most dangerous infectious diseases. The Ministry of Health requires doctors and health officials from local health authorities to report any suspected cases of CJD to the health authorities of the region and to the Ministry and the SHI. In 2002, the first case of a person with variant CJD was diagnosed in Italy.

• Communication within the surveillance system

Several experts have commented that the BSE emergency revealed a structural limitation to the Italian surveillance system, which is organized as a control (i.e. passive surveillance) system rather than a surveillance system per se. They maintain that the numerous changes made over the years — the last of which was made on the emergence of BSE — did not change the basic culture of the system, which remained one of control, not of health protection. As one vet from a Regional Health Office put it:

> We have a long tradition of control, our system has eradicated serious diseases (...) but we

found ourselves in a crisis over a disease against which we had no weapons. If we had been able to diagnose the disease in live animals, it would have been easy to control the situation in a short space of time. However, we had to base our work on reporting animals with 'strange' symptoms and on taking samples and making analyses (which took 20 days prior to the recent introduction of faster tests) when an animal died and in the meantime you didn't know what to do with the carcass.

> (interview, veterinary officer).

Therefore, in the face of BSE, the only "weapons" public veterinary officers had were their training and conscientiousness — like the Sicilian vet who recognized the first clinical case of BSE to be diagnosed in Italy, one of the two English cows found to be infected in 1994.

In addition to these structural limitations, existing regulations were not being applied. Twenty years after the introduction of major health reforms, the principles underlying state health policies had still not really been put into practice, nor had decisions been acted upon or funded even when designated as priorities.[9] These aspects probably influenced the way in which the lower echelons of the surveillance system interpreted their superiors' messages about paying attention to the symptoms of BSE, to the use of animal-based bone meals, to controls on slaughtered animals, etc.

their information and communication practices

Quite apart from any cases of people acting in bad faith, it is commonly held that the base of the surveillance system accepted these messages passively, in a certain sense. They fitted them into established work routines and thus prevented any such messages from modifying their usual day-to-day activities.

Among the experts interviewed, some thought that this occurred because the messages were not sent to the right correspondents. A manager of a regional veterinary office, for example, thought that the surveillance system should have addressed private veterinary surgeons and that future reforms would have to include these players more directly in surveillance work. That expert was of the opinion that, during the BSE crisis, the public system should have offered free training to these private professionals to involve them in surveillance activities. They would have been better at performing those activities because of their more direct knowledge of the livestock farms.[10] Another manager in the regional veterinary services said that, in reality, vets had received the necessary information but they had not been given any new procedural

guidelines or resources to reinforce their powers vis-à-vis the producers.

Until 1996, Italian controls on the application of the European ban were the responsibility of the Ministry of Agriculture's Inspectorate for the Suppression of Fraud, which clearly paid close attention to commercial interests. When surveillance authority passed to the EAHIs, alarming data began to emerge on illegal substances present in animal feed.

Pressure exerted on the Government and the public administration by the powerful producers' interest groups constitutes a major problem. However, various respondents asserted that this situation is facilitated by the fact that the majority of experts and the entire surveillance system have not yet sufficiently considered the question of risk. A research manager at the SIH, a vet who has personally followed the BSE problem from the start, states:

> In Italy there is a total lack of understanding of what risk analysis means, at least in our field. Risk analysis involves a series of stages: identification, evaluation, management and communication — a pathway completely foreign to us. At each of the stages I have mentioned there are precise functions and responsibilities and each of us must fulfil our own. Risk identification is a typically scientific role while for management, the political role is the most important. Communication involves

---

[9] Law 833/1978 reorganized the health system and, amongst other things, established the National Health Service (the NHS). This law lays down the principles to be respected by the regional legislatures so as to ensure a uniform standard of health services throughout Italy.
[10] The question of the relationship between public veterinary officers and private vets has revealed itself to be rather controversial and complex. Veterinary officers often practise privately as well and so do both jobs in adjoining districts.

Surveillance systems:

various levels: the scientific world, the decision-makers and consumers themselves. In Italy, everything to do with the mad cow situation has been confused.

(interview, veterinary officer).

The issue of risk was raised by other respondents, notably a SIH researcher who followed the problem of controlling animal feed and a regional veterinary office manager. They observed that working in the framework of risk surveillance raises questions about the objective of that surveillance beyond those on the techniques and means to be used. In other words, what must risk surveillance policies monitor, which kind of information have they to collect, and from where? The experts replied that, in order to assess risk, it is necessary to carry out surveillance and monitoring of the entire production cycle, and it is essential to acquire full information. The same SIH researcher recalled:

> From the beginning of the 1990s we saw it was likely that the BSE problem had been transferred from the UK to the rest of Europe. ... It is true that the scientific world also tended to minimize the problem. But it is also true that it was extremely difficult to know how much bone meal we had imported from the UK, and it was impossible to make a reliable estimate of our risk exposure.

The bone meal question clearly highlights the kind of problems a surveillance system has to address if it

wants, as a regional veterinary office manager put it, "to work in such a way as to protect health in fields such as that of the animal feed and the meat industry, where the economic implications are enormous". That manager concluded that, "A public surveillance system will never be effective if it tries to make external controls on production processes". He argued that the primary objective should be the reorganization of production methods and the introduction of systems that favour certain choices and render others too expensive (i.e. built-in incentives and disincentives).

• Communication problems between the state and the regions

In order to understand how information about BSE risk was passed through the surveillance system, it is necessary to understand the difficult relationship between the state and the regions.

There were two main sets of reasons for these communication difficulties. First, some regions tended to make maximum use of their own autonomy in relation to central government, especially in the areas in which responsibility was shared between the state and the regions. Then there were regions that had a tradition of weak public institutions in their territory: for example insufficient health services and schools in terms of number and quality. This first approach is typical of some of the northern regions, but is also apparent elsewhere, in the Region of Sicily for example, which has a special statute regulating its areas of autonomy. The second approach is predominantly the case in southern regions although

their information and communication practices

there are big differences between one region and another and even within the same region, and there are also significant variations from sector to sector.

The Lombardy Region is a useful example of the tension between the state and the "strong" regions. In 1997, the Ministry of Health issued a decree creating the National BSE Surveillance Centre with headquarters at the EAHI in Turin and arranging for the opening of corresponding local units at all EAHIs. Lombardy applied to the Constitutional Court claiming that this decree was in violation of articles 5, 97, 117 and 118 of the Italian Constitution, which define the Region's autonomy. But the Constitutional Court found against Lombardy, arguing that "regional autonomy must take account of the need to maintain links with primary public interests in the veterinary, food and consumer protection field in order to prevent infectious disease entering from abroad ...
Maintaining such links is surely the responsibility of the State and its organs."

In the case of these southern regions, there was no real resistance to central government provisions. The provisions were simply not applied, i.e. they were formally accepted but only partially and superficially so, or just were not applied because of lack of the means to do so. In these regions, governance of community life is conducted through so-called "informal" institutions rather than through public ones. Community life is regulated according to procedures and cultures that are very closely tied up with the specific local situation, rather than to state objectives and public policies.

In such a national context, characterized on the one hand by strong regions that tend to act independently and on the other by regions with weak institutions that do not work properly, the central authority did not take the BSE situation in hand. The central authority's establishment of a provision or a programme is not enough to activate the structures of the surveillance system in a relatively fast and uniform way throughout the country. Given this situation, the state Government creates bodies endowed with special powers in response to specific situations with the objective of giving the national authority more weight in relation to the decentralized institutions.

The BSE crisis provides an example of this. From the first commission of May 1993 up to the present-day surveillance structure, a series of institutions have been created which, except for the National Centre of Reference, have not had any operational duties. They mainly function to strengthen the head of a system that finds it difficult to coordinate its work and to move in a consistent and uniform way.

• Dissemination of BSE surveillance data
From "no communication strategy"
to "communication with no strategy"

Until the media started a vast information campaign about the possibility that endogenous BSE could exist in Italy, the surveillance system did not communicate to the general public that it was experiencing and addressing a situation of risk to community health. Respondents have different opinions about this decision not to release any information, even if it is generally held that the institu-

Surveillance systems:

tions' silence may have contributed to the serious crisis of trust on the part of the citizens. In the opinion of many, this is perhaps the most unfortunate legacy of the BSE crisis.

Nevertheless, at the head of the surveillance system, there are still those who do not consider it to be their responsibility to communicate with citizens. They argue that the surveillance system is a technical organ of the state administration and its job is supervision: politicians are responsible for communication with citizens and also for deciding on the content of any communication. A high-ranking official in the Ministry of Health stated:

> We are a country that has fulfilled its duty of immediate communication within the system of international organizations. Communication to the public is important but, with all due respect, it is secondary. The important thing, given our role, is that those who must be informed — the international organizations and other countries — do not even harbour a single doubt that Italy may be hiding health problems. A country's credibility depends above all on this, and Italy, from this point of view, has always enjoyed complete credibility. Whenever there has been a health problem we have always communicated the fact immediately.

These observations illustrate how the culture of the Italian surveillance system is still based on a principle of control, i.e. of the passive surveillance of phenomena that the system has already identified and classified.

They also confirm the extent to which public health is still considered in a very traditional way as a technical function of some professionals. The citizens are seen as simple subjects of this technical work and later as users of it.

The same officer recognized that it is crucial to have a relationship of trust between the surveillance system and the citizens, and that, in the case of BSE, this was seriously compromised. He concluded that, in addition to acting, the state administration had to make sure that such acting was witnessed:

> To better honour our responsibilities we must learn to communicate. As we know, the government has a department devoted to communication and information located at the Prime Minister's Office. And then all the ministries have press offices. The administration must move in this direction ... You see, we believed in giving the fullest information. Then if there are individuals at different levels who take this information and want to use it for good or for bad, this is a problem that must be addressed in other places, within the communication system as well.
>
> (interview, Ministry of Health official).

All those interviewed recognized that, at least from October 2000 onwards, a phase of chaotic communication had started. The study team did, however, encounter two different explanations for this. At the head of the Ministry of Health, senior officials and the Ministry's press office

their information and communication practices

considered that the problem should have been addressed by trying to provide a sort of "official communication". In the last stage of the BSE crisis, the Minister's press office was very active and it tried to issue consistent information. A Ministry spokesperson stated in an interview:

If you want to make a parallel study of the news emerging from the daily papers over the last few months and our press releases, you will see that in response to any piece of news being printed that had not been released by us, we sent a comment or a clarification that the papers always printed ... This began when the problem was at its most acute. Starting in December 2000, we have been a daily presence in the newspapers with information or a press release on BSE.

(interview, Ministry of Health official).

In contrast, the Commissioner for BSE considered that the idea of trying to centralize information was unrealistic, noting that different governmental players had specific powers in their particular areas and were therefore legitimate sources of communication:

I am convinced that the administration must take responsibility, above all in emergencies, but it must not try to control the organs of information that would be counterproductive in the long run ... In my opinion, the administration must have clear points of reference as far as information is concerned.

For example, in Italy we have the SIH which, far more than a minister, is the institution able to say if something is bad for us or not. We must therefore protect the authority of this kind of institution.

(interview, Commissioner for BSE).

But this does not seem to have been done. There is a rather striking example, quoted in the newspapers and confirmed by some officials from the SIH. On 17 November 2000, the Ministry of Health had called a press conference at the SIH to give an update on the BSE situation. At that date, information was already circulating on the results of the European Commission's enquiry into geographical risk, which placed Italy among the countries in which BSE was presumed to be present, even though it had not yet been diagnosed owing to insufficient testing. Among the documents prepared by the SIH for the journalists were parts of the Commission's report, but shortly before the start of the press conference this information had not been distributed. In the same period, the Ministry requested the SIH researchers not to give any interviews unless they had been given prior permission. Journalists were to fax the questions they intended to ask to the Ministry beforehand. The same rules applied to researchers at the Centre of Reference.

Provisions such as these continued to be applied through 2001 as well. Eventually they created a "boomerang" effect because the information still reached the media in one way or another surrounded, however, by an aura of scandal.

• Risk communication by stakeholders

During the stage of chaotic communication described above, there were many different attempts to deal with the public's concerns, which had been expressed not only verbally but as a sharp drop in consumption of bovine meat. There were numerous examples of initiatives promoted at the local level by producers' and veterinary associations in collaboration with the local health authorities, involving vets, biologists and neurologists from the EAHIs and the universities. Travellers in Italy at the end of 2000 and in the first few months of 2001 could see posters everywhere inviting people to debates and seminars, and local newspapers printed information and interviews on the issue.

Two examples of such initiatives serve to illustrate the different approaches at work. One is a national campaign run by a farmers' association, while the other is the attempt of a local school canteen service to provide safe food to students in state schools.

The food producers' "Friendly Countryside" campaign

The "Friendly Countryside" was a nationwide campaign run by Coldiretti, the leading Italian farmers' association, in collaboration with the Ministry of Agriculture and the Ministry of Health. On 3 and 4 December 2000, stands were set up in 100 Italian towns and in the most important squares such as the Piazza Venezia in Rome. The stands offered the citizens products from the local countryside and region, and in the large cities additional stands were set up representing all the regions of Italy. The overall message of the campaign was that the quality and safety

of Italian products was threatened by risks coming from other countries, and that Italian agriculture was good simply because it was Italian.

Visitors to the stands were invited to taste sample products free of charge, to buy them, and to take information regarding their origins. They were also asked to sign a document called the "Pact with the consumer", which included text describing the "rights and duties" of farm enterprises. The list of duties reflected a generic promise by the farmers to supply consumers with healthy, genuine and safe food products, while the list of rights contained a detailed series of requests for the Government to support Italian firms. Although much was made of the importance of buying meat from Italian pedigree cows, there was complete silence in the documents on issues such as the use of bone meal to feed these cows. Questions about this issue brought only irritated denials from those giving out information at the stands.

The authorities that attended the campaign's inauguration did not try to give any message other than of a generally patriotic nature. Furthermore, the day before the "Friendly Countryside" event, the Minister of Agriculture had issued a press statement expressing his satisfaction with Coldiretti's decision to suspend its block on imports at the borders, which had been going on for weeks. The blockage had allowed Italian producers to grab newspaper headlines, and supported the same message as that contained in the "Pact with the consumer".

It is difficult to assess the impact of this striking if elusive

their information and communication practices

campaign. The end-of-year holidays saw a slight increase in bovine meat consumption (that had otherwise been falling) but the final blow arrived only a month after the campaign, when on 13 January the first case of BSE of Italian origin was discovered.

Debate in the school canteens

Italian state schools often have canteens organized by the local authorities. Families make a contribution to the cost of meals on the basis of a means test. There is a parents' council in every school that meets periodically and that also monitors the canteen. The local health authorities are responsible for health controls on the canteens that are carried out by the Public Hygiene Service. From November 2000, the canteens of state schools in many Italian towns, beginning with Milan and Rome, decided not to serve bovine meat to the children. The media gave it considerable coverage, and national health authorities were quite concerned.

San Benedetto del Tronto (in the Marche Region), is a town of approximately 50 000 people, and is the largest fishing port in Italy. Faced with "mad cow disease", the local council and the local health authority decided to carry out an experiment in risk communication, with the aim of turning the BSE crisis into an opportunity for improving the citizens' participation in community health management. A councillor for education, Renato Novelli, describes the experience (sources for the research on this also included articles from the local paper, letters sent by the local council to parents and schoolchildren, and information leaflets published by the councils). The

richness of his commentary in reflecting the experience from the local point of view deserves quoting *in extenso*:

> Every day our canteens produce about 4000 meals. We have seven kitchens and 21 members of staff (cooks and kitchen assistants). When the 'mad cow' emergency came to the attention of the public in November 2000, four of the seven cooks came to me and said, 'Look, Mr Novelli, the parents are worried'. I immediately advised the Mayor to withdraw all bovine meat from the canteens. We had four meals with bovine meat on our weekly menus and we removed three of these, leaving only thin cutlets since the Ministry of Health had said these were safe and we then explained what we had done in a letter to the parents.
>
> It seemed important to involve the parents right from the start. Some colleagues advised against this, saying that it was a time of great confusion and no one had a very clear idea and that if we called a parents' meeting we would not be creating any real participation but only a generalized irresponsibility. In the end, we decided that debate and clarity were important. So, after having consulted each canteen one by one, we promoted a general meeting, open to all parents, of the parents' school canteen committees and we gave an update on the situation. At that time, a television programme was

aired in which the Rome and Milan city councils announced they had taken bovine meat off the school menus as well, and we later found out that many other councils had done the same. So with the support of the parents, at the local council meeting we decided unanimously to leave only one meat dish on the menu with the agreement of the local health authority doctor who must be consulted even if you are only changing a single ingredient in a school meal.

Then the first Italian cases of mad cow disease began to be reported, and when rumours began to circulate about cows "made younger" [cows whose ear identification-tags had been changed], we decided to ban also veal from animals under 30 months of age.
We wrote to the parents to explain that this was a temporary decision and a meeting was called to discuss it. At the meeting, the parents arrived en masse. The local health authority doctors, who were also present, contested our decision saying that they had agreed to withdraw meat only because they had been requested to do so by an important authority such as the local council, but they had been in total disagreement. During the meeting, on two occasions they had spoken out about the dangers inherent in other meats, chicken, pork and fish as well. The parents held different opinions.
In the end, we were able to adopt three

decisions unanimously. The first was immediately to start using firms that employed organic production methods for foods most at risk, such as meat. We could not change over to organic products entirely, as some parents wished, because of existing contracts with suppliers and because it is not easy to find organic products. The second decision was to obtain regional funds for courses for parents to train them to understand the question of organic products better, to teach them how to evaluate the quality of food, etc., and the courses should also talk in overall terms about nutrition making use of the experts who already work for the council and the local health authority. The third decision was to consider what to do at the end of the provisional period and study ways of changing over to organic products.

I think that we did the right thing. We pointed out that we didn't have a magic wand and we didn't know any more than the parents. We could try to understand the situation together and we assured them that we would give out correct information. I asked a doctor to help me, and then a nutritionist. This was a small task force with a single objective — to work things out together with the parents. Nobody gave me any help in interpreting what was happening and I think that we — the local health authority and the persons responsible for the canteens —

their information and communication practices

should have been given detailed information by national authorities. But perhaps the truth is that we are living in a period of great uncertainty, a moment of transformation, and it is very difficult to find our way and understand how to react. We did not want to be the ones to hand out certainties we do not have, but nor did we want to leave people on their own.

• Surveillance of public attitudes

There was no attempt, on the part of the national authorities, to involve citizens in what was happening, or to monitor public opinion. Senior officials at the Ministry of Health think that this lack of contact with the public was a mistake but it is clear from their statements above that, in their minds, the objective of communication with the public was to prevent the authorities being seen as the guilty party, rather than to improve public awareness and participation in health protection policies.

It is then realistic to assume that, with this kind of goal, any monitoring of public opinion (i.e. surveys on the public perception of risk) may give rise to the simple manipulation of the public, with positive results in the short term perhaps, but fragile and inconsistent ones in the long term. This point was made by one of the interviewees, the mayor of Grugliasco, one of the towns where school canteens had to take beef off the menu:

> The problem of communicating the risk presupposes a relationship of trust between the person giving out the information

and the person receiving it. This relationship can only be built up over a relatively long period of time. If communication is not part of a relationship of trust it has no sense and is of no use ... This means you have a harder job, but afterwards a result is reached that endures.

Among the national authorities, the BSE Commissioner, Mr Alberghetti, was more interested in the search for communication tools geared to public participation. When interviewed he gave the positive example of the campaign on the AIDS risk, run by the local and regional health authorities and later by the Ministry of Health as well:

> I am convinced that as was done in that case, there should be a big increase in the amount of information released to the public, both on what the administration is doing and on what should be done to reduce or eliminate the risk. Because if this is not done, if the public institutions do not take on this responsibility, communications become alarmist and desperate.

The Commissioner suggested further research on the perception and communication of risk, since the Italian case showed just how easy it is to swing between negation and exaggeration of the risk, especially when there are such vast and complex interests involved. The Commissioner concluded:

> It would therefore be most useful if

Surveillance systems:

authoritative international organizations would take the lead on the subject of risks. Their intervention is important especially in those countries or those situations where, for one reason or another, the hold on public opinion is weaker.

▼ Finland

Finland's BSE surveillance system is integrated with the general surveillance system for animal health, feed and food. Several organizations are involved.

- The Food and Health Department of the Ministry of Agriculture and Forestry (MAF) is responsible for animal health policy and therefore for BSE.

- The National Food Agency is the technical body responsible for surveillance of food safety and quality, as well as for giving guidance to the provincial and municipal levels on issues concerning quality assurance and risk management.

- The National Veterinary and Food Research Institute (NVFRI) is responsible for risk assessments and surveillance of animal health and safety of food of animal origin, as well as for relevant scientific research and information guidance to consumers, producers, veterinarians, the food industry and civil servants at various levels. However, in the case of BSE, scientific risk assessments have been made by consultants engaged by the European Commission.

Operationally, the surveillance system is to a large extent carried out by the municipalities. The current system of self-regulation by enterprises and producers was established when Finland joined the EU and covers all surveillance on food safety.

Before that time, animal imports were subject to permission given by the MAF, while surveillance of imported feed was the responsibility of the Board of Customs and its Customs Laboratory. After joining the European Economic Area (EEA), local food control authorities were given the responsibility for surveillance of foodstuffs imported from other EEA countries at the first point of arrival. However, the ability of local administrations to monitor new and potential human exposure to food risks and their capacity to respond to emerging issues remains limited (Valtiontalouden tarkastusvirasto, 1997; Niemi, 2002).

• CJD surveillance

The National Public Health Institute, which comes under the authority of the Ministry of Social Affairs and Health, takes care of official statistics and reporting on infectious diseases. For most diseases, information on incidence and mortality is monitored through death certificate information and routine disease surveillance, and through hospital reporting systems. In the case of certain infectious diseases, however, there is obligatory reporting to the National Public Health Institute, which collects the information and publishes it in a detailed form in its newsletters and on its web site (http://www.ktl.fi). In the case of prion diseases such as CJD, until 1999 the

their information and communication practices

main route of official surveillance was through the routine disease registration system. Since that year, the disease has had obligatory reporting status and has been included as part of the list of infectious diseases to be followed up routinely. The European measures on CJD surveillance systems further enhanced the build-up of a specific surveillance system for the disease. In practice, CJD surveillance in Finland has been functioning as part of a national research project since 1974 and of a European Community research project since 1997, but it gained a more official status as the national focal point of the surveillance system in 1999. It may thus be claimed that, while official obligations to monitor and report CJD were launched only in 1999, research project-based surveillance had been going on for much longer.

• BSE surveillance policy

Prior to 1994, Finnish policy on BSE consisted of banning cattle imports from the United Kingdom, banning all imported meat and bone meal, and surveillance of the health of the cattle that had already been imported into the country. In 1995 the use of domestic meat and bone meal was banned. Between 1990 and 1996 the annual number of cattle brains tested for BSE varied between 5 and 23, and only voluntarily reported cases of suspected BSE were tested. Beginning in 1997, the number of BSE-screened cattle rose somewhat to 57 in 1997 and 78 in 1998.

After joining the EEA in 1994 and the EU in 1995, measures to control BSE were largely driven by European Community requirements. In 1996, Finland adopted the EU-wide BSE measures, including the exclusion of cattle

of British origin from food and feed chains. Since 1998, the national authorities have provided detailed instructions on BSE measures to be taken by Finnish producers. For example, producers are required to report to municipal veterinarians all cases of cows over 20 months of age that have suspected symptoms of BSE.

Also as the result of EU legislation, Finland started active BSE testing in 2001. However, it was allowed an exemption by the EU, and thus was not required to screen all cattle slaughtered at the age of more than 30 months. During 2001, a total of 20 000 cows were tested for BSE, including all cows that had neurological symptoms, as well as those slaughtered prematurely due to sickness and those dying prematurely of "natural causes". In addition, a sample of about 5000 healthy, non-suspect cows was tested. All ruminants imported from countries in which BSE has been found were subject to special surveillance measures. By the time the first BSE case was detected at the beginning of December 2001, more than 23 000 ruminants had been tested, including more than 6000 healthy ones (*Helsingin Sanomat*, 2001).

Although the Finnish authorities have implemented EU measures as required under its legal and administrative obligations, at least some of the authorities have often felt some of the measures to be unnecessary. According to the study team's interviews, the attitudes of the surveillance authorities have ranged from seeing BSE measures as exaggerated, to seeing them as necessary to maintain consumers' trust in the EU exemption, to seeing them as necessary to food safety. Press and TV discussions of BSE reflected the same kind of range of attitudes (see, for example, *Helsingin Sanomat*, 2000).

After the first case of BSE in a Finnish cow was reported in December 2001, the EU exemption was lifted and all cows of more than 30 months were required to be screened. By September 2002 there had still been only one case detected in the Finnish national herd.

• Dissemination of BSE surveillance data

Responsibility for communication about BSE surveillance activities in Finland has always resided firmly with the MAF's upper administrative and political levels. Officials have argued that it was difficult to engage in communications activities about a disease that was not seen as a potential domestic risk and had not been detected in the country. In fact, an imaginary domestic BSE case was used in administrative workshops on risk communication and assessment during 2000.

In 2000, as EU monitoring requirements and controls on specified bovine offal began to be introduced, the MAF initially considered such measures as costly and as having a negative impact on the agricultural and commercial sectors, especially on slaughterhouses (see Chapter 9). The Ministry lobbied for exemptions from what were considered unnecessary control measures.

The official message was that Finnish meat was safe and that the surveillance system worked. This message was evident in many press releases by the MAF, and in press interviews with officials (see, for example, *Helsingin Sanomat*, International Edition, 2000a and 2000b). During 2001, the fact that rapid tests had been introduced was used in official communications to emphasize the low risk from BSE and the fact that Finnish authorities were doing their best to ensure that Finnish meat was safe. Detailed information became available on the MAF's web pages devoted to BSE (http://www.mmm.fi/el/art/bse. html), and two-way communication Internet sessions with the public were organized in February 2001. The MAF also carried out a campaign of information exchange with the public through seminars, public lectures, and radio and television discussions. Experts were available to the media whenever requested.

The authorities have also stepped up their provision of technical information to those directly involved in meat production. This reflects the fact that the BSE surveillance system largely depends on farmers being able to recognize symptoms of the disease. Until 2000 the main channel of information to the cattle producers was the MAF's official journal *Eläinlääkintötiedote* (Veterinary communication) covering animal health matters. Since 2000, the MAF has produced information booklets entitled *BSE-opas tuottajille* (BSE guide for producers) and *BSE hullunlehmän tauti* (BSE, the mad cow disease) and made them available to veterinarians and cattle producers, a group that had not previously directly received any information from the Government about BSE.

The lack of risk of BSE in Finland was still being emphasized by the higher administrative and political levels in 2000, and some civil servants in the MAF felt that

their information and communication practices

Finland's inclusion in Risk Category II by the Commission was unfair (interviews, MAF officials). Others, however, including those closer to the operational levels of the surveillance system and risk assessment activities, were more open to expressing uncertainty. Issues such as the costs and benefits of surveillance, legal (i.e. European Commission) requirements, and cost concerns were discussed by the Minister in radio interviews, and were also addressed in official press releases.[11]

The basic policy framework seems to have been predominantly based on:

- risk assessment and scientific factors
- calculations of the costs of safety measures
- concerns of producers.

This framework reflects an implicit emphasis on the scientific basis of risk assessment, expert advice and mostly unidirectional communication. Since 2000, however, there has been an evident intention to move towards two-way communication, in which the authorities respond to questions and concerns raised by the public. This has included provision of information through various channels and especially the web site, as well as ensuring the availability of high-level civil servants with expertise on animal health and responsibility for communication on BSE in the MAF to respond to the media swiftly.

In the NVFRI, which is responsible for risk assessment and analysis in this area, risk communication has been defined as part of the risk analysis function. The NVFRI web site defines risk communication as "two-way com- munication of information and views of risk assessment and risk management between those responsible for these activities, consumers and other interested parties" (http://www.eela.fi). However, at the time of writing (summer 2002) the unit was still concentrating solely on risk assessment and management, indicating that risk communication has not yet been fully integrated in its ongoing work.

The concentration of responsibility for external communication at the level of the highest authorities in the veterinary and foodstuffs section (i.e. director level) was an explicit communication strategy of the MAF.

• Surveillance of public attitudes

Public perceptions of BSE have not been systematically monitored by the Finnish authorities. For the most part, monitoring has been indirect and passive, with an emphasis on media reports or reactions by parliamentary representatives. This was not surprising given the apparent absence of BSE in Finland until 2001 and the fact that

---

[11] For example: "Maa- ja metsätalousministeriön selvitys päivittäistavarakaupalle BSE-kriisin aiheuttamista kustannuksista" [The MAF's account of the costs of BSE crises for trade in perishable goods], MAF press release, 30.3.2001, http://www.mmm.fi/tiedotteet/tiedote.asp?nro=425; "Ohjelman laajentamisesta muihin yli 30 KK:n ikäisiin nautaeläimiin päätetään kesäkuussa. EU:n BSE valvontaohjelmasta päätetty riskinautojen osalta" [the decision over extending the programme to other ruminants of more than 30 months will be made in June. The decision over EU surveillance of ruminants with BSE risk has been made]. MAF Press release 22.11.2000, http://www.mmm.fi/tiedotteet/tiedote.asp?nro=286.

Surveillance systems:

it did not represent a crucial problem in animal health and food safety before 2000. This approach seems also to be partly associated with the expertise-based orientation of those working in the surveillance system.

A survey financed by the meat industry was conducted in 2001 after the first BSE case was announced (Finnish Food and Drink Industries' Federation, 2001). This indicated that 85% of consumers were satisfied with the actions of the meat industry and government officials, and that 88% considered Finnish beef to be safe. It also indicated that consumer trust in the food control authorities and on the safety of domestic beef had remained essentially the same as before the first BSE case.

• A successful strategy?

In comparison to other European experiences, the Finnish strategies can be considered relatively successful — at least from the administration's point of view. In 2001, the Finnish Association of Communicators gave its annual communications award to the MAF's BSE communication activities. In 2002, the person responsible for the MAF's animal health and risk communication was appointed as a Deputy Director-General of the EU's Directorate of Health and Consumer Protection (see Chapter 9).

However, this study's analysis does not reveal a huge difference in risk communications between Finland and other countries, or in the precautionary measures taken by the surveillance system. The strategy of making commentators available and ample provision of information

to the media may have helped, but the Finnish case may also reflect the fact that citizens felt a relatively stronger trust in the national surveillance system and government authorities. Also, the simple fact that the first Finnish BSE case was found much later than in many other countries may have diminished the media attention to it.

▼ Conclusions

Systematic epidemiological surveillance of BSE in Germany, Italy and Finland started only in 1998 after EU Decision 98/272/EC established the obligation to implement a monitoring programme in each Member State. The European Commission's decision in 2001 to require mandatory use of rapid postmortem tests in active surveillance programmes considerably strengthened BSE surveillance programmes in all jurisdictions, including the United Kingdom.

In all countries, the information gathered by surveillance institutions focuses primarily on monitoring for disease and regulatory compliance, throughout the food-chain, with existing regulations. Other types of non-veterinary or non-food surveillance data, for example, regarding media or public perceptions of BSE are in general not systematically monitored, either by surveillance institutions or by the regulatory regimes. Nor have those data been thought to be worth gathering.

The veterinary, health and compliance information that is collected by surveillance institutions has been viewed primarily as a way of supporting animal disease control policies at the national level or as a means of complying

their information and communication practices

with EU-level obligations. Thus communication activities by the surveillance institutions have been designed for the most part to inform government and the scientific community (including the specialist public, such as journalists and science editors), but not the wider public.

Moreover, since current surveillance systems have been planned primarily to help avoid transmission of diseases through contaminated foods or animals, they are staffed by scientists and other personnel who are specialized in detecting these diseases and contamination but who have no background or training in dealing with public perceptions. The importance of perceptions of food risks in expanded and globalized food markets was made evident by the BSE saga, but there is so far no corresponding shift in the skills and agendas of the surveillance institutions.

Since 2000, most countries have nevertheless made greater efforts to disseminate veterinary surveillance data to the public, especially data on regulatory compliance. The shift from passive to active veterinary surveillance and the need to report those activities to the European Commission's Food and Veterinary Office has had a noticeable effect on domestic information dissemination patterns.

The benefits of this shift towards greater public disclosure of surveillance data are evident from historical practices. British communication practices before 1996 restricted the dissemination of raw surveillance data, which were therefore unavailable to the broader scientific community and the general public. This contributed to slowing down the pace at which scientific experts, policymakers and the general public learnt about the BSE epidemic. Those restrictions diminished awareness amongst the public about the number of infected animals they were consuming, and it meant that advisory scientists and other stakeholders were often not aware of the extent of regulatory noncompliance.

Similarly, the German Government's BSE risk communication strategy had serious adverse consequences. Most directly, a low priority was given to BSE surveillance — and hence communication — in most regions because most authorities believed the official federal line (shared by most states) that Germany was free of BSE. Thus, they saw no need to address this issue in a broader German context, in contrast to the vigorous discussions of the BSE problem in the United Kingdom following the events of 1996. As there was little surveillance, BSE was not detected and thus Germany maintained its ostensibly BSE-free status. The first domestic BSE cases to emerge in November 2000 triggered a deep crisis of credibility and public trust regarding the risk assessment and risk management abilities of German regulatory institutions. In particular, complaints were raised in public that, with very few exceptions (see below), there was no BSE risk communication in Germany by scientists and policymakers.

The major exception was the communication practices adopted in North Rhine-Westphalia, which acknowledged, at a relatively early stage, the possibility that BSE

Surveillance systems:

might be present in the domestic herd. North Rhine-Westphalia policy-makers did not, as a consequence, find themselves in the position of having to deny that there was any need for a monitoring programme. On the contrary, the Agriculture Minister actively sought to initiate an active monitoring programme at the earliest possible stage (i.e. the introduction of a rapid postmortem test). Once the presence of BSE in the domestic German herd became apparent, North Rhine-Westphalia did not suffer the same political consequences that faced the federal government and other *Länder*.

In Italy, regulatory authorities initially chose not to disseminate information to the public about BSE. As BSE rose up the political agenda, officials began disseminating information. However, the strategy was marred by conflicting information about the nature of the risks, the location of regulatory responsibilities and the proposed policy responses to the threat. Many of those involved now believe that those practices contributed to a serious crisis of trust.

The Finnish strategy seems to have worked reasonably well, even in the aftermath of the first BSE case. BSE did not lead to a crisis of public trust such as occurred in Germany. However, the messages communicated by the authorities were similar to those in other countries, and there is no evidence that Finland was more comprehensive in its BSE control and surveillance measures than the rest of the countries in this study. It is possible that the public's continued trust may owe something to the fact that only one case of BSE was found, and that this

occurred later than in other countries. The media and the public may have become used to hearing about BSE, the administration to dealing with media on the matter, and the lack of a larger "epidemic" may have diminished the dramatic sense of crisis. Another factor may be the (to date) positive "track record" of Finland's public administration in the field of animal health and food safety. It is possible that a relatively positive public perception of the overall state of the surveillance system and animal health in the country may have been a more important factor than previously assumed.

Several institutions have begun to recognize the importance of obtaining information about public views of food safety risks and of involving the wider public in policy-making. Some have also been developing communication mechanisms to facilitate that process. In those cases, however, it has been the policy divisions rather than veterinary and health surveillance institutions that have undertaken that task. One example is the British Food Standards Agency, which has, for example, encouraged stakeholder and public involvement in setting the priorities for a review of the risks and regulations on BSE. This is a dramatic contrast to the British risk communication strategy prior to 1996, under which public involvement in policy was non-existent.

Whilst the importance of involving the wider public in policy-making is increasingly recognized, policy-makers appear unsure as to how practically to proceed. For example, officials in the British Food Standards Agency and members of its main expert committee on BSE agree

their information and communication practices

that information on public attitudes is relevant to policy, but were not always explicit as to how that information could be gathered and incorporated into decision-making processes. As some of the risk communication practices taking place at national level (e.g. the British Food Standards Agency), regional level (e.g. North Rhine-Westphalia in Germany) and local level (e.g. San Benedetto del Tronto in Italy) indicate, there is considerable innovation taking place. There remains an important opportunity for collective learning, both about how to engage with the publics' beliefs, aspirations and knowledge over issues such as BSE, and about the implications of such engagement for policy-making.

References

Anderson R (2000) *Statement No. 9 to BSE Inquiry*. In: Phillips et al. (2000) op. cit.

Breakwell G, Purkhardt C (1993) *Risk perception and communication audit, final report*. BSE Inquiry, M55 Tab 10. In: Phillips et al. (2000) op. cit.

DEFRA (Department for Environment, Food and Rural Affairs) (2001) *The interim response to the report of the BSE Inquiry*, para. 6.4. (http://www.defra.gov.uk/animalh/bse/general/inquiry.pdf.)

Dressel K (1999) *BSE and the German national action system*. (http://www.upmf-grenoble.fr/inra/serd/BASES/report.)

Dressel K (2002) *BSE – the new dimension of uncertainty. The cultural politics of science and decision making*. Berlin, Edition Sigma.

European Commission (1996) *Report of a veterinary mission to Germany concerning the assessment of protection measures against Bovine Spongiform Encephalopathy* (18 to 22 November 1996). Directorate-General for Agriculture, Office of Veterinary and Phytosanitary Inspection and Control – Unit 2.

European Commission (2000a) *Report on the assessment of the geographical BSE-risk (GBR) of Germany*, July 2000. (http://europa.eu.int/comm/food/fs/sc/ssc/out120_en.pdf.)

European Commission (2000b) *Report of a mission carried out in Italy from 17 to 21 January 2000 with regard to certain protective measures against BSE, in particular implementation of Commission Decisions 98/272/EC, 94/381/EC, and on animal identification (Council Regulation 820/97)*, DG(SANCO)/1024/2000 – MR, Final.

European Commission (2001) *Draft report of a veterinary mission to Germany with regard to the implementation of Commission Decisions 98/272/EC and 94/381/EC and Council Regulation 1760/2000/EC*. Health & Consumer Protection Directorate-General, Food and Veterinary Office: 9.

European Commission (2002) *EC funds new wave of TSE-related research projects and extends inventory of TSE research to Eastern and Central European countries*, Press release. Brussels, 10 April 2002. (http://europa.eu.int/comm/research/press/2002/pr1004en.html.)

Surveillance systems:

Finnish Food and Drink Industries' Federation (2001) *Kuluttajien luottamus Suomen liha-alaan ja naudanlihan turvallisuuteen on sailynty ennallaan [Consumer reliance on Finnish meat industry and beef has been maintained].* Helsinki, Finnish Food and Drink Industries' Federation [Elintarviketeollisuusliitto] (Press Release, 20.12.2001 http://www.pressi.com/fi/julkaisu/41625.html.)

Fisher C (undated) *Statement No. 307 to BSE Inquiry*, Para. 19. In: Phillips et al. (2000) op. cit. (http://www.bseinquiry.gov.uk/files/ws/s307.pdf)

FSA (2000a) *The Food Standards Agency's approach to risk, consultation document.* London, Food Standards Agency: paras. 6.1 & 6.2.

FSA (2000b) *Food Standards Agency review of BSE controls: Final report, 20 December 2000.* London, Food Standards Agency. (http://www.food.gov.uk/bse/what/about/report/repcontents.)

FSA (2000c) *The Food Standards Agency's approach to risk. Consultation document.* London, Food Standards Agency. (http://archive.food.gov.uk/pdf_files/openness_risk.pdf.)

FVO (Food and Veterinary Office) (2001) *Final report of a mission carried out in the United Kingdom (Great Britain) from 25 to 29 June 2001 in order to evaluate the implementation of certain protective measures against bovine spongiform encephalopathy (BSE)*, (DG(SANCO)/3266/2001 – MR final).

Goodman R, Remington P, Howards R (2000) Community information for action within the public health system. In: Teutsch SM, Churchill RE, eds. *Principles and practice of public health surveillance*, 2nd ed. Oxford, Oxford University Press: 168–175.

Government of Finland (2000) *Hallituksen esitys eduskunnalle Elintarvikeviraston ja elainlaakinta ja elintarviketutkimuslaitoksen perustamista koskevaksi lainsaadannoksi [Government proposal for new institutional structures in food and animal health surveillance and research].*

Government of Finland [Suomen Hallitus], HE 114-2000VP. (http://www.finlex.fi.)

Helsingin Sanomat (2000) *Hullun lehmän tauti jakoi EU:n riiteleviin leireihin [Mad cow's disease divides the EU into fighting parties].* 22 November 2000.

Helsingin Sanomat (2001) *Tänä vuonna tehty yli 23000 pikatestiä [Over 23000 tests done this year].* Helsingin Sanomat, 11 December 2001.

Helsingin Sanomat International Edition (2000a) *EU criticises Finland for lax monitoring of BSE,* 29 October 2000.

Helsingin Sanomat International Edition (2000b) *Agriculture Minister argues testing of cattle would be excessive and absurd,* 20 October, 2000.

MAFF (Ministry of Agriculture, Fisheries and Food) (1999) *The tool kit for managing food related risks,* memo submitted by MAFF to the BSE Inquiry, M66, tab 10. In: Phillips et al. (2000), op. cit.

MAFF (2000a) *Veterinary surveillance in England and Wales: a review.* London, Ministry of Agriculture, Fisheries and Food.

MAFF (2000b). *Veterinary surveillance in England and Wales: report of a consultation.* London, Ministry of Agriculture, Fisheries and Food.

MAFF (2001) *BSE in Great Britain: a progress report, December 2001.* London, Ministry of Agriculture, Fisheries and Food.

Ministry of Agriculture and Forestry (2001) *BSE hullunlehmän tauti* [BSE: Mad cow disease]. Helsinki, Ministry of Agriculture and Forestry.

Ministry of Agriculture and Forestry (2001) *BSE-opas tuottajille* [BSE Guide for Producers]. Helsinki, Ministry of Agriculture and Forestry.

Ministry of Agriculture and Forestry (undated) *Eläinlääkintötiedote* [Veterinary communication], series.

MURL (Ministry for the Environment, Environmental Planning, and Agriculture) (1998) Press Release: *Umwelt- und Landwirtschaftsministerin Bärbel Höhn: BSE-Schnelltest für Nordrhein-Westfalen [The Minister for the Environment and Agriculture Bärbel Höhn: Rapid BSE testing for North Rhine Westphalia].* Ministry for the Environment, Environmental Planning, and Agriculture, 22 November.

MURL (Ministry for the Environment, Environmental Planning, and Agriculture) (1999). Press Release: *BSE-Schnelltest abgeschlossen/ Schutz der Verbraucher in*

their information and communication practices

Europa. Sprechzettel Landwirtschaftsministerin Bärbel Höhn, NRW, 28 June 1999. Pressefrühstück, 11 Uhr im Stadttor, Düsseldorf *[Rapid BSE testing finished/consumer protection in Europe*. Draft paper of the Agricultural Minister Bärbel Höhn, NRW, 28.6.1999. Breakfast with the media, 11 o'clock in the Stadttor, Dusseldorf]. See also: Staatliches Veterinäruntersuchungsamt Krefeld (1999), Jahresbericht: 7.

National CJD Surveillance Unit (undated). *The European and Allied Countries Collaborative Study Group of CJD (EUROCJD) plus the Extended European Collaborative Study Group of CJD (NEUROCJD)*. (http://www.eurocjd.ed.ac.uk.)

Niemi V-M (2002) *Selvitysmiehen raportti. Kuntien ja Valtion tehtävänjako elintarvikevalvonnassa [Report of the Government Counsellor on the state of food control*. The distribution of labour between the state and municipalities]. Maa- ja metsatalousministerio [Ministry of Agriculture and Forestry].
(http://www.mmm.fi/julkaisut/muut/2002etvselvitys.pdf; http://www.mmm.fi/tiedotteet2/tiedote.asp?nro=903.)
Noelle-Neumann E, Köcher K eds (1997) *Allensbacher Jahrbuch der Demoskopie 1993–1997* Vol. 10. Munich, KG Saur.

Phillips N, Bridgeman J, Ferguson-Smith M (2000) *The BSE Inquiry: Report: evidence and supporting papers of the inquiry into the emergence and identification of Bovine Spongiform Encephalopathy (BSE) and variant Creutzfeldt-Jakob Disease (vCJD) and the action taken in response to it up to 20 March 1996.* London, The Stationery Office. (http://www.bseinquiry.gov.uk/index.htm.)

Pickles H (1999) *Statement No. 115 to BSE Inquiry*. In: Phillips et al. (2000) op. cit.

Swann W (1998) *Statement No. 158 to BSE Inquiry*. In: Phillips et al. (2000) op. cit. (http://www.bseinquiry. gov.uk/files/ws/s158.pdf.)

Valtiontalouden tarkastusvirasto [State Audit Office] (1997) *Elintarvikevalvonta Tarkastuskertomuksia* [Food Control: Performance audit reports 3/1997.]

WHO (undated). *Surveillance and control.* Geneva, World Health Organization (http://www.who.int/csr/disease/bse/surveillance/en/.)

Chapter **9**

**Evolution and implications
of public risk communication strategies on BSE**

Evolution and implications of public risk communication strategies on BSE

Erik Millstone, Patrick van Zwanenberg, Reimar von Alvensleben, Kerstin Dressel, Pier Paolo Giglioli, Meri Koivusalo, Eeva Ollila, Maria Rusanen, Timo Rusanen

Risk communication strategies are interesting and important for several reasons. The conclusions of the British Public Inquiry into BSE suggest that almost everything that went wrong in British BSE policy-making occurred as a consequence of failures of communication (Phillips et al., 2000, Vol. 1). Risk communication problems may not have been the only kinds of problems, but they certainly have been, and remain, extremely important. Risk communication has not, however, just been a problem historically in relation to BSE; it remains a formidable challenge to public policy-makers with respect to the entire gamut of policy-making, and especially in relation to science-based risk issues.

It is widely acknowledged that there is a crisis in science and governance (House of Lords, 2000; Commission of the European Communities, 2000). Old ways of conducting, or at any rate of representing, science-based public policy-making have become scientifically and democratically unsustainable. Historically, a dominant assumption, from a "technocratic" perspective (see Chapter 7), has been that risk communication was a strictly downstream or "tertiary" activity, because it arose only once scientific and policy deliberations had been completed. Such a conception of risk communication is not one that can readily account for the history of BSE policy-making in the United Kingdom or in other EU Member States, and has lost much of its plausibility across the entire spectrum of policy-making. There is now a growing recognition that policy-making processes need to be more consultative and participative, especially in the light of scientific uncertainties. Risk communication is therefore increas-

ingly seen not just as a tertiary consideration, but rather as a fundamental challenge and one that is coupled directly with risk appraisal and policy decision-making. One key challenge for this project has been to identify what would be the main characteristics of a viable and constructive risk communication strategy for BSE, or in other science-based risk policy issues, and how considerations of risk communication can most effectively contribute to overall risk policy-making.

The concept of a risk communication strategy can be interpreted narrowly or widely. A narrow interpretation would focus essentially on the communicative activities of government departments in their relationship with consumers and the general public. In this study, however, the team has chosen to interpret the concept more widely. Communicative activities between government policy-makers and members of their general publics are important, but the focus needs to be broader. Within the four countries covered in this book (the United Kingdom, Germany, Italy and Finland) BSE policies have been decided by senior government ministers in collaboration with their senior officials. Their decision-making processes have, however, been embedded in broader advisory and administrative structures, including, for example, official veterinarians, laboratories, those responsible for veterinary and clinical surveillance, advisory committees, and officials and institutions responsible for regulatory enforcement.

To deal with a policy challenge like BSE, the public sector policy regime also has to engage with representatives of farmers, the slaughterhouse industry, the rendering industry, the animal feedstuffs industry, the food processing industry, butchers and food retailers, not to mention representatives of consumers and public health professionals. The study team interpreted the concept of official risk communication strategies in a broad sense to include communication within the broader public policy community and between public officials and key industrial, technical and scientific stakeholders and their representatives, as well as with consumers and citizens. Ensuring effective communication between policy-makers, their scientific advisers, senior officials, enforcement officers, abattoir managers, food processing companies and veterinarians may be no less important than communication between policy-makers and citizens.

The central unit of analysis of this chapter is what the study team refers to as a "risk communication strategy". It is important therefore to clarify the meaning ascribed to this concept. Firstly, the main actors whose risk communication strategies are being analysed are national governments (in this study, the governments of the United Kingdom, Germany, Italy and Finland). A government has a risk communication strategy to the extent that there is an underlying systematic pattern to the selection and orientation of the messages it disseminates concerning what is known, and what is being done, about a risk. While many aspects of a risk communication strategy will be deliberate, a strategy may also have unintended characteristics. Since it is clear that risk communication strategies have changed over time, this study's descriptions and analyses will refer to the evolu-

tion of those strategies as much as to their characteristics during particular periods.

The study team conducted empirical research into the risk communication strategies of the governments of the United Kingdom, Germany, Italy and Finland. In each jurisdiction, documentary material was gathered and interviews were conducted with representatives of government departments responsible for BSE policy, expert advisory committees, the media, industry and consumer groups. For the analysis in the United Kingdom, the empirical evidence made available by the Phillips Inquiry was a rich source of information on the historical characteristics of BSE risk communication strategies. Since BSE policy-making began in the United Kingdom in the mid-1980s, but became salient in the other jurisdictions at later dates, the temporal scope of the study team's studies and analyses differ between the four countries. BSE policy-making gained salience in Germany in the late 1980s, but in Italy salience developed only in the 1990s. In the Finnish case, BSE hardly had any salience whatsoever until after 20 March 1996, although that date transformed the BSE risk communication challenge in all jurisdictions.

The phase structure of official BSE risk communication strategies in Germany, Italy and Finland has been rather different to that in the United Kingdom. In each of these countries, there was an early relatively tranquil phase when BSE was presumed not to represent a hazard, just so long as British beef was not consumed. The second phase erupted once domestic cases of BSE emerged,

Evolution and implications

while later phases correspond to the introduction of active BSE surveillance in place of the previously more passive regime.

▾ The United Kingdom

BSE has primarily been a British problem, although it has been and remains a policy challenge for many jurisdictions. In one of its few barbed comments, the report of the Public Inquiry into BSE policy in the United Kingdom characterized official risk communication strategy on BSE (at least up to March 1996) as having been one of attempted "sedation" (Phillips et al., 2000, Vol. 1, para. 1179: 233). Nothing that the study team has found during research has led it to contradict that judgement, but it will supplement that statement with a more detailed account of changing tactics within the overall strategy. The study team suggests four discrete phases of the evolution of the British Government's BSE risk communication strategy.

• Phase I: concealment

The initial phase began when staff in the Pathology Department of the Central Veterinary Laboratory (CVL) of the Ministry of Agriculture, Fisheries and Food (MAFF) first identified a novel cattle disease in November 1986. It came to an end in October 1987 when the first public reports of BSE emerged. During this first phase, MAFF's strategy was to prevent any information whatsoever about BSE from being disclosed to anybody outside a relatively small circle of senior staff in MAFF and at the CVL. The very existence of the disease was deliberately concealed from all other parts of the British Government,

as well as from the broader veterinary community, farmers, consumers, the medical profession and the rest of the world.[1]

The strategy was adopted firstly by senior officials at the CVL, but then adopted even more vigorously within MAFF. Senior officials in CVL were concerned about protecting the laboratory's reputation for scientific and veterinary competence, and were therefore anxious that the existence of the disease should not be disclosed until the CVL's scientists could properly characterize the novelty. The decision (by the Chief Veterinary Officer) to tell the Secretary of State for Agriculture was not taken until he learnt that an independent veterinarian working in private practice, who had discovered a case of BSE, was planning to reveal the existence of the disease to a meeting of the British Cattle Veterinary Association in July 1987 and was about to accuse MAFF of a cover-up (Phillips et al., 2000, Vol. 3, para. 2.51: 24).

By late June of 1987, senior CVL staff were anxious that, if they failed to inform professional colleagues in the State Veterinary Service, veterinary practitioners and the relevant parts of the scientific research community, CVL would lose credibility with its peers. Officials at MAFF, however, were far more anxious about the vulnerability of

---

[1] The fine details of the process by which that policy was decided and implemented are set out in the discussion of "Dissemination of information — a chronology" in Vol. 3 *The Early Years, 1986–1988*, of the Phillips Inquiry Report.

# of public risk communication strategies on BSE

export markets and the reputation of the department, or as one official euphemistically said: "... the veterinary political viewpoints must be respected" (Phillips et al., 2000, Vol. 3, para. 2.68: 29).

Academic papers on the early cases of BSE were eventually published by MAFF scientists in the *Veterinary Record* in October and November 1987 — one year after the first cases were diagnosed (Wells et al., 1987). By then, with the numbers of cattle that had been diagnosed as having BSE rising rapidly, the media began to take an interest in the new disease (Phillips et al., 2000, Vol. 3, paras 2.111–2.116). During this initial phase, non-disclosure was justified in part by reference to the severity of the underlying scientific uncertainties. It is ironic, therefore, that one of the key characteristics of the second phase was that officials at MAFF radically understated the scientific uncertainties.

During Phase I, the British Government imposed no regulatory restrictions on meat from cattle with BSE, or on the composition of animal feedstuffs or the human food-chain. It remained entirely lawful in the United Kingdom to sell meat from animals known to have died from BSE. The covert risk communication policy adopted by MAFF during this first phase also involved deliberately not informing or involving the staff of MAFF's own specialist scrapie research institute known as the Neuro-pathogenesis Unit. The consequences of that decision included delaying collaborative research between the staff at CVL and the United Kingdom's leading experts in transmissible spongiform encephalopathies and

inhibiting the detection, diagnosis and reporting of the disease in British herds.

• Phase II: understatement

Phase II of the United Kingdom's official BSE risk communication strategy commenced once the existence of BSE became known outside the small closed circle of senior staff at the CVL and MAFF. The transition from Phase I to Phase II can be dated to the weekend of 23–25 October 1987, when media articles reporting BSE appeared for the first time. (See, for example, *Farming News*, 23 October 1987; *Sunday Telegraph*, 25 October 1987.) During this second phase, the British authorities introduced some important regulatory restrictions, starting in July 1988 with a ban on the use of potentially contaminated ruminant protein (i.e. slaughterhouse waste from cattle and sheep) in the feed of other ruminants and a ban on the use of clinically affected cattle in the human food-chain.

Once those regulatory restrictions had been introduced, MAFF's primary BSE risk communication strategy was to try to transmit a consistently reassuring narrative to the British public and to representatives of all other markets. MAFF also, however, tried to adopt a slightly different strategy internally within the confidential parts of the British Government. The external message was constructed from two main elements. One key component was to claim to possess robust scientific knowledge about BSE, while the second was to claim that the risks to human consumers were nonexistent, or negligibly slight. On the other hand, MAFF and especially CVL

Evolution and implications

officials were very concerned about the limitations of their knowledge about BSE, and the risks that it might pose.

The predicaments of MAFF and the CVL were complicated by the fact that, under the British Government's macroeconomic strategy at that time, there was an overall goal of reducing public expenditure, and this was being applied vigorously to support for scientific research. The resources of MAFF and the CVL were insufficient to invest in the necessary research on BSE that would rapidly have diminished the key scientific policy-relevant uncertainties about issues such as pathogenesis and inter-species transmissibility. MAFF assumed that it could only have invested heavily in BSE research by cutting other food safety research budgets. Extensive cuts had already been made in the early 1980s, and MAFF was being criticized for underinvestment in other areas of food safety research. MAFF therefore needed to try to obtain extra funding to support BSE research, and to that end submitted a written case to the Treasury in 1988 (MacGregor, 1988). That document, which at the time was secret, indicated that it would be premature to presume that BSE posed no risk to human consumers. That message may have been correct, but it was directly at variance with the messages that were being transmitted to the general public.

A key step in the implementation of the second phase of MAFF's BSE risk communication strategy involved the creation and management of the Southwood Working Party, which was the first attempt to provide external independent scientific assessment of the risks that BSE might pose. Expert advisers played a complex role in the implementation of the Government's risk communication strategy. That role involved both the communication relationships between advisers and the wider public as well as those between advisers and the policy-making community. These are addressed below.

• Expert advice and risk communication

Many British expert committees, among which the Southwood Working Party was no exception, play an important role in risk communication. Indeed, for government, drawing on expert advice has advantages in so far as policy decisions appear to be endorsed by an independent and highly credible authority. As one senior MAFF official recalled:

> … people do not believe what ministers say, inherently they [the people] do not believe what they [the ministers] say, therefore you have to turn to external bodies to try to give some credibility to public pronouncements …
>
> (BSE Inquiry transcript, 29 June 1988: 79. In: Phillips et al., 2000).

The Southwood Working Party members were clearly aware that their report would be a public document. They recalled that they were "… mindful of the disastrous consequences of an alarmist report …" (Southwood et al., 1999, para. 4). By "disastrous" the Committee members explained that they meant, in part, the possible economic consequences for farmers and those involved in the livestock industry (BSE Inquiry transcript, 21 July 1999: 7, in Phillips et al., 2000).

# of public risk communication strategies on BSE

When the Southwood Working Party was first set up it initially appeared reluctant to contribute to, or to endorse, the Ministry of Agriculture's risk communication strategy. For example, the chair of the Southwood Working Party was explicit in his concerns about the absence of evidence regarding BSE. He told journalists that: "If the agent has crossed from one species to another there is no reason why it should not cross from cattle to man" (Erlichman, 1988b).

Soon after the Working Party started to meet, however, it began, in effect, to acquiesce with the Government's risk communication priorities. The first draft of the committee's report, written a few weeks after the comment to journalists, described the risks of transmission to humans as "remote", but that phrase had been provided by civil servants (BSE Inquiry transcript 21 July 1999: 27– 28. In: Phillips et al., 2000). Similarly, in its published report, the committee decided deliberately to downplay discussion of the risks from consumption of asymptomatic cattle tissues, especially since there were no restrictions on consumption of asymptomatic animals and because the committee did not recommend any such restrictions. In private correspondence, the Chair of the advisory committee acknowledged that his committee had decided "not to press the point" about the possible risks from asymptomatic animals on the grounds that it did not want to cause excessive alarm, given the likelihood that BSE would behave like scrapie and be harmless to humans (Phillips et al., 2000, Vol. 4, para 10.66).

Another more specific manifestation of the intention not to be alarmist was in relation to non-food sources of exposure to the BSE pathogen. The Chair of the committee recalled, for example, that the committee members "really thought the medical problem was severe" because of the use of bovine materials in the manufacture of pharmaceutical products such as vaccines (Phillips et al., 2000, Vol. 4, para. 10.83). Early drafts of the Working Party's report had drawn attention to those concerns but the members were persuaded by the Department of Health secretariat to modify the relevant passage of the committee's report on the grounds that public confidence in the vaccination programme might have been put in jeopardy (and because the authorities had already privately been alerted to the possible risks). Indeed, the Working Party adopted verbatim the Department officials' suggested wording for the relevant section of their report (Phillips et al., 2000, Vol. 7, para. 5.21).

The Southwood Working Party also played an important role in communicating risks to the BSE policy-making community, i.e. policy officials, ministers and the agricultural and food industries. In at least two respects that role was problematic. First, there is evidence that the Southwood Working Party was initially set up, under slightly fraught conditions in the spring of 1988, so as to transmit and to endorse the views of officials to their ministers (Millstone & van Zwanenberg, 2001). By early 1988, with reported cases of BSE increasing rapidly, MAFF officials had become concerned that, unless ministers introduced a policy to slaughter and destroy clinically affected animals in order to keep their meat out of

Evolution and implications

the food-chain, ministers would be held responsible if it later transpired that BSE was transmissible to humans (Phillips et al., 2000, Vol. 3, para. 5.41). Senior MAFF officials therefore recommended in February 1988 that the Minister of Agriculture, John MacGregor, should authorize the introduction of a slaughter policy with compensation payments to the farmers. MacGregor resisted that advice because he was anxious that any regulatory action would undermine confidence amongst domestic consumers and in export markets too. MAFF officials then insisted on consulting the Chief Medical Officer (located in the Department of Health) who, in turn, insisted on the creation of an external expert advisory group — the Southwood Working Party — not because he doubted that MAFF or the Department of Health possessed the requisite expertise, but because he judged that advice from eminent external experts would significantly contribute to changing the ministers' minds.

The first step taken by the Southwood Working Party was to recommend that animals clinically affected with BSE should be excluded from the food-chain for both humans and animals. That advice was reluctantly accepted by MacGregor. The Southwood Working Party did not provide scientific expertise that was unavailable within the civil service. It was established primarily to provide officials in MAFF and the Department of Health with a political resource with which to persuade MAFF ministers of the importance of introducing consumer protection regulations. They believed that agricultural ministers and the Treasury would not otherwise have accepted those regulations. Second, Southwood has

indicated that the Working Party's decisions were influenced not just by its scientific judgements but also by assumptions it was making about what might or might not be politically acceptable to government ministers. In 1996, Southwood explained: "We felt [a ban on bovine brain material from food products] was a no-goer. They [MAFF] already thought our proposals were pretty revolutionary" (Pearce, 1996). That remark implies that direct pressure from officials had not been required, in this case, to influence the committee's eventual recommendations — anxiety about upsetting ministers seems to have been sufficient. It is important to recognize that the members of the Southwood Working Party did not make explicit the political judgements that they had made when deciding not to recommend restrictions. Instead they chose to provide the impression, in public, that the risks were negligible, and as if their decision not to recommend restrictions was purely scientific. They stated, for example, that the risks of consuming bovine brain and lymphatic tissues from asymptomatic cattle would not even justify labelling of products containing central nervous system tissue (MAFF/Department of Health, 1989, para. 5.3.5). One consequence was that many policy actors did not think that there was any scientific case whatsoever for restricting the consumption of asymptomatic animals.

Third, although the Southwood report sometimes attached caveats to its more reassuring statements, the fact that the underlying scientific evidence was so fragmentary, fragile and indirect was not always made explicit. Privately, however, the committee acknowled-

# of public risk communication strategies on BSE

ged, in correspondence with medical colleagues, that their scientific assessment was essentially "guesswork" (Phillips et al., 2000, Vol. 4, para. 10.33). Several ministers and officials have claimed that they were largely unaware of the fragility of Southwood's conclusions (Phillips et al., 2000, Vol. 4, para. 11.6). It would appear that the frank advice from the Southwood Working Party about the risks from BSE was not communicated beyond the small circle that initially received it.

In general, the members of the Southwood Working Party and the relevant government departments failed to acknowledge explicitly the policy contexts in which they developed their advice and within which their appraisal was conducted. Political framing commitments clearly shaped the production of the advice from the Southwood Working Party, even though its report was presented in ways that concealed those factors and suggested that the risk assessment was purely scientific and entirely apolitical. That subterfuge suited MAFF officials and ministers because it allowed them to argue that they were doing what, and only what, their scientific advisers recommended, and it allowed officials to use the ostensible scientific authority of the committee to persuade the public, the Treasury, other government deparments, ministers and the beef industry to accept some of their policy preferences. It also served to flatter the scientists by representing them as authoritative and influential. The study team's analysis indicates, however, that those arrangements not only allowed political deci-

sions to be taken under the guise of science but also that the spectrum of policy choices available on BSE was rendered opaque to ministers, the broader policy community and the general public.

• A strategy of sedation

After the publication of the report of the Southwood Working Party, MAFF's overt risk communication message was a narrative of reassurance. The comment from the Southwood Working Party that the risk to humans from BSE was "remote" was interpreted by senior MAFF officials, ministers and many in the meat industry as showing that the risk was nonexistent or entirely negligible. By representing the provisional judgement of Southwood and his colleagues as if it were final and definitive, MAFF officials embraced a strategy of pretending to be in possession of fully certain science that had established that risks were nonexistent or negligible. Nevertheless, some senior officials were being told, both by the scientific experts on whom they claimed to be relying and by many in the wider scientific community, that it was impossible to be certain that consuming meat, milk and dairy products from animals with BSE posed no risk to consumers, that evidence definitely to answer such questions could not be expected for many years, and that one could not demonstrate the absence of the BSE agent from the human food-chain. The contrast between the following private and public statements is singularly revealing.

Evolution and implications

In private, 1988: "We cannot answer
the question 'is BSE transmissible to humans'"
(MAFF scientist).[2]

In public, 1989: "I am totally and completely
sure that there is no risk to man from eating
beef"
MAFF Chief Veterinary Officer).[3]

In private, 1990: "It would not be justified
to state categorically that there was no risk
to humans"
(Scientific adviser).[4]

In public, 1990: "... clear scientific evidence
that British beef is perfectly safe"
(MAFF Minister).[5]

In private, 1990: "Such agent that does remain
may ... still accompany some preparations
of meat"
(Scientific adviser).[6]

In public, 1992: "It isn't possible for BSE
to enter the human food-chain"
(MAFF Chief Veterinary Officer).[7]

The Department of Health, which had a subordinate role
in BSE policy-making generally, also adopted a low profile on BSE risk communication. As one Department of
Health official explained to a colleague, in 1990: "We decided
some time back to leave MAFF in the lead in providing
information on BSE since there was a real chance any

subtle differences in material provided by the two departments would be exploited by the media" (Phillips et al.,
2000, Vol. 6, para. 4.680). Nevertheless, there were several
occasions on which public statements on BSE risk were
made by the Department of Health, in particular by the Chief
Medical Officer. Most of those statements were similar to
those of MAFF officials and ministers in so far as they
were intended to reassure consumers that beef was safe.

The Government's statements about the safety of British
beef were echoed by the farming and meat industries.
The main industry body to take an active role in risk communication about BSE was the Meat and Livestock
Commission — a partially publicly funded body. The
Commission repeated the same messages being given by
the British Government but also issued statements that
were inaccurate and misleading. For example, in May
1990, in the wake of intense press interest in BSE, the
Commission issued a press release that stated:

> All the scientific evidence — as opposed to con-
> jecture, rumour and guess — provided by leading
> veterinary surgeons and scientists in the United

---

[2] Bradley R, BSE research projects, Minute dated 19 July
1988. BSE Inquiry Year Book, reference number
88\07.19\2.1-2.2. In: Phillips et al., 2000. Available at:
http://www.bseinquiry.gov.uk/index.htm
[3] BBC Television, Panorama "The BSE Story, pt. II", 1996.
[4] BSE Inquiry transcript, 24 March 1988: 71. In: Phillips
et al., 2000, op. cit.
[5] Hansard, 8 June 1990, column 906.
[6] Phillips et al., 2000, op. cit. Vol. 11, para. 4.120.
[7] Radio Times, 31 May 1992.

# of public risk communication strategies on BSE

Kingdom and the rest of the EEC has indicated that British beef is perfectly safe to eat. Even if no further action had been taken following the outbreak of the disease there was considered to be no risk to consumers from eating beef
(Meat and Livestock Commission, 1990).

From the publication of the Southwood report in February 1989 until March 1996, MAFF ministers and senior officials endeavoured to remain loyal to, and indeed were locked into, the narrative that risks from BSE were non-existent or negligible. In that intervening period, however, the scientific case, the policy case and the British Government's communication strategy unravelled. That process of unravelling was driven by four sets of forces.

• The narrative unravels

Firstly, Southwood and his colleagues had expressed the hope that the risks to humans from BSE were "remote" on the basis that BSE would behave in exactly the same way as scrapie and would not therefore transmit to humans. On numerous occasions, however, evidence emerged showing that BSE could be, and had been, transmitted to a far wider range of different species than had previously been assumed.

In 1990, for example, domestic cats began to be diagnosed with a spongiform encephalopathy. The cases of feline spongiform encephalopathy not only indicated that BSE was transmissible across species, and by a feed route, but they also indicated that BSE had a host range that was evidently different from that of scrapie because

cats were not thought to be susceptible to scrapie. That point was clearly recognized by the Government's scientific advisers (BSE Inquiry transcript, 24 March 1998: 128. In: Phillips et al., 2000). In public, however, MAFF's Chief Veterinary Officer responded by representing the cases of FSE as inconsequential (Phillips et al., 2000, Vol. 5, para. 3.149). Other evidence also indicated that BSE and scrapie had different transmission properties and a different pathogenesis (Phillips et al., 2000, Vol. 2, paras. 3.48–3.61). Taken together, this evidence did not indicate that BSE would pose a risk to human health but it did suggest that an analogy with scrapie could not be relied on to provide reassurance.

Secondly, critical analyses of MAFF's reassuring narrative were articulated by a handful of independent scientific experts, including a retired neurologist (Helen Grant), a Leeds University professor of microbiology (Richard Lacey), a clinical physician (Stephen Dealler) and a microbiologist at the Government's Public Health Laboratory Service (Harash Narang). Even though many of the arguments advanced by that group of experts were subsequently shown to have been well grounded and entirely legitimate, between 1989 and March 1996 they were repeatedly ridiculed and discredited by officials from MAFF, CVL and the Department of Health. The Agriculture and Health Select Committees of the House of Commons also contributed to the attacks on these scientists in ways that, at the time and in retrospect, did them no credit.

The official response of MAFF to the arguments of these scientific critics was, in effect, to insist on interpre-

Evolution and implications

ting the absence of proof that BSE posed a risk to human health as if it amounted to proof that BSE was perfectly safe (Phillips et al., 2000, Vol.1, para. 1180). Moreover, having asserted that the science of BSE was adequate, robust and entirely reassuring, MAFF's risk communication strategy put the department into a corner because officials and ministers could not readily respond constructively to new data or critical comments without fundamentally undermining the narrative and the reassurance.

A third source of information that contributed to the unravelling of MAFF's reassuring narrative came from some members of the domestic news media. A journalist on the *Guardian* newspaper, James Erlichman, played a key role in questioning and challenging many of the weaker aspects of the official narrative, as did Andrew Veitch on the television programme *Channel Four News*. While some newspapers did articulate the Government's reassuring narrative, it was evident to many in the United Kingdom that the majority of media personnel with a professional interest in BSE found the Government's account unconvincing.

The fourth source of problems for the British Government's attempt to maintain confidence in the market for British beef came from regulatory decisions taken by countries outside the United Kingdom — in particular Austria, France, Germany, the United States of America and eventually the European Commission. Many non-EU countries such as Australia, Finland, the Russian Federation and Tunisia banned the import of all British cattle in the period between late 1988 and 1990 (MAFF, 1990). Within the EU, the European Commission strug-

gled to maintain a market in British beef but unilateral controls were temporarily imposed by France and Germany in 1990. The European Commission responded by implementing slightly stricter controls on exports of British beef than those that existed domestically.

The evident reluctance of countries outside the United Kingdom to accept British beef and bovine animal products or the reassurances articulated by the British Government contributed to undermining such confidence as the British public may have had in MAFF's risk communication strategy. This reluctance also provided the British Government with an opportunity to interpret and domestically represent those restrictions as symptomatic of anti-British prejudice and of narrow nationalistic trade protectionism on the part of foreign governments. The fact that official criticisms from the United Kingdom were directed towards other European countries, rather than to the United States, implies that nationalistic and strategic considerations also influenced British policy-makers.

The British Parliament had a nominal role in scrutinizing government policy. In respect of BSE policy, however, Parliament was noticeably ineffective. A very small number of parliamentarians did ask a few difficult questions, particularly in 1988, but once the Southwood report was published most parliamentarians ceased to question or challenge MAFF's risk communication narrative. After the emergence of FSE in 1990, the level of media reportage on BSE in the United Kingdom rose rapidly. The response of the House of Commons Agriculture Select Committee was to hold a set of hearings, and to publish a

# of public risk communication strategies on BSE

report in 1990. That report endorsed MAFF's narrative almost entirely, representing the absence of proof of a risk as if it amounted to proof of the absence of any risk (House of Commons, 1990).

In the middle of this second phase of MAFF's risk communication strategy, i.e. in 1993, MAFF employed academic consultants to provide a confidential assessment of MAFF's own risk communication strategy (Breakwell & Purkhardt, undated). The document remained confidential until after March 1996 and it is not difficult to see why MAFF chose not to publish it. The Breakwell & Purkhardt report concluded that MAFF completely lacked a risk communication strategy, or at any rate a coherent one, and it possessed no mechanisms for evaluating the effectiveness of its risk communication. Breakwell & Purkhardt also reported that none of the officials in MAFF's Animal Health Group accepted the proposition that the public should be given a full explanation of food risks. Instead the officials believed that the public did not need any detailed explanations of risks or of the reasons for Ministry actions. Staff in the Animal Health Group did not believe that the public could distinguish between hazard and risk, and assumed that the public only understood safety as an absolute concept. That implies that MAFF's risk communication strategy was intended to tell the public what MAFF officials wanted them to believe, not to provide a frank, full or accurate account of the science or of regulatory policy.

In the autumn of 1995, however, the rate at which MAFF's reassuring narrative unravelled accelerated. On 1 December 1995 the BBC Radio 4 consumer programme

You and Yours broadcast an interview between James Erlichman and Professor Sir Bernard Tomlinson, a very senior clinician and government adviser on the future of London's hospitals. Tomlinson remarked:

> Until we can say quite positively there really is no evidence now that BSE transfers to humans, until we can say that, I believe we've got to pay that price and all offal should be kept from public consumption. But I certainly don't eat any longer beef pies, for instance, or puree, I wouldn't eat a burger"
>
> (Phillips et al., Vol. 6, para. 6.273: 623).

Tomlinson was by no means the first or last to express such doubts about the safety of British beef (prior to 20 March 1996), but he was one of the most authoritative, influential and eminent experts to contradict the MAFF risk communication narrative.

The response of the British Government to the unravelling of its reassurances and sedating narrative was to assert them with ever-greater vigour. On 3 December 1995, the Secretary of State for Health, Stephen Dorrell, agreed during a television interview that it was "inconceivable" that BSE posed any risk to human health (Phillips et al., Vol. 6, para 6.280: 625). A pivotal moment occurred on 8 March 1996 when the CJD Surveillance Unit informed the Spongiform Encephalopathy Advisory Committee (SEAC) of findings of 10 cases of what appeared to be a new variant of CJD. None of those internal exchanges were open to public scrutiny until the

Evolution and implications

Daily Mirror revealed the imminent crisis on the morning of 20 March 1996. On that day Dorrell was obliged to go to the House of Commons and announce that a new variant of Creutzfeldt-Jakob disease had emerged in at least 10 young people in the United Kingdom, and that the most likely source of infection was BSE-contaminated foods (*Hansard*, 1996, col. 375–376). The events that culminated in Dorrell's statement to the House of Commons mark the end of the second phase of the British official BSE risk communication strategy and the start of phase three.

• Phase III: belligerence and the "Beef War"

The third phase began on the afternoon of 20 March 1996. With the previous reassuring narrative having disintegrated, the MAFF shifted to a new narrative, the primary feature of which was that, if there had ever been a significant risk from eating British beef, then it had occurred during the mid- to late 1980s. Now that all regulations were being fully enforced, and tightened, British beef was as safe as any other European beef.

The persuasiveness of the British Government's new reassurances after March 1996 was not evident in continental European countries, or in the United Kingdom's other potential export markets. The European Commission, in collaboration with all other EU Member States, prohibited British exports of live cattle, meat and meat products from cattle and mammalian-derived meat and bone meal to any part of the world (European Commission Decision 96/239/EC). At a time when domestic confidence in the British Government's ability properly to manage food safety risks was vulnerable, it responded by arguing to its domestic audience that the refu-

sal of continental European countries to accept British beef (that was *now* as safe as any in Europe) was the product of anti-British prejudice and was totally devoid of any scientific legitimacy. It was during this phase that commentators in both France and the United Kingdom started to talk about what came to be known as the "Beef War". As in almost all Member States (including particularly Austria, Finland and Germany), the British Government tried to emphasize what it represented as the dangers of foreign beef and the safety of the domestic supply.

In Chapter 6 of this book, Bauer et al., characterize this period as one during which MAFF focused on external blame management, damage containment, and national interests and identities. Public information did play some role in the Government's risk communication strategy, but it was a somewhat ambiguous role. In the aftermath of the March 1996 crisis, MAFF was more open with many kinds of information about BSE than had previously been the case, but not with all. It was not until the intervention of the President of the Royal Society, in collaboration with a handful of equally eminent scientific experts, that MAFF reluctantly disclosed much of the basic epidemiological data about BSE that eventually allowed Anderson et al. (1996) to construct a remotely plausible model of the past, present and future of the epidemic of BSE in British herds.

In the immediate aftermath of the March 1996 crisis, the British Government threatened to disrupt a broad range of business at the European Council of Ministers unless barriers to continental imports of British beef were rapidly dismantled. Much of that belligerence may have

# of public risk communication strategies on BSE

been for domestic consumption, but it contributed very little to resolving disputes or reassuring domestic consumers (see Chapter 5). That approach was, however, echoed extensively in parts of the British press.

Over a relatively brief period in late 1996, when the British Government was trying to persuade domestic and international consumers that British beef was safe, it started to talk about adopting policies to eradicate BSE. The word "eradicate" had been virtually absent from official British public discourse during the preceding ten years. It is ironic, therefore, that the report of the Phillips Inquiry (Phillips et al., 2000) retrospectively — and it might be said rather generously — misrepresented MAFF's approach as if it had aimed at eradicating the risk, when in practice it had only ever aimed at reducing infectivity in cattle and the human food supply. The Phillips Inquiry cites several occasions when, behind closed doors, MAFF, CVL and SEAC considered the feasibility and costs of eradicating BSE, but the term was noticeably absent from all public discourse.

• Phase IV: enter the FSA

The final phase of the British BSE risk communication strategy is the one that endures at the time of writing, and which was accomplished by the creation of the British Food Standards Agency (FSA). Food safety policy had been so badly handled by the outgoing British Government that, on the day Tony Blair became Prime Minister in May 1997, he received in person a report from Professor Philip James recommending the creation of a Food Standards Agency. The FSA, which operates under the auspices of the

Department of Health, did not become fully operational until 1 April 2000. Over the intervening period a transition occurred during which responsibility for the post-farm gate aspects of food safety policy-making were taken away from the Ministry of Agriculture, Fisheries and Food and transferred to the FSA. In the immediate aftermath of the general election in May 2001, Blair abolished MAFF and created the Department for Environment, Food and Rural Affairs (DEFRA) in its place. Since that date the United Kingdom has been the only EU Member State not to have a designated minister of agriculture.

Unlike MAFF, the FSA has a primary focus on the protection of consumers and public health. While it is supposed to "have regard" for the consequences of its decisions for the food trade, the FSA is not responsible for promoting the economic interests of farmers or the food industry. The primary responsibility for SEAC now lies with the FSA rather than with MAFF. The FSA also has a policy of thorough openness, quite unlike the policy of secrecy that was endemic in MAFF. The Board of the FSA holds its meetings in public. Under the direction of the FSA, SEAC now holds its meetings in public, and members of the public have an opportunity to raise questions and contribute comments. The BSE risk communication strategy adopted by the FSA is significantly different from that adopted by MAFF, even during what the study team has termed Phase III.

The FSA has abandoned any pretence that there are no risks from BSE. A recent leaflet entitled *BSE and beef* published by the FSA explicitly points out that "the risk from BSE cannot be removed completely" (FSA, 2001). SEAC has

Evolution and implications

estimated that fewer than one infected animal per year is entering the British food supply, and SEAC and the FSA judge that the residual level of infectivity is low enough to justify allowing British beef to be sold, just as long as it satisfies the requirements of the Over-Thirty-Month scheme and the other prevailing restrictions. The FSA Board interprets the evident stability of the level of beef sales in the United Kingdom as providing a reliable indication that British consumers are persuaded that British beef is now acceptably safe. The FSA has also ceased to pretend that the science of BSE is secure, let alone complete. SEAC and the FSA now acknowledge far more of the scientific uncertainties than was ever the case with MAFF.

The FSA has been actively and openly conducting a review of BSE controls. The FSA did not simply ask SEAC for its opinion, or consult wider stakeholders only after it had definitive proposals to publish, as MAFF might have done. The FSA has sought detailed advice from SEAC, but it has also been actively soliciting, and receiving, views and information from a broad range of stakeholder representatives and members of the general public (see, for example, the "Correspondence" web page at http://www.food.gov.uk/foodindustry/Consultations). The resultant risk communications narrative has emphasized the case for exercising precaution in the face of uncertainties, and the need to provide consumers with reassurances.

In this latest phase, the FSA Board has been critical of standards and regulatory enforcement in some EU Member States because, on a few occasions, residual spinal cord

material has been present in imported beef (FSA, undated). The FSA has argued that, because regulations are tighter in the United Kingdom than in some other EU Member States, and because enforcement is more consistent and reliable, British beef is probably safer (in respect to BSE) than beef from other EU countries. A nationalistic dimension remains an ingredient, however, in the BSE risk communication strategies of all the EU Member States.

▼ Germany

The German authorities' risk communication strategies for BSE can be divided into four phases. The first phase began in the late 1980s and culminated in the crisis of March 1996. The overall narrative during that period was that BSE was not a domestic challenge and that the German Government had adopted a precautionary and successful policy of excluding BSE-contaminated material from the country. During the second phase, which ended in November 2000, the German Government actively sought to reassure domestic consumers, insisting that Germany was BSE-free. The third phase began in November 2000 when the first genuine German BSE case was detected, triggering confusion and a major crisis in Germany. The fourth phase began in January 2001, after the Agriculture Ministry was replaced by a new Ministry for Consumer Protection, Food and Agriculture, and collective responsibility for the crisis was taken by politicians, scientists, and producers of feed and food.

• Phase I: someone else's problem
The first phase of the official BSE risk communication strategy in Germany began in the late 1980s and ended in

# of public risk communication strategies on BSE

March 1996. Over that period BSE was seen by most federal German officials and ministers as an external problem deriving from the United Kingdom, and not as a domestic challenge. The clash of priorities between promoting domestic industrial interests and protecting public health was consequently less stark than in the United Kingdom. German policy-making has traditionally been a fairly opaque process, so while it has been possible to identify the BSE risk communication strategy it has not been possible to detail the underlying process through which that policy was negotiated within and between the agriculture and health ministries.

The evidence suggests that officials in the German health ministry were never persuaded by British reassurances that BSE posed no threat to human health. A consensus emerged around a narrative that argued firstly that BSE might potentially pose a risk to human health, but secondly that BSE was not present in German herds, and thirdly that all necessary measures should be taken to exclude cattle, beef and any bovine materials that could introduce the BSE pathogen into Germany (Dressel, 2002). That narrative was widely welcomed by German farmers, the meat industry and by some of the consumer groups. It was, however, always vulnerable to the emergence of evidence of BSE in Germany.

As described in Chapter 2, the German Government was at the forefront of countries calling within the EU for tighter and more precautionary restrictions on bovine exports from the United Kingdom, to prevent the spread of the disease. Those efforts were not always entirely

successful. For example, in November 1994, at a meeting of the EU Scientific Veterinary Committee, Professor Arpad Somogyi, head of the Federal Institute for Health, Consumer Protection and Veterinary Medicine (*Bundesinstitut für gesundheitlichen Verbraucherschutz und Veterinärmedizin*), expressed his concern that BSE might be transmissible to humans by food. He was, however, warned by a senior Commission official not to "continue the debate" because it risked undermining public confidence about food safety (European Parliament, 1997: 111).

By the end of Phase I, in the spring of 1996, German policy-makers therefore came to think of themselves as having adopted a pre-eminently precautionary, and successful, policy regime. When the crisis of March 1996 erupted, the official German policy of precaution was widely seen as having been fully vindicated. The discreet response of the German expert advisers on public health, however, was to argue that it was then more important than ever to ensure that BSE was absent from, and excluded from, Germany (interview, German official). The narrative adopted by the German Agriculture Ministry was to emphasize the steps that were being taken to exclude BSE from Germany, but to discount arguments calling for active surveillance. In other words, policy-makers discouraged scientists from actively trying to find BSE within Germany's domestic herd.

• **Phase II: reassurance**
Phase II of Germany's risk communication strategy began as a response to the key event of the crisis of 20

Evolution and implications

March 1996. On the one hand, Germany's precautionary approach seemed to have been vindicated, but on the other hand the demand for beef in Germany fell abruptly. A concern with agricultural economics became at least as influential in the Federal Government as the protection of public health. The German Government, strongly supported by the German beef industry, sought to reassure domestic consumers, both by issuing reassuring statements and by setting tighter regulations. That expressed itself in the dominance of the narrative affirming that Germany was BSE-free.

The first animal to succumb to BSE in Germany after 20 March 1996 was diagnosed in early 1997, but the provenance of that animal was difficult to establish. Although some alleged that it had been born in Germany, it became eventually known that it was of Swiss origin. The Federal Government responded to that single particular BSE case by ordering the slaughter of over 5000 imported cattle, reinforcing the narrative that BSE was an alien pathogen. In February 1997 Germany, together with several other EU countries, applied for the status of being "BSE-free". The Commission's Scientific Veterinary Committee did not support that application because too few data were available to support the classification (*Süddeutsche Zeitung*, 1997a).

On 26 June 1997, the European Commission announced that it would initiate legal proceedings against 10 Member States, including Germany, for only partially implementing European Commission decision 96/449/EC (on heat-treating abattoir waste) and decision 94/381/EC

(prohibiting the use of mammalian tissue for ruminant feed). At least 200 000 tonnes of bones from German beef cattle were processed annually and substantial amounts of bone meal were still being used in the German animal feed industry. In the summer of 2000, the European Commission's Food and Veterinary Office issued a report on the possible risks of BSE in Germany (geographical BSE risk assessment). The Commission warned that there probably was some undetected BSE infectivity in German cattle, given the limitations of the German passive surveillance system (European Commission, 2000a).

There was also some domestic criticism of German BSE policy during this phase. For example, in January 1997, the Minister of Environment and Forestry of the Rhineland-Palatinate, Klaudia Martini (of the Green Party), accused the Federal Ministers for Agriculture and Health of being too slow in responding to the threat of BSE (Ministry for the Environment and Forestry of Rhineland-Palatinate, 1997) whilst in the same month the Bavarian Consumer Association stated that eating beef sausages might result in a risk to humans (*Süddeutsche Zeitung*, 1997b).

Important differences between the German *Länder* also emerged. As noted in the previous chapter, in North Rhine-Westphalia the Green Party's agriculture minister argued that it was important to test asymptomatic German cattle with the then newly available Prionics test, even though the test had not been fully "validated" at that time (interview, North Rhine-Westphalia official).

# of public risk communication strategies on BSE

Despite finding no evidence of BSE, the official narrative was not that North Rhine-Westphalia had no BSE, as the Federal Government and some other *Länder* insisted, but that it was only possible to say that the incidence of BSE was lower than 1:5000. The policy was described by an interviewee:

> We have deliberately distanced ourselves from [reassuring] statements and have said: 'There is always a risk, but we don't know for sure how big it is, but we try hard to minimize it'. But we've never tried to lead somebody to believe that there is a safety that cannot exist in reality. That was quite decisive, I think, and that contributed to credibility at the end.
>
> (Interview, North Rhine-Westphalia politician).

• Phase III: confusion

The second phase of Germany's BSE risk communication strategy ended (abruptly) in November 2000 when the first unambiguously German case of BSE was identified and officially acknowledged. It was this disclosure, and similar revelations in France, Italy and Spain that triggered a major continental crisis, and necessitated the introduction of a new BSE risk communication strategy. The ramifications of that discovery were complicated by the fact that the German Government had recently been especially emphatic in its insistence that Germany was BSE-free.

The political controversy in Germany arose not so much from the kinds of concealment and sedation that had taken place in the United Kingdom, but from a dispute about the precautions that needed to be taken to prevent the further spread of BSE. In mid-November 2000, after the results of rapid tests had started to reveal previously hidden cases of BSE in German cattle, the Agriculture Minister (Karl-Heinz Funke, himself a farmer) delivered a speech to the cabinet of Chancellor Schroeder, insisting that no further restrictions should be imposed on the use of meat and bone meal in animal foodstuffs before "the full facts were known", and opposing a ban on the use of meat and bone meal in feedstuffs intended for pigs and poultry (Anon, 2001).[8] Veterinary and political problems subsequently arose because evidence emerged, in Germany as it had previously in the United Kingdom, showing that farmers were not always scrupulously careful about which species received which feedstuff; cross-contamination could and did occur during production, distribution and storage of feedstuffs. Furthermore, because the labelling procedure for feed producers had been changed, it was impossible for farmers to identify whether protein added to the feed was of an animal or plant origin (such as soya bean). Even though Funke could claim that 16 000 tests for BSE infectivity in German cattle had all proved negative (the vast majority of which were conducted in North Rhine-Westphalia), his position was undermined one week later when BSE was found in an animal exported to Portugal from Germany. The German Government responded by proposing to

---

[8] EU-wide rules prohibit the use of meat and bone meal in cattle feed, but their use was still permitted in feed intended for non-ruminant species.

Evolution and implications

ban meat and bone meal from all animal feeds, and extending cattle testing.

Funke's position was weakened further when the European Commissioner for Health and Consumer Protection, David Byrne, said at the end of November 2000 that Germany had been too complacent about the risks of BSE, especially when German ministers had consistently opposed his plan for a complete ban on all use of meat and bone meal (European Commission, 2000d). In mid-January 2001, as Germany's BSE crisis deepened and domestic demand for beef slumped, both Funke and Health Minister Andrea Fischer — who resigned in order to force Funke's departure — departed from the German Federal Government.

Prior to that crisis, German federal officials responsible for BSE policy had not seen public attitudes to BSE or the safety of the beef supply as problematic, or particularly worthy of concern or surveillance (see Chapter 8). Similarly, officials had not seen media coverage of BSE as having been particularly problematic. However, since November 2000, ministers, senior officials, farmers and the food industry have seen both as intensely problematic. This crisis was widely interpreted as a crisis of credibility and public trust in the risk assessment and risk management abilities of official German risk regulation institutions (see, for example, Böschen et al., 2002; Dressel, 2002).

Subsequently, the attitudes and beliefs of the German public towards policy-makers and food safety has become a matter of active concern to the new Ministry for Consumer Protection. The crisis led not only to substan-tial reorganization and restructuring of various political institutions, but also kicked off a continuing public debate about farming practices, consumption issues, and the application of the precautionary principle in questions of risk and scientific ignorance.

• Phase IV: collective responsibility

The fourth phase of Germany's official risk communication strategy began when the Agriculture Ministry was abolished in January 2001 and replaced by the *Bundesministerium für Verbraucherschutz, Ernährung, und Landwirtschaft* (Ministry for Consumer Protection, Food and Agriculture) under the stewardship of Minister Renate Künast from the Green Party. Künast defined the new top priority of the new ministry as being consumer safety (Künast, 2001).

Künast and her fellow ministers have repeatedly referred to what they term "the magic hexagon". That hexagon is defined as a set of six policy actors, namely consumers, farmers, the animal feed industry, the food industry, the retail sector and policy-makers (Künast, 2001). The new narrative asserts that these six groups are collectively cooperating in the creation of a new form of consumer-oriented quality-based agricultural and food system. It will reconcile the long-term interests of all those groups of actors, and provide a long-term, sustainable, safe food supply and agricultural economy. It is striking how similar this narrative is to that emerging from the European Commission (in relation to the European Food Safety Authority), the British Government's Food Standards Agency and the French Government's AFSSA.

# of public risk communication strategies on BSE

There are a few *prima facie* indicators that public confidence in the safety of the German food supply may be improving, but it would be premature to try to evaluate the consequences of the adoption of this narrative. An assertion that German beef is entirely safe or free from BSE is, however, noticeably absent from this narrative. A majority of German experts on TSEs and public health anticipate, however, that eventually cases of vCJD will emerge in Germany, and it is difficult to predict the impact that such news might have (interviews, several German scientists and officials). Policy-relevant scientific uncertainties are being acknowledged to a greater extent than hitherto, but it is still not always clear how policy-makers are coping with those uncertainties.

▼ Italy

The Italian authorities' risk communication strategies for BSE can be divided into three phases. The first phase began in the late 1980s and culminated in the crisis of March 1996. The second phase began in response to that crisis. Phase III occurred once the result of active surveillance and data from a new set of rapid tests began to reveal in late 2000 a hitherto unacknowledged epidemic of BSE in cattle.

• Phase I: keeping Italy BSE-free

As described in Chapter 2, after BSE first emerged in the United Kingdom, regulatory restrictions to reduce the risk from BSE were introduced by the Italian Government as European directives were adopted, but the disease was not considered by the Italian Government to represent a public health hazard in Italy. It was seen as a British veterinary problem. Italian policy therefore was to try to exclude British cattle and feedstuffs containing any meat and bone meal. At that stage, the official Italian BSE risk communication narrative asserted that BSE was a British problem, and that enough was known about BSE, and enough was being done about BSE, to ensure that Italians were not at risk from the disease. That narrative was transmitted to the Italian public by the Italian media, and it was effectively uncontested — at least in public. Some scientific and medical experts in the public sector and private practice were unconvinced, but they tended to keep their doubts out of public debates.

Although, in the early 1990s, the Italian Government began constructing an institutional framework to try to manage the risks posed by BSE, it did not engage in extensive risk communication about BSE with the Italian public or with key agricultural and food industry stakeholders. The assumption in official circles, however, was that it would be premature to assume that BSE posed no risks to public health, and therefore that it was important to try to exclude BSE-contaminated bovine products from Italy. The public narrative emphasized the steps being taken to keep Italy BSE-free rather than discussing the risks that might be posed if BSE were to reach Italy.

When the two first cases of BSE in Italy were diagnosed in 1994, in animals that had been imported from the United Kingdom, that episode did not provoke much public debate or concern. The disclosure did not have a significant impact on the sale of beef in Italy, and the Government's risk communication strategy of empha-

Evolution and implications

sizing that BSE was an alien problem that had to be, and was being, excluded remained uncontested.

• Phase II: reassurance

The announcement on 20 March 1996 of a probable link between the consumption of BSE-contaminated foodstuffs and the occurrence of a new variant of CJD provoked a significant social, political, economic and agricultural crisis in Italy. Sales of beef in Italy fell quite sharply and media coverage reinforced consumer concerns. Some television programmes even suggested that the anticipated epidemic of vCJD could be even more serious than that posed by AIDS. Some leading Italian scientific experts were so uncomfortable with the approach adopted by parts of the Italian media that they refused to appear on television, and restricted themselves to newspaper interviews and to contributions to professional conferences. The 1996 BSE crisis was represented as a challenge from outside Italy. To cope with that crisis, however, the Italian Government had to change its risk communication strategy and its regulatory regime.

The crisis persuaded the Italian Ministry of Health to initiate a marginally more open and inclusive debate about how to respond to the policy challenge of BSE — at least, there was a marginal shift in official rhetoric although this was not entirely matched in practice. A wider range of scientific and public health researchers and institutions were involved than had been the case before March 1996. Prior to that date, the Italian Government's attitude towards consumer groups was based on the view that they had no significant role to play in regulatory delibera-

tions on BSE; in 1997, that approach was modified by the recognition, at least in principle, that consumer organizations might have a legitimate contribution to make to policy deliberations.

By the end of 1998 the Italian Government had strengthened its regulatory structure with which to manage the risks posed by BSE, and articulated a narrative insisting that Italy remained BSE-free. Policy officials and expert scientific advisers on BSE in Italy between March 1996 and November 2000 adopted, in practice, a predominantly unidirectional risk communication strategy, with a reassuring nationalistic narrative. They saw little need for more public dialogue on BSE policy-making with key industrial stakeholders public health or consumer groups.

The crisis of March 1996 initially had a strong impact in Italy. The Italian media gave great prominence to the stories about BSE and sales of beef fell sharply (see Chapter 6). By the end of the summer of 1996, the crisis had subsided and media attention had rapidly diminished. The campaign by the Italian Government to reassure the public that BSE was being kept out of Italy, and that beef on sale in Italy was safe, appeared to have been successful until November 2000 when the situation changed abruptly, once again.

• Phase III: confusion and contradiction

The discovery of cases of BSE in cattle in France and Germany, and the detection of the cases of BSE in Italian animals starting in January 2001, created what might be

# of public risk communication strategies on BSE

described as "a wave of panic". Media coverage of BSE rose rapidly, and much of it was focused on the alleged shortcomings of the Italian policy-making and enforcement systems. During the second half of November 2000, beef purchases fell by almost 36% and remained at that level until mid-December. At the end of January 2001, sales of beef in Italy were 60–65% down on the levels seen one year earlier (ISMEA, 2001).

During the post-November 2000 BSE crisis, the Italian Ministry of Agriculture frequently joined in debates on BSE policy with the Ministry of Health, and numerous tensions between the two ministries emerged. That occurred partly because the ministers had different political affiliations but also because they separately developed conflicting opinions about the risks that BSE posed. The Minister of Health, Umberto Veronesi, was not a professional politician but a well known oncologist who had only recently assumed political office. Several times during that crisis he argued publicly that worries about the threat to public health were greatly exaggerated and were giving rise to pointless alarm among consumers. The Minister of Agriculture, Pecoraro Scanio, on the other hand, was a professional politician and member of the Green Party. He repeatedly took the side of consumers, claiming that "mad cow disease" had extremely worrying implications for public health. The contrast, in that respect, between Italy on the one hand and Germany and the United Kingdom on the other is quite striking.

In order to remedy the consequences of having the ministers of health and of agriculture openly contradicting each other in public about the risks that BSE might pose, in mid-December 2000 the Prime Minister appointed an Extraordinary Commissioner for BSE in the person of Senator Alborghetti (see Chapter 8). His appointment was not, however, sufficient to ensure that the Italian Government spoke with one voice on the risks posed by BSE. A general election was rapidly approaching and the ministers were members of competing political parties, so unanimity was hard to achieve.

Many Italian policy officials have argued that responsibility for communicating about the risks of BSE should have been given exclusively to the expert scientific advisers and to top officials at the Ministry of Health (interviews, Ministry of Health Officials). In practice, that did not happen. The view of those officials and advisers is that risk communication should furnish the general public with prudent and responsible information and that information should flow in only one direction, from the top downwards, i.e. from the technical-bureaucratic apparatus to the public.

They adopted moreover a model of public opinion that represented the Italian public as essentially irrational and easy prey to irresponsible elements of the media. Those officials appear to have assumed that it was always vital not to alarm the public, even if that meant keeping information out of the public domain, or disclosing it as cautiously as possible. While the expert scientific advisers often made it clear to ministry officials that they were not certain that BSE posed no risk to Italian consumers (interviews, Italian scientists), the narrative

Evolution and implications

that the Ministry had been disseminating had asserted that Italy was BSE-free and that therefore beef in Italy was entirely safe.

From the point of view of policy-makers in the health ministry, the post-November 2000 crisis was manufactured by irresponsible elements of the media (interview, Ministry of Health official). Policy-makers argued that the media were primarily interested in bad news, and that they tended to create panic without a sound scientific basis. The media, they alleged, were intent on boosting their audiences and circulation by irresponsibly sensationalizing the issues rather than by providing serious information.

Government scientific advisers tended rather to emphasize the shortcomings of policy enforcement on the part of local authorities, and complacency on the part of national authorities about the use of meat and bone meal in animal feedstuffs. Scientists working for official government bodies were also very critical of what they saw as attempts to restrict their freedom of expression, especially when they were banned from talking to journalists in early 2001 (interview, Italian scientist). Unlike the ministry officials, government scientists maintained that the public should be treated like responsible adults, not as irrational children. They argued that the public should be properly informed without the truth being varnished, and they should be told that there were no absolute safeguards against BSE. The measures taken by the Government should be explained to them, and they should not be fobbed off with reassurances and rash statements that the available evidence could not sustain.

Although criticisms of sensationalism on the part of the press and television may not have been entirely unwarranted, they indicate some naivety and complacency on the part of some key public officials about contemporary news media. Officials appear to have just followed the agenda set by the media — denying stories in the press, accusing journalists of distorting the facts, blaming them for emphasizing emotional aspects of the problem — rather than being able to articulate an agenda of their own (interviews, various officials). Officials in the health and agriculture ministries were, following the discovery of BSE in Italy in January 2001, unable to cope effectively with the contemporary formats of mass communication. They were disconcerted by talk shows, round tables and sound-bite interviews. They wanted and expected the media to be deferential and only to present them as reliable and authoritative, and give them all the time they needed for what they took to be calm and rational explanations. The extraordinary commissioner for BSE acknowledged that the public officials' scant familiarity with the media may have seriously hampered risk management and communication (interview, BSE Commissioner).

When the policy-makers became aware of their inability to handle the media they concluded that it was impossible to communicate their view of the risk of BSE. Rather than intervening actively, they preferred to wait for the issue to disappear from the front pages of the newspapers and from prime-time television. When top-down risk communication failed, they failed to identify the need for open dialogue with consumers and social and economic stakeholders. In the words of a ministry offi-

# of public risk communication strategies on BSE

cial, "It's our job to produce health, not to read opinion polls" (interview, Ministry of Health official). The beliefs, attitudes and aspirations of the Italian public were considered largely irrelevant to decisions on BSE policy. Officials thought that it was necessary to come to terms with the concerns expressed by the public and the media, but to do so only *ex post*, as a follow-up once policy decisions had been taken. The decisions were not themselves influenced by those concerns.

While policy officials were substantially indifferent towards public opinion, they were evidently preoccupied with the domestic economic consequences of BSE. The interests of the large agro-food companies, cattle farmers and animal feed producers were well represented, not only at the Agriculture Ministry but also at the Ministry of Health. As a Health Ministry official explained, those interests influenced decisions concerning BSE:

> We have always tried to ensure the safety of consumers, but when deciding between two options we have always chosen the one that did least damage to the economy. We'd be crazy to do otherwise. When you choose, you evaluate these things as well, and decisions on health matters always have positive or negative consequences for the economy.
>
> (interview, Ministry of Health official).

▼ Finland

The phase structure of the Government of Finland's BSE risk communication strategy can be divided into three parts. Phase I evolved slowly from the first emergence of BSE in the United Kingdom until the end of the 20th century. The overall narrative during that period was that BSE was predominantly a British problem, but that the Government of Finland knew enough about the possible risk of BSE, and had taken sufficient steps to exclude BSE-contaminated material from Finland, to ensure that beef sold in Finland was safe.

This phase of quiet confidence had already started to crack in the autumn of 2000, when new BSE cases were found in France and new EU requirements concerning slaughtering practices and feed quality were put in place. Nonetheless, the strategy of quiet confidence that there was "no domestic problem" lasted until early 2001, when official rhetoric came to acknowledge the possibility of a minor risk and recognize the necessity of doing everything, including testing more animals for TSEs, to ensure food safety in the country.

The third phase started when the first case of BSE was detected in late 2001. This changed the message into one that emphasized that the finding of the first case proved that Finnish surveillance was effective and that risk was still very low.

• Phase I: quiet confidence

Until it joined the EEA in 1994 and the EU in 1995, Finland's policy on BSE was based on banning both the importation of cattle from the United Kingdom and the importation of meat and bone meal for feeding to ruminants. Those measures were represented in Finland as

Evolution and implications

prudent and sufficient. Finnish expert advisers and public policy-makers never assumed that BSE would be innocuous. Policy was always predicated on the assumption that BSE was a risk to veterinary health and might be a risk to human health, and therefore (as far as possible) it should be kept out of Finland. The official narrative was that Finland was BSE-free and that eating beef in Finland was therefore safe, and that narrative passed uncontested.

In spite of the recognition of BSE as a possible risk, the belief that BSE was not a Finnish concern was reflected in the lack of precautionary measures in the country for many years. As noted in Chapter 2, until 1995 it was lawful for farmers in Finland to use domestically produced ruminant protein in animal feed. Under those conditions, therefore, if BSE had entered Finland, it might have been amplified domestically through the closed loop of the food-chain. Until 2001, it remained lawful to feed ruminant proteins to non-ruminant farm animals and consequently cross-contamination may also have occurred. Those practices have subsequently been prohibited under EU rules. In 2001, when Finland implemented the European guidelines and initiated a programme of active surveillance using the Prionics Western Blot test, it negotiated an exception to the rule that applied in most other EU Member States, and was not obliged to screen all cattle slaughtered above the age of 30 months. At the beginning of 2000, the Finnish Government started testing meat from some 20 000 cattle, including all animals with neurological symptoms, all those slaughtered prematurely, and unexpected fatalities. The costs incurred in the process were officially deemed acceptable, but it was widely assumed amongst senior officials that they served only to reassure Finnish customers and were not required for veterinary purposes (*Helsingin Sanomat*, International Edition, 2000).

The study team's interviews suggest that, within the different parts of the food safety policy-making system in Finland, information about BSE risk was always provided quite freely, and that active exchanges of ideas occurred. Senior officials in the MAF had frequent consultations with experts in the National Public Health Institute on human risk-related issues (interviews, MAF officials). Official information on BSE and its diagnosis was first given to veterinarians in 1988 when they were told to track cattle imported from the United Kingdom. In addition, a rabies epidemic in 1988–1989 triggered seminars and other information dissemination on the diagnosis of neurological veterinary pathology, including BSE. The MAF issued information leaflets on animal diseases to veterinarians and the media.

From the late 1980s until autumn 2000, the official approach to BSE risk communication in Finland was based on a fairly traditional top-down, expert-derived model. Policy-makers argued that consumers and their organizations could always have been involved in BSE policy discussions but in practice they never chose to do so. Policy-making was therefore routinely represented as science-based and precautionary, given some of the uncertainties. While BSE risk communication later became more active, it remained unidirectional. The Government of Finland discussed BSE policy with repre-

# of public risk communication strategies on BSE

sentatives of farming and food industry interests, but until the first case of BSE emerged in Finland, little dialogue took place with representatives of consumer and public health groups.

Accountability and communication responsibilities for BSE and CJD were divided between the MAF and the Ministry of Social Affairs and Health (MSAH). The primary responsibility for information and communication strategies on CJD was assigned to the MSAH and the National Public Health Institute, while the upper levels of the MAF were given responsibility for BSE.

In 1997 the Finnish authorities established a coordinating group on risk communication, to bring together all the different organizations involved. The aim was to improve risk communication and ensure that, should a crisis arise, the authorities' response would be coherent. In 2000, two seminars on risk communication and risk assessment were organized by those responsible for BSE surveillance of both animals and the human food supply. They brought together public health experts with representatives of the food industry and meat and dairy trade interests. The discussions included a study looking at how the different parties could and should respond in the event of a BSE case in Finland.

• Phase II: increased caution

Some increased caution began to be visible in Finnish public life in the early months of the new millennium. In March 2000, a written question was asked in Parliament regarding consumer protection and BSE. In particular,

the questioner referred to possibly contaminated meat from Denmark, and asked why Finland had not joined the other Nordic countries in measures to protect consumers against this possible risk (Räsänen, 2000). Another cause for increased attention was the fact that Finnish surveillance measures in slaughterhouses had received critical comments in a European Commission FVO report (European Commission, 2000b). The report queried whether surveillance measures had been appropriately understood in municipalities and farms, suggested that the efficiency of the monitoring programme in slaughterhouses was being diluted, and found that during 1998 and 1999 only the Commission's minimum required samples were taken.

The authorities' response to the FVO report, however, highlighted mostly that the Commission's overall assessment was excellent (see, for example, *Helsingin Sanomat*, 2000). Nonetheless, in response to the FVO report, a leaflet on BSE was reprinted in 2000 and sent to all cattle farmers, and more information was also sent to veterinarians (European Commission, 2000c).

In the autumn of 2000, rising numbers of BSE cases in continental Europe and growing demands for EU safeguards prompted energetic discussion in Finland. With the increased number of ruminants to be tested by the beginning of the year 2001, official communications started to be more open about the risks of finding some BSE cases in the country. This more cautious line may also have been prompted by criticism raised over the previous approach, including a statement by the parlia-

Evolution and implications

mentary opposition leader that the Government had been understating the risks of BSE in Finland. The criticism, presented in an editorial of the Centre Party's journal, stated:

> ... the way in which the Minister of Agriculture has emphasized the costs of the testing of the animals and understated the problem has been wrong; in addition in Finland BSE tests need to be done extensively and reliably. Costs are not a reason to lower quality or safety of food. In the context of public health policies and national economy the costs of testing are bearable.
>
> (Jäätteenmäki, 2001).

The importance of the Centre Party's statements and its influence on official policies is difficult to assess. However, as the Centre Party has always been one of the three largest national parties (with the Social Democrats and Conservatives) it cannot be ignored. Furthermore, as it is the main party in most rural areas and has broad support amongst farmers, the relevance of its views cannot be ignored in the policy process of BSE communication at national level.

Further parliamentary questions related to BSE were asked concerning issues such as the occupational safety of persons carrying out BSE testing, the use of gelatin in foodstuffs, and "BSE hysteria" in general (Vistbacka, 2000; Aittoniemi, 2001; Syvärinen, 2001; Tiura, 2001). However, as the Minister of Agriculture and Forestry,

Kalevi Hemila, made clear in a report to Parliament in late January 2001, the government line was still one of implementing minimal required procedures, although there was more emphasis on the importance of maintaining trust (Hemila, 2001).

In February 2001, a possible case of BSE was provisionally identified, but subsequent histopathological tests on that animal were all negative. This appears to have increased the authorities' awareness that a BSE case might eventually be found in Finland.

• Phase III: reassurance

On 7 December 2001, the Ministry of Agriculture and Forestry announced Finland's first (and so far only) case of BSE. The disease was detected in a dairy cow born in Finland in 1995. No meat or bone meal had reportedly been used in that herd for more than 20 years. No evidence of BSE was found in any of the other animals in that herd. The Finnish authorities remain uncertain about how that animal came to be infected. Officially, the prime suspect for the source of infection remains contaminated fat in milk-replacer feeds used to feed calves.

The role of contaminated fat and the possibility that use of animal fat in feeding calves (so far, a permissible practice) was a problem that was also debated. At the time of the first BSE case the Finnish authorities were reported to have been aware of the concerns in Denmark about the practice but to have considered them safe (*Helsingin Sanomat*, 2001; YLE, 2001).

# of public risk communication strategies on BSE

Although a report emerged on 24 December 2001 indicating that a second animal was suspected of having BSE, the results of subsequent tests contradicted that diagnosis (Meatnews, 2001). Since 7 December 2001, the authorities in Finland have had to further modify their risk communication strategy in favour of one that is somewhat more cautious. The fact that the BSE case was found was argued to show that the safeguards in place were, indeed, working. This message was voiced strongly by the food industry representatives, but also articulated clearly by the MAF representatives. According to Jaana Husu-Kallio, the head of the MAF's veterinary and foodstuffs section and the person with overall responsibility for BSE communication, the finding of the first case of BSE actually supported the view that surveillance had been effective (*Helsingin Sanomat*, 2001). The more recent narrative has avoided assertions that all possible risks of BSE have been eliminated; instead it has focused on arguing that all statutory and practical measures are being taken and that if there is a residual risk it is extremely slight, and diminishing.

The identification of more BSE cases in other EU countries and the one case of BSE in Finland (the cause of which could not readily be explained) necessitated a shift in risk communication strategy. The new strategy changed from one of emphasizing that Finnish meat was safe and that EU measures were unnecessary to one of emphasizing that everything necessary was being done to ensure that meat remained safe.

This strategy appears to have been successful. Compared to other countries, Finnish demand for beef has remained stable since the first BSE case in December 2001, suggesting high levels of consumer confidence in domestic meat supplies (Finfood, 2001; Finfood, 2002; MAF, 2002). Another indicator of the success of Finnish BSE communications — as perceived within the country — can be seen in the awarding of two prizes by national associations in the course of 2002. The first was the annual prize of the Finnish Association of Communicators, awarded for carefully planned and effective communication efforts, which lauded the Government's communications on the issue as "open and clear" (Finnish Association of Communications Professionals, 2002).[9]

The second was awarded by the national Consumer Association to the abovementioned official, Jaana Husu-Kallio, in recognition of how consumer and citizen viewpoints were reflected in official communications on food and veterinary matters (including the first BSE case), and these communications' rapidity and openness. The Consumer Association judged that her work had enhanced consumer influence, and that consumers could continue to put their trust in food quality in Finland (Finnish Consumers' Association 2001).[10]

---

[9] Vuoden viestintöteoksi valittiin BSE-tiedotus. [BSE communication awarded the annual communication prize], information available from MAF's web site, http://www.pressi.com/fi/release/48331.htm.
[10] Ms Husu-Kallio was appointed Deputy Director-General of the European Commission's Directorate General of Health and Consumer Protection in June 2002 (European Commission, press release, 19 June 2002).

Evolution and implications

However, in spite of the awards and apparent satisfaction amongst some media and consumer representatives, it is difficult to say whether consumers' views were really addressed better than in other European countries. While some communications practices in Finland were different to those in other countries, it seems unlikely that the content of the messages per se were more influenced by consumer viewpoints or that communications practices were more geared towards taking consumer or citizen opinions into account as a starting point. To the study team's knowledge, no analysis of consumer or citizen views was ever carried out as part of the communication process before the crisis.

In short, it is difficult to claim that the success of Finnish communications on BSE was due to better awareness of consumer and citizen viewpoints. Rather, it may represent (a) the relatively broader trust that Finns have in both the honesty and the accountability of those in charge, and (b) the fact that the first case of BSE in Finland occurred later than in other countries and after the EU regulations had been implemented.

▾ Conclusions

The evidence from the comparative study of the evolution of four national BSE risk communication strategies strongly suggests the following.

- All jurisdictions, at almost all stages in the evolution of their risk communication strategy, have tried to use concerns about BSE to promote the reputation of domestic beef supplies and to diminish confidence in foreign supplies.

- Public policy-makers have routinely represented risk communication as if it were a purely tertiary activity. However, the study team's research shows that, in practice, risk communication considerations have often played a far more fundamental, but unacknowledged, role in BSE policy-making. To the extent that an aspiration to reassure consumers about the safety of beef has been a dominant concern of public policy-makers responsible for BSE, risk communication policy has been a primary or a secondary consideration rather than a tertiary one.

- Risk communication practices in most jurisdictions have sometimes been less than frank, and have misrepresented and/or concealed the objectives of policy and oversimplified and exaggerated the reliability of the available knowledge and the rationality of their actions.

- Public policy-makers have been operating with distinctive models of the beliefs, attitudes and wants of their citizens, but those models have had virtually no empirical support whatsoever, and have often been unrealistic. Furthermore, governments have seen public opinion as an object of policy, and as a problem that may need to be managed, rather than as a primary input to policy (as shown amply in Chapter 8). Risk communication strategies have therefore typically been unidirectional and top-down with little or no effort to engage in reciprocal communication activities.

- The risk communication strategies of all four countries ran into unanticipated difficulties when evidence emerged showing that they had been premised on false assumptions, both about science and about public beliefs and attitudes. Further difficulties occurred

# of public risk communication strategies on BSE

because it became evident that the authorities of all jurisdictions were at least as concerned to reassure consumers (so as to maintain stability in agricultural markets) as they had been to protect public health.

In the United Kingdom, at several stages of the BSE saga, official risk communication messages suggested that public authorities had a secure scientific understanding of the putative risks of BSE and that such risks were zero, or virtually zero. British policy-makers also represented science as the exclusive determining factor in the decision-making process. The effect of adopting that strategy was that it allowed British ministers and officials to conceal their policy objectives and their trade-offs between risks, costs and benefits, and to hide behind a cloak of "scientificity". German policy-makers never asserted full certainty with respect to the risks posed by BSE and British beef, but they did assert that German beef was perfectly safe. Italian and Finnish policy-makers insisted that BSE was a "foreign" problem and that BSE was being kept out of their jurisdictions, and that beef on sale in those countries was entirely safe.

The experiences described in this chapter suggest that risk communication strategies that assert full certainty when significant uncertainties remain are unlikely to be sustainable in the long run. Risk communication strategies that assert risks to be zero, or virtually zero, are also unlikely to be sustainable in the long run. Any risk communication strategy that combines those two shortcomings is likely to become especially problematic, particularly as and when new evidence emerges.

The British Government's pre-March 1996 risk communication narrative backfired dramatically after evidence emerged showing that such claims had been premised on false assumptions about both the science of BSE and policy-making processes. Trust, on the part both of domestic consumers and of international consumers, in British regulatory institutions and their expert advisers evaporated. Prior to March 1996 those risk communication practices had also had an adverse impact on the substance of policy, by diminishing the scope for policy-makers to appreciate the need to make judgements about the extent to which precaution was appropriate, and the scope for exercising precaution. Having started with a risk communication strategy of consumer reassurance that asserted that British beef was safe, policy-makers were inhibited from learning about the risks or responding to new evidence.

The reassuring, and nationalistic, risk communication narratives adopted by German and Italian policy-makers in the 1990s were also ruined by the discovery of cases of BSE in cattle in German and Italian animals in late 2000 and early 2001; these events were closely followed by dramatic and abrupt reductions in beef sales within those jurisdictions. In Germany it became evident that, despite the rhetoric about having a pre-eminently precautionary policy regime, agricultural policy-makers had been at least as preoccupied with promoting the interests of the cattle farmers and animal-feed producers as with protecting public health. In Italy, once the domestic crisis broke, the authorities were unable to provide a coherent or consistent message about the risks that BSE

Evolution and implications

posed in Italy, or to deal effectively with the media. Consumers therefore drew the conclusion that they had not been, and were not being, properly informed about BSE.

The risk communication narrative adopted by Finnish policy-makers has proven to be more sustainable than in Germany, Italy or the United Kingdom (again, this is in a context of far fewer reported cases of BSE than in most other European countries). Although, like the German and Italian governments, the Finnish authorities had characterized domestic beef as reliably safe, the Finnish narrative began to shift well before the first domestic case was discovered in late 2001. At the beginning of that year, policy-makers began to emphasize the possibility of a risk from Finnish beef; once the first domestic case had been discovered, policy-makers then insisted that it demonstrated the effectiveness of Finnish safeguards. The fact that demand for beef in Finland did not follow the pattern in other jurisdictions may also represent a relatively high degree of public trust in Finnish policy institutions.

Of all the strategies examined, the approach adopted in North Rhine-Westphalia seems to have been the most robust and sustainable. The authorities of that *Land* acknowledged many of the scientific uncertainties, and adopted a more open rhetoric and practice than any of the other jurisdictions. North Rhine-Westphalia consequently initiated a programme of active surveillance for BSE at the earliest possible opportunity. The adoption of that strategy appears to have been exceptionally effective

in maintaining public confidence in at least the relative effectiveness of their BSE policy.

In both Germany and the United Kingdom, following the creation of new food safety institutions in 2000 and 2001, respectively, risk communication strategies shifted significantly. The new institutions abandoned the traditional pretence that the science of BSE is secure or complete, or that the risks have been entirely eradicated. They have both also introduced a new emphasis on collective, consumer-orientated and precautionary decision-making and, in the United Kingdom at least, have been experimenting with innovative forms of reciprocal communication and deliberation. It will be fascinating to see how these initiatives will be refined in the longer term.

References

Aittoniemi S (2001) *BSE hysteria, written question*. Finnish Parliament, KK 242/2001.

Anderson RM et al. (1996) Transmission dynamics and epidemiology of BSE in British cattle. *Nature*, 382:779–788.

Anon. (2001) The agricultural policy crises in the UK and Germany. *Oxford Analytica*, 3 April.

Böschen S, Dressel K, Schneider M, Viehhöver W (2002) Pro und Kontra der Trennung von Risikobewertung und Risikomanagement - Diskussionsstand in Deutschland und Europa. Im Rahmen des TA-Projekts "Strukturen der

# of public risk communication strategies on BSE

Organisation und Kommunikation im Bereich der Erforschung übertragbarer spongiformer Enzephalopathien"
[Pros and cons of the separation between risk assessment and risk management – state of discussion in Germany and Europe. In the context of the technology assessment project: Structures of the organization and communication on the exploration field transmissible spongiform encephalopathies]. Berlin, TAB-*Hintergrundbericht*, No. 10.

Breakwell G, Purkhardt C, (undated). *Risk perception and communication audit, Final Report*. Department of Psychology, University of Surrey.

Commission of the European Communities (2000) *Science, society and the citizen in Europe* . Brussels, Commission of the European Communities.

Dressel K (2002) *BSE – the new dimension of uncertainty*. Berlin, Edition Sigma.

Erlichman J (1988a) Brain-disease in food. *Guardian*, 4 June.

Erlichman J (1988b) Butchers selling diseased meat. *Guardian*, 29 June.

European Commission (2000a) *Report on the assessment of the geographical BSE-risk (GBR) of Germany, July 2000*:36. (http://europa.eu.int/comm/food/fs/sc/ssc/out120_en.pdf.)

European Commission (2000b) *Report of an FVO Mission to Finland with regard to implementation of Commission decisions 98/272/EC and 94/381/EC and Council Regulation (EC) No 820/97 (8–12 May 2000), DG(SANCO)/1127/2000-MR, Final*. (http://europa.eu.int/comm/food/fs/inspections/vi/reports/finland/vi_rep_finl_1127-2000_en.pdf.)

European Commission (2000c) *Comments on the draft report of the FVO mission to Finland concerning implementation of Commission decisions 98/272/EC concerning epidemiosurveillance on TSEs, Commission decision 94/381/EC concerning certain protective measures against BSE (feed ban) and animal identification (Council Regulation No.820/97/EC)*. (http://europa.eu.int/comm/food/fs/inspections/vi/reports/finland/vi_rep_finl_1127-2000cm_en.pdf.)

European Commission (2000d) *David Byrne on BSE – developments in Germany and Spain*. Health and Consumer Protection Directorate, press release, 27 November.

European Parliament (1997) *Report on alleged contravention or maladministration in the implementation of Community law in relation to BSE, without prejudice to the jurisdiction of the Community and national courts*. Doc_EN\RR\319\319544 A4-0020/97A, 7 February.

Finfood (2001) *Kuluttajien luottamus suomen liha-alaan ja naudanlihan turvallisuuteen on säilynyt ennallaan [Consumer trust in Finnish meat industry and safety of beef has remained]* Press release, 20.12.2001. (http://www.pressi.com/fi/julkaisu/41625.html.)

Finfood (2002) *Kuluttajien luottamus naudanlihan turvallisuuteen on vahvistunut [Consumer trust in safety of beef has strengthened]* Press release, 12.3.2002. (http://www.nettikeittio.fi.)

Finnish Association of Communications Professionals (2002) *Vuoden Viestintäteko on BSE-tiedotus [BSE Communication awarded the annual communication prize]*. (http://www.pressi.com/fi/release/48331.html.)

Finnish Consumers' Association (2001) *Vuoden Kuluttajateko - tunnustuspalkinnon saavat osastopäällikkö Jaana Husu-Kallio Maa-ja metsätalousministeriöstä sekä Kuluttjayhdistysd Korson Linkki [The annual Consumer action award is awarded to Jaana Husu-Kallio from the Ministry of Agriculture and Forestry and to Consumer Association Korson Linkki]*. (http://www.kuluttajaliitto.fi/Kuluttajateko2001.htm.)

FSA (2001) *BSE and beef*. (http://www.food.gov.uk/multimedia/pdfs/bse-and-beef.pdf.)

FSA (undated) Seizures of SRM in imported meat. *BSE controls review*. (http://www.food.gov.uk/bse/facts/srm.)

Groschup M, Kramer M. (2001) Epidemiologie und Diagnostik der BSE in Deutschland [Epidemiology and diagnosis of BSE in Germany]. *Deutsches Tierärzteblatt*, 5:510–517.

Hansard (1996) 20 March.

Helsingin Sanomat (2000) *Suomi joutuu kiristämään BSE-valvontaa. [Finland had to tighten up BSE surveillance]*. *Helsingin Sanomat* 29 November.

Helsingin Sanomat (2001) *BSE tautia ensi kertaa Suomessa [First BSE case in Finland]. Helsingin Sanomat* 8 December.

Evolution and implications

Helsingin Sanomat International Edition (2000) *Agriculture Minister argues testing of cattle would be excessive and absurd*. November 20.

Hemila K (2001) *SuV-tiedotteet [Report to Grand Committee, Finnish Parliament]* 15 January.

House of Commons (1990) *Bovine Spongiform Encephalopathy (BSE), Fifth report of the Agriculture Committee*. House of Commons Paper No. 449.

House of Lords (2000) Select Commitee on Science and Technology, Third Report, HL Paper 38, *Science and Society*. London, Her Majesty's Stationery Office.

Isaacs D, Fitzgerald D (1999) Seven alternatives to evidence based medicine. *British Medical Journal*, 319:1618.

ISMEA (2001) *Indagine sull'acquisto di carne bovina nel periodo di crisi BSE, [Survey on purchasing beef during the period of the BSE crisis]*. ISMEA (Istituto di Servizi per il Mercato Agricolo Alimentare). Rome, Osservatorio Consumi.

Jäätteenmäki A (2001) *On valittava puhtaan ja terveellisen ruoantuotannon linja [Finland must choose healthy and safe food production practices]*. Verkkolehti Apila, 18 January. (http://www.keskusta.fi/apila/paakirjoitukset/?article_id=3039.)

Künast (2001) *Remarks at TAFS Conference on 'BSE and food safety'*. Basle 19 April. (http://www.tseandfoodsafety.org/startseite.htm.)

MacGregor J. PES (1988) Agriculture, Fisheries and Food, Letter to John Major dated 8 September 1988. BSE Inquiry Yearbook Document No. YB 88/9.8/6.1–6.6. In: Phillips et al (2000) op. cit.

Maclean D (1990) Comments in *This Week*, transmitted on 17 May.

MAF (2002) *Kotimaisen naudanlihatuotannon elvyttamista selvittava tyoryhma. Loppuraportti [Final report of the working group on enhancing of beef national beef production]*. Helsinki, MAF.

MAFF/DoH (Ministry of Agriculture Fisheries and Food/Department of Health) (1989) *Report of the Working Party on Bovine Spongiform Encephalopathy*. London, Ministry of Agriculture, Fisheries and Food.

MAFF (Ministry of Agriculture, Fisheries and Food) (1990) *Bovine Spongiform Encephalopathy (BSE)*. London, Ministry of Agriculture, Fisheries and Food. (Memorandum by the Ministry of Agriculture, Fisheries and Food, Consumer Panel document No. CP(90)3/9, Annex F.)

Meat and Livestock Commission (1990) *BSE scare overblown says MLC scientist*. MLC press release, 18 May. (http://www.bseinquiry.gov.uk/report/volume6/chapt413.htm.) (see para. 4.537–4.540)

Meatnews (2001) *Finland finds second BSE case*. (http://www.meatnews.com/index.cfm?fuseaction=article&artNum=2373.)

Meldrum K (1995) Comments in *BSE the hidden epidemic*. World In Action, television programme, transmitted on 13 November.

Millstone E, van Zwanenberg P (2001) The politics of expert advice: lessons from the early history of the BSE saga. *Science and Public Policy*, 28:99–112.

Ministry for the Environment and Forestry for Rhineland Palatinate (1997) *Martini: Borchert und Seehofer laufen der BSE-Gefahr seit Jahren hinterher [Martini: Borchert and Seehofer run the risk of BSE danger for years in the future]*. Ministry for the Environment and Forestry for Rhineland Palatinate, press release, 22 January.

Pearce F (1996) Ministers hostile to advice on BSE. *New Scientist*, 30 March: 4.

Phillips N, Bridgeman J, Ferguson-Smith M (2000) *The BSE Inquiry: Report: evidence and supporting papers of the Inquiry into the emergence and identification of Bovine Spongiform Encephalopathy (BSE) and variant Creutzfeldt-Jakob Disease (vCJD) and the action taken in response to it up to 20 March 1996*. London, The Stationery Office (http://www.bseinquiry.gov.uk/index.htm).

Räsänen P (2000) *Kuluttajien suojelu hullun lehmän taudilta [Protection of consumers from BSE]*. Written question, Finnish Parliament, KK204/2000.

Southwood R (2000) *Witness Statement No 1 to BSE Inquiry*. In: Phillips et al., op. cit., Disc 11.

# of public risk communication strategies on BSE

Southwood R, Epstein A, Martin W (1999) Lord Walton, Witness Statement No. 483A. In: Phillips et al., 2000, Disc 11.

Süddeutsche Zeitung (1997a) *EU-Ausschuß: Keine Gelatine von Rinderknochen aus BSE-Gebieten [EU-Committee: No gelatin from beef bones coming from BSE areas]*. 23 February 1997.

Süddeutsche Zeitung (1997b) *Weil die Herkunftskontrollen nach wie vor lückenhaft sind. Verbraucherschützer warnen vor Rindfleisch [As the control of the origin is still incomplete, consumer protection organisations warn about beef]*. 30 January 1997.

Syvärinen K (2001) *BSE-tautiriskin vaikutukset työsuojeluun. [The impact of BSE risk on occupational health and safety]*. Written question, Finnish Parliament, KK 134/2001.

Tiura M (2001) *Gelatiinin kayto elintarvikkeissa. [The use of gelatin in foodstuffs]*. Written question, Finnish Parliament, KK 202/2001.

Vistbacka R (2000) *Ranskalaisen naudanlihan tuonti. [Imports of French meat]*. Written question, Finnish Parliament KK 864/2000.

Wells G et al (1987) A novel progressive spongiform encephalopathy in cattle. *Veterinary Record*, 121:419.

YLE (2001) *Pallo hallussa: Eläinperäisestä juottorehusta varoitettiin*. YLE *(Finnish Broadcasting Company)*, 16 December 2001. (www.yle.fi/pallohallussa/arkistot/t161201a.html.)

chapter 10

**Improving communication strategies
and engaging with public concerns**

Improving communication strategies and engaging with public concerns

Erik Millstone, Patrick van Zwanenberg, Martin Bauer, Carlos Dora, Elizabeth Dowler, Alizon Draper, Kerstin Dressel, Giancarlo Gasperoni, Judith Green, Meri Koivusalo, Eeva Ollila

As the previous chapters have indicated, within many jurisdictions the BSE saga has provoked changes in the ways in which risk policies are made and legitimated. New and reformed institutions are adopting new risk communication strategies, both in an attempt to diminish what is widely seen as a crisis of public trust and confidence in food regulation and also to engage with public concerns more adequately than has historically been the case. Although there has been much procedural innovation in risk communication, there is far less clarity about precisely why such innovations might be necessary or desirable and how they might best be undertaken. Drawing on the BSE case, this chapter provides a framework for thinking about which aspects of, and topics within, risk appraisal and decision-making might be subject to communication. It identifies particular forms of communication that might be appropriate for those different topics.

One key assumption informing this chapter is that risk communication cannot be and should not be reduced to public relations exercises. As argued in Chapter 9, historical risk communication strategies in the United Kingdom, Germany and Italy, in particular, were designed to persuade their citizens to accept those governments' preferred risk management decisions. The adoption of those particular strategies ultimately undermined public confidence in BSE policies and risk governance more generally.

The preceding chapters show that more sophisticated attempts simply to persuade the public of the acceptability of risk-policy decisions are neither desirable nor possible. Nor should risk communication be concerned solely with consumer preferences, equating stable levels of beef demand with broader support for BSE policies and food policy more generally. Rather, risk communication should be concerned with supporting and enhancing democratic processes and accountability, i.e. with helping to render explicit the politics of risk decision-making, and promoting democratically legitimate policy creation and decision-making.

The key interest of this chapter, therefore, is in how communication processes — be they information dissemination practices, surveillance procedures or deliberative processes — can support those objectives. It begins by drawing on the "co-evolutionary" model of policy-making discussed in Chapter 7. Within that model, a set of distinctions are described between the three sequential stages of the policy process and the types of issues or topics that typically need to be identified and resolved at each of those three stages. The purpose is to identify those issues or topics within risk decision-making that could be subject to broader forms of communication with representatives of the public and key stakeholder and public interest groups. Three sets of issues are identified: framing assumptions issues, risk assessment policy issues, and risk-cost–benefit trade-off issues.

After discussing a range of techniques that have been developed for public deliberation and communication on issues of risk, the chapter returns briefly to the empirical material on BSE discussed earlier. Finally, several issues are identified where different forms of communication and engagement might enhance the democratic acceptability and scientific robustness of policy-making.

Stages of policy-making and their inputs

Chapter 7 outlined a co-evolutionary model of the inter-action between science and policy-making. Figure 7.2 represents that model, suggesting a fairly straight-forward but useful distinction between three sequential stages of the policy-making process, termed upstream, midstream and downstream. The model can be used to focus on the different topics to be considered and the different kinds of scientific and policy inputs that are appropriate to those stages and topics.

• Upstream: dealing with framing assumptions

To recapitulate: the upstream stage of the decision-making process involves what are appropriately called framing assumptions in the scholarly literature (Jasanoff & Wynne, 1998). Sometimes implicit and often opaque, these decisions and assumptions have important implications for the scope and conduct of subsequent risk appraisal and decision-making processes. They concern, for example, the general goals, objectives and commitments of particular policy regimes. These, in turn, can influence the policies and practices that affect the potential production of risks, and the degree of commitment to possible alternative technological systems that might mitigate the risks in question. More specifically, they can also influence judgements about the type and range of risk issues and regulatory options under scientific and policy consideration by those responsible for risk assessment and management. Values do not just influence the selections made from a range of technically determined options; they influence which options are addressed in the first place.

In relation to BSE policy-making, upstream framing assumptions have been concerned with broad policy objectives. For example, are policy-makers aiming primarily to protect public health, or primarily to maintain stability in domestic and export markets for beef? Or is some form of intermediate balance between those competing objectives being sought? The ranking of such objectives has implications for whether policy might be seeking to eradicate the disease and consequent risks entirely, or just to diminish risks to levels deemed to be the lowest practically achievable at reasonable cost.

Such alternative objectives have consequences for the types of policy options and risks that will be subject to scientific and socioeconomic/political scrutiny, and the ways in which those options and risks are appraised. These derivative issues constitute a further set of important framing assumptions. For example, will the practice of recycling animal slaughterhouse wastes into the animal feed-chain itself be evaluated, or are policy options limited to different ways in which such recycling (or indeed other aspects of intensive animal production) could be rendered safer? Will the relevant risks be defined as those that might arise for people consuming beef from potentially affected herds, or will they also extend to the possible risks from consuming milk, or from potential exposure to infectivity from pharmaceutical products manufactured using bovine materials, or from occupational exposure to cattle? Which potential routes of infection will be included in analysis and subsequent policy deliberation: all possible routes or only those that are judged to be the most significant sources of exposure? Should risk assessments include exposure through products manufactured using bovine materials such as cosmetics

Improving communication

or fertilisers? More subtly, by reference to what baseline will possible risks to human health be analysed? Should they be compared to the background rate of CJD or to a rate set at zero? Or should risks be measured absolutely or relatively to the risks that already exist in other jurisdictions?

While some framing assumptions may be explicitly articulated, for example in the terms of reference of an expert advisory committee, others tend to be privately decided upon. Others still are taken for granted; they exist as part of the unspoken rational or even operational culture of regulatory institutions. What they all have in common, however, is that they are primarily policy or value considerations. Scientific considerations may help to identify and shape particular framing judgements in the light of evidence about possible risk, but such judgements are not in themselves scientific in nature. This implies that policy-makers, as opposed to expert advisers, should take explicit responsibility for articulating those assumptions, rather than pretending that they either do not exist or that they are purely scientific, even though their articulation may require dialogue with scientific experts. It also implies that policy-makers should take explicit responsibility for justifying those assumptions in democratically legitimate ways. It follows therefore that, at a minimum, information about those framing assumptions should be communicated to those both within and outside a policy regime, so that those responsible for policy-making can be held accountable for the decisions that they have made. There may also be scope for more deliberative forms of communication over the choice of framing assumptions. As Stirling (1998: 97) has argued, since

there is no uniquely rational way of framing risk issues "... public participation is as much a matter of analytical rigour as it is of political legitimacy".

• Midstream: risk assessment policy questions
The midstream stage of the co-evolutionary model consists of a scientific appraisal, conducted within the terms set by the upstream framing assumptions. Although deliberations at this stage are primarily technical in nature (that is, they are concerned with identifying the existence of risks, their probability and severity, and some of the scientific uncertainties), several evidential framing assumptions have to be invoked at this stage. Many of those evidential assumptions can in principle be codified as a risk assessment policy. Such policies refer, for example, to the procedures and processes by which expertise and advice are procured. For example, will risk assessors be expected to provide scientific advice or policy advice? If the latter, which assumptions will be used to translate their understanding of science into policy advice?

Risk assessment policy also refers to decisions about the ways in which uncertainties are handled within assessment and the extent to which identified uncertainties should be acknowledged. Do policy-makers wish advisers to adopt a precautionary approach to appraising risks, and if so, what does that imply? Risk assessment policy is complex because it often takes the form of hybrid judgements that comprise both scientific and non-scientific elements. Such hybrid judgements are often difficult to separate into their policy and scientific components. They may concern decisions about issues such as the

strategies and engaging with public concerns

types of disciplinary approaches to bring to bear on a problem, and which types of evidence are deemed relevant to any particular risk issue.

In relation to BSE policy-making, risk assessment policy has been concerned with decisions such as whether all possible uncertainties should be acknowledged, or only those that appear to be relevant to the policy options under active consideration, or only those that current research could diminish. Should best-case, worst-case, or most-likely-case risk scenarios be explicitly articulated, or a spectrum of possible scenarios? Will expert advisers be responsible for risk communication to the wider public? Other risk assessment policy decisions may concern the mix of expertise required to perform adequate and appropriate appraisal (e.g. TSE researchers, veterinarians, virologists, public health specialists, etc.). Finally, risk assessment policy might consider assumptions about whether policy options under evaluation will in practice be fully complied with, or how they might be enforced.

Many aspects of risk assessment policy are entirely non-scientific in nature. For example, should expert advisers provide a single assessment of their most likely estimates of risks, or multiple assessments of a range of risk scenarios? Such decisions, as with the upstream framing assumptions, are properly the responsibility of policy-makers and in principle could be subject to broader deliberation and communication with key stakeholder and public interest groups. Other risk assessment policy judgements, of a more hybrid nature, can also in principle be subject to broader forms of deliberation and communication. Here it is experts from the broader scientific community rather than the lay public in general who might be the key participants. Yet even in this situation, some subsections of the public may possess knowledge that is relevant to the conduct of expert appraisals.

• Downstream: trading off risks, costs and benefits

The downstream stage consists of the judgements that are necessary once expert scientific risk assessors have reached conclusions about the probability and severity of risks and the nature of any associated uncertainties. These evaluative judgements, or risk-cost–benefit trade-offs, refer to (a) the kinds of risks and levels of uncertainty that might be deemed acceptable in exchange for some presumed or evident benefits, and (b) the nature and level of costs and restrictions that would be socially acceptable in order to achieve certain kinds of reductions in risks, or even their elimination. Such trade-offs are especially difficult to make when the risks, and the possible benefits of any reduction in risk, are unknown or highly uncertain. Risk-cost–benefit trade-offs also involve decisions about the type of policy intervention appropriate for any desired level of risk reduction. Different forms of intervention may have varying consequences for the effectiveness of compliance, for example, or for the distribution of costs as between public and private actors, or for the civil liberties of those required or expected to change their behaviour.

In relation to BSE, risk-cost–benefit trade-offs have most obviously been concerned with the level of contamination in the food supply that is deemed to be socially acceptable, given the private and public costs of regulatory

Improving communication

restrictions. In some instances these judgements have also taken the form of "risk–risk" trade-offs. For example, consider decisions about what to do with an existing stock of vaccine supplies produced using potentially contaminated bovine material; such decisions would involve not only setting the possible risks against the costs of producing new stock but also the risks that vaccine uptake rates amongst the general population may diminish, even if new stocks were produced. Risk-cost–benefit trade-offs in BSE policy-making have also involved decisions about assumed compliance. For example, a decision to outlaw the use of ruminant protein in ruminant feed implies that such feed will be available and used in the feed of other farm animals. If policy-makers wish to minimize opportunities for illegal use of ruminant feed for ruminants, a more appropriate policy might be to ban the sale of ruminant feed for all farm animals.

Risk-cost–benefit trade-offs are primarily policy judgements, although they may require supporting technical, scientific and/or economic information. As such, risk-cost–benefit trade-offs should be the responsibility of democratically accountable policy-makers, not technical experts. While such policy-makers may feel that the public needs to be persuaded that risk management decisions are prudent and fair, that can only be accomplished if policy-makers understand public perceptions of prudence and fairness as they apply to the issues at stake. Communication about risk-cost–benefit trade-offs may therefore require more than a one-way explanation of why certain regulatory measures have been adopted. It also has to facilitate information in the other direction, to enable policy-makers to understand the conflicting concerns and interests of different social groups and their varying willingness to tolerate different kinds of risks in exchange for different kinds of benefits.

▾ A framework for engaging and communicating with the public

Before considering different forms of communication and public deliberation in the light of the stages and topics described above, it is useful to reflect on the various purposes or rationales for public deliberation, of which three have been identified by Fiorino (1990). These are to obtain democratic consent (which Fiorino calls the "normative rationale"), to increase legitimacy (the "instrumental rationale") and to identify relevant knowledge and values (the "substantive rationale").

• **The normative rationale** derives from the democratic principle that government ought to obtain the consent of those it governs. The right to be fully informed about, and to be able to influence, collective decision-making implies that the basis for policy decision-making (that is, the value judgements and policy decisions that shape decisions about issues such as BSE) should be made explicit and that methods for influencing the choice of such decisions and judgements should be available.

• **The instrumental rationale** for public deliberation is that opportunities to be informed about, participate in, and influence risk policy-making should increase the legitimacy of public decisions. They may also serve to reduce social conflict over risk policy issues, or at least diminish conflict over the process of decision-making, even if reasonable consensus over specific policies is not achieved. In

strategies and engaging with public concerns

addition, public deliberation processes may provide early warning of potential problems, or provide elected representatives with intelligence about the values, views and attitudes of lay publics, thus increasing the likelihood that decision-making processes will be better informed.

• **The substantive rationale** holds that knowledge and information from non-specialists (or at least those outside the small policy communities of officials and selected experts) is pertinent and indeed essential for effective decision-making. Participation by key stake holder groups in risk policy-making may, it is argued, identify aspects of risk that would otherwise be neglected, or provide key facts and information that are pertinent to technical risk assessments, for example, by providing empirical support to the numerous assumptions that are inevitably part of risk appraisal.

These three rationales can usefully be tabulated against the three stages of policy-making identified earlier, as shown below in Table 10.1.

Table 10.1. Rationales for public deliberation at different stages of the policy process

Stages in the risk policy decision-making process	Rationales for public deliberation on risk issues		
	To obtain democratic consent	To increase legitimacy	To identify relevant knowledge and values
Upstream framing assumptions (e.g. concerning overall policy objectives and options, and the scope of risk assessments)			
Midstream risk assessment policy (e.g. concerning the ways in which uncertainties are managed in appraisal)			
Downstream risk-cost–benefit trade-offs (e.g. concerning risk acceptability and the distribution of risks, costs and benefits)			

Improving communication

For any particular row in this matrix, and perhaps any particular cell, a variety of different communication and deliberation techniques or methods may be more or less applicable and more or less important. The choice of communication strategies and tactics depends in large part on the policy stage, policy issue and rationale for deliberation. Below, various kinds of methods are considered which might be suitable at each of the three policy stages when communicating with, learning about or engaging with key stakeholder groups.

• Clarifying what is at issue

At each particular stage in the policy process it is important to clarify precisely what is at issue. If, for example, policy institutions are planning to communicate with the public about upstream framing assumptions, the publication of information about policy objectives and the range of policy options under consideration may not be sufficient. Nor may it be sufficient to enter into a process of consultation about the choice, or ranking, of those published policy objectives and options. The nature of framing assumptions is such that citizens may have concerns about a risk issue that are not necessarily the concerns that policy-makers think that the public are, or should be, articulating.

In relation to BSE policy, for example, it may be that significant sections of the public have ethical reservations about the practice of recycling animal protein into animal feed, in addition to harbouring concerns that government should properly appraise the technical safety of such practices. It may also be the case that those ethical con-

cerns derive in part from beliefs about how adequately or inadequately policy institutions will, in practice, appraise and control the physical risks of recycling animal protein. Yet public policy-makers may not have placed such public concerns on their policy agenda; indeed they may not even be aware of the nature of those concerns.

Adequate and appropriate methods for communication about upstream framing assumptions may therefore need to be designed in such a way that citizens, stakeholders and specialists, as well as government, are able to define the meaning, components and boundaries of the issue in question (Burgess et al., 2002). Such methods may also need to ensure that stakeholders can articulate what they want to, or need to, know to help them arrive at an informed definition of, and judgement about, the issue in question.

• Upstream methods

Deliberative methods for addressing upstream framing assumptions include focus groups, citizens' panels and consensus conferences, all of which, if appropriately facilitated, may be used to elicit people's own definitions of what matters about particular issues. (Focus group methodologies are described in Chapters 3 and 5.)

One example of an ambitious process of public deliberation about the framing assumptions that guide risk policy-making stems from the ongoing public debate, which began in 2002 in the United Kingdom, about the possible commercialization of genetically modified crops (Agriculture and Environment Biotechnology

strategies and engaging with public concerns

Commission, 2002). The objective is to inform decision-making on this issue by assessing the publics' views on possible commercialization, and the conditions under which commercialization might or might not acceptably proceed. Normative, instrumental and substantive justifications for such an exercise are all apparent. The proposal specifically recognizes that the policy issues regarding commercialization should be framed by the public itself, prior to stimulating an informed debate about those issues.

Under the proposed process, the identification of framing issues will be sought by recruiting groups of citizens, and facilitating cross-examination by those citizen groups of representatives of external organizations and experts. In a subsequent stage, debate will be stimulated about that set of framing issues using both focus group discussions and consensus conferences. The objective will be to explore the extent of people's agreements about possible ways forward in dealing with the commercialization of genetically modified crops. The outputs of these exercises will then be used to inform ministerial decision-making. It is expected that ministers will respond to the public debate by identifying what they have learnt, and how they plan to take this into account in decision-making.

• Midstream methods

Communication and engagement regarding midstream issues and risk assessment policy could take several forms. Firstly, much of what constitutes risk assessment policy can be codified. Thus, procedures for selecting advisers, organizing and conducting their deliberations,

forms of transparency, and presentation of findings can be explicitly specified in policy documents. Many jurisdictions provide such general guidelines. For example, the British Food Standards Agency has recommended that all its expert advisory committees should conduct their business in open session. It has stipulated that unorthodox and contrary scientific views should be considered, and that advisory committees should always provide a clear audit trail showing how and why they reached their decisions, where differences of opinion had arisen, and which assumptions and uncertainties were inherent in their conclusions (FSA, 2002).

More specific policy guidance about how scientific data and evidence should be produced, selected, disclosed and interpreted for particular risk issues can sometimes be established too. Regulatory authorities in Sweden and the United States, for example, produce science policy guidelines stipulating how distinctions between sufficient and insufficient evidence of chemical carcinogenicity, for example, can be established for regulatory risk assessment purposes. The production of such guidelines could be subject to consultation and broad review within relevant scientific and policy stakeholder communities.

Risk assessment policy guidelines will not be able to stipulate generic rules for selecting, interpreting and representing evidence, partly because decisions about how to handle uncertainty, for example, are necessarily specific to each assessment. Nonetheless, the need for transparency requires that such decisions be explicit, and that responsibility for those decisions ultimately should

Improving communication

rest with policy-makers and not experts. One way to do this is to insist that scientific experts provide and publish advice based on a spectrum of possible risk scenarios, and that their deliberations are subject to (or at the very least accessible for) peer review.

Expert advisers have normally provided single, integrated interpretations of the risks in question and concluded with specific policy recommendations. Where sufficient evidence and theory are available, scientific advisers can often form relatively straightforward judgements about the magnitude of particular risks, and advise accordingly. In dealing with many risk issues, however, such empirical evidence may be equivocal or incomplete. Scientific opinion about risk and uncertainty tends to be quite diverse. In the absence of explicit and widespread knowledge of that diversity, policy-makers and other stakeholder groups tend to be unaware of the extent to which risk assessments are partial or incomplete. They may be unaware of the full scope for exercising precaution.

Conveying that diversity of scientific opinion effectively would mean that, instead of providing a single estimate of the existence and likely significance of a risk, expert advisers would present a range of alternative risk scenarios. Responsibility for deciding what constitutes an appropriate response to uncertainty would then rest with policy-makers rather than with experts. This would not only help policy-makers to exercise their risk-cost–benefit trade-offs further downstream, but policy-makers would also find it more difficult to draw a veil over their judgements concerning the risk-cost–benefit trade-offs.

Furthermore, plural advice would create a clear point of engagement for different public and professional perspectives on any given risk regulatory issue.

• Downstream methods

As far as communication and deliberative methods concerning downstream issues (i.e. risk-cost–benefit trade-offs) are concerned, an effective communication strategy, at a minimum, would require an explanation of (a) which regulatory measures are being proposed, (b) the reasons for those proposals, and (c) a consultation process about which of those proposed measures would be most acceptable, practical and enforceable. Such strategies are often routinely practised by regulatory institutions but they face two shortcomings if policy-makers responsible for risk-cost–benefit trade-offs are properly to understand the various concerns of different social groups and their willingness to tolerate different kinds of risks.

First, the range of stakeholders included in consultation is typically quite narrow. They tend to comprise firms, trade associations, and scientific and professional bodies. Consumer or environmental nongovernmental organizations may also be included in consultation processes, but such bodies may not adequately represent the views of citizens. Second, consultation processes rarely encourage or allow stakeholders and citizens to articulate measures other than those identified by policy-makers, or to allow those groups to specify what kinds of criteria that identified policy options should be assessed against, and how those various criteria should be ranked.

strategies and engaging with public concerns

Stakeholder dialogue is one method for broadening the range of social groups normally involved in consultation processes, and for encouraging identification of policy measures and the criteria by which they could be assessed. This technique covers a range of processes that bring together interested parties to deliberate and negotiate on a particular issue or set of issues.

The review of BSE controls conducted in 2000 by the British Food Standards Agency provides an example of a stakeholder dialogue process. During the review, several open meetings were organized in different locations with a wide range of stakeholders and interested members of the public. The meetings allowed for input over the terms of the review and the type, and choice, of policy measures that were to be recommended to ministers. Furthermore, draft reports of the review were published and deliberated on, prior to the production of the final review document.

▾ Lessons learnt from the BSE saga about risk communication

In the light of the generic discussion above concerning the different forms of communication and deliberation in risk decision-making, this chapter returns briefly to the historical analysis of BSE. What was learnt about how BSE risk communication was handled in the four jurisdictions? What was learnt about the extent of divergence and convergence between the beliefs and aspirations of public policy-makers as compared to European publics and the media? Can the way in which different forms of communication and engagement might lead to improved policy-making on BSE be assessed?

• Risk communication strategies

The research for this study has indicated that, in every country studied (the United Kingdom, Germany, Italy and Finland), and at several stages of the BSE saga, governments have seen public opinion as an object of policy, and as a problem that may need to be managed, rather than as a primary input to policy. As such, risk communication strategies have typically aimed at "one-way" dissemination of information to the general public. Until relatively recently, there has been little or no effort to engage in reciprocal communication activities, or even to monitor public attitudes. Surveillance of public attitudes has not been deemed necessary; information exists only in the form of a few fragments of evidence of homeopathic doses, and statistics on levels of demand for beef. Indeed, in each country, stable sales were and are interpreted as an indication that the prevailing levels of risk are acceptable.

As well as adopting unidirectional forms of communication, the information that has been disseminated in most jurisdictions has been primarily "technical" in nature. Risk communication activities did not make explicit official policy objectives, the necessity of making trade-offs between risks and benefits, or the actual trade-offs themselves. Indeed, in many cases, risk communication activities have actively sought to conceal policy objectives and the need to make risk-cost–benefit trade-offs, especially by representing science as the determining factor in the decision-making process.

Improving communication

Not only has risk communication been predominantly unidirectional and technocratic, but in some jurisdictions it has also tended to represent science as reliable and decisive. At several stages of the BSE saga, especially in the United Kingdom, official risk communication messages have suggested that public authorities had a secure scientific understanding of the putative risks of BSE and that they were zero, or virtually zero, at least within particular jurisdictions. German policy-makers never asserted full certainty with respect to the risks posed by BSE and British beef, but they did assert that German beef was perfectly safe. Italian and Finnish policy-makers insisted that BSE was a "foreign" problem and that BSE was being kept out of their jurisdictions, and that beef on sale in those countries was entirely safe.

Such strategies were not sustainable in the long run, and they have contributed significantly to what some commentators have called "a crisis of science and governance" (House of Lords, 2000; Commission of the European Communities, 2000). Claims of certainty and zero risk in some countries were misleading and backfired dramatically after evidence emerged showing that such claims had been premised on false assumptions about the science of BSE. Furthermore, in Germany and the United Kingdom, risk communication practices have constrained the ways in which policy regimes have been able to respond to new evidence, learn about the risks, and ensure that policy actors are aware of the scope for exercising precaution. Only in Finland has the official risk communication strategy appeared to be sustainable, although in a context of far fewer reported cases of BSE than in most other European countries. Notably, Finnish authorities modified their strategy of insisting that Finnish beef was safe well before a domestic case of BSE was actually discovered.

The unique approach to communication adopted in North Rhine-Westphalia seems to have been the most robust and sustainable of all the strategies examined in the study. The authorities of that *Land* acknowledged many of the scientific uncertainties, and adopted a more open rhetoric and practice than any other jurisdiction. North Rhine-Westphalia consequently initiated its programme of active BSE surveillance at the earliest possible opportunity. The adoption of that strategy appears to have been effective in maintaining public confidence in BSE policy (at least relative to other jurisdictions).

Risk communication practices in most jurisdictions have sometimes been less than frank, have concealed or misrepresented the objectives of policy, and have oversimplified and exaggerated the reliability of their knowledge and actions. This is because the authorities in those jurisdictions have been at least as concerned with reassuring consumers, and maintaining stability in agricultural markets, as they have been with protecting public health. Furthermore, all jurisdictions, at almost all stages in the evolution of their risk communication strategy, have tried to use concerns about BSE to promote the reputation of domestic beef supplies, and to diminish confidence in foreign supplies.

• Incorrect assumptions about the public
Traditionally, many policy officials and media commenta-

strategies and engaging with public concerns

tors have assumed that the public wants simple answers to simple questions, and at the same time demands zero risk and robust certainty. That assumption, given the dominant policy objective of maintaining stability in domestic beef markets, implies the delivery of uniformly reassuring narratives of the type that many jurisdictions promulgated. Yet, public policy-makers have been operating with models of the beliefs, attitudes and wants of their citizens that have had virtually no empirical support, and have often been unrealistic.

The study's focus group research (see Chapter 4) showed that the public are not in any state of panic, even though they recognize that there are unknown and uncertain risks. It is the media, not their audience, that polarize discussions into "totally safe" versus "totally dangerous". The research for this study indicates, not surprisingly, that consumers operate from somewhat more sophisticated assumptions than policy-makers and the media give them credit for.

The focus group data also indicated indifference to many non-safety issues that preoccupied policy-makers, namely the economic interests of their beef producers and food industry, departmental and ministerial reputations, or impacts on public expenditure. There was, in addition, little nationalism, although in all countries greater faith was placed in food from known and local sources. Public officials and lay publics both had framing assumptions that were wide in some areas and narrow in others, but in opposite senses.

Neither the public nor the policy-makers were aware of, or particularly interested in, each other's framing assumptions, and the media did little to bridge that gulf. As demonstrated in Chapters 8 and 9, public authorities often interpreted media coverage of BSE as if it provided a suitable proxy for some key indicators of public attitudes, beliefs and wants. In fact, as suggested in Chapter 6, media coverage was influenced as much by the risk communication strategies of the public authorities, or the editorial policy of the paper, as by the concerns of consumers and citizens. It offered a cut-down representation of the public to the policy-makers and vice versa.

• Fitting the communication strategy to the policy decision
It is not possible to say what would have happened historically if policy-making institutions had adopted different risk communication strategies and known more about public beliefs and attitudes, or if they had engaged in deliberation with the public on various issues and at various stages of BSE policy-making. Comment can, however, be made on key issues where different communication strategies might be relevant to policy decision-making in the future.

One historical and ongoing set of policy decisions that might usefully be subject to deliberative forms of communication concerns the choice of overall regulatory strategy in relation to BSE. The policy choices involved are fundamental: should the current strategy be to eradicate the BSE agent from European beef and European cattle or only to diminish the levels of infectivity in food and animals? If the former, then how rapidly and at what

Improving communication

cost should eradication be pursued? If the latter, then what level of infectivity is tolerable, given all the uncertainties about the effects of different regulatory instruments on the level of infectivity, and the risks associated with those levels of infectivity?

Such strategic decisions, both at the European and Member State level, have been and continue to be taken with almost no dissemination of information, let alone deliberation, as to how those decisions have been taken, or indeed what precisely the decisions have been. To the extent that regulatory strategy has taken public attitudes into account, they have only been understood by policy-makers in terms of aggregate levels of demand for beef (i.e. the public as consumers, rather than as citizens, as discussed in Chapter 3). Responsibility for taking strategic decisions about BSE belongs with ministers, but the resulting strategies might be more socially robust if (a) ministers were transparently accountable for their decisions, and (b) if those decisions were informed by intelligence about what different fractions of the public and key stakeholders considered to be a reasonable and fair distribution of risks, costs and benefits.

That lack of clarity and communication about overall BSE policy objectives has been reflected in several subsidiary issues. For example, one major source of recent tension has concerned the European Commission's decision in 1999 (on the basis of advice from its scientific experts) to lift the export ban on British beef and the French Government's decision (on the basis of its own body of scientific advisers) not to accept that decision. That dispute

has been complex, but one important reason for the dispute is that the two jurisdictions were asking slightly different questions, because they framed the issue in slightly different ways. Both jurisdictions agreed that exported British beef in 1999 could not be assumed to be pathogen-free. However, the EC assessed the risks of British beef relative to the risks present in other European jurisdictions, and concluded that they were broadly similar, whereas the French authorities assessed the absolute risks posed by British beef and concluded that they were not negligible.

On this issue, communication and deliberation about the appropriate choice of baseline against which to assess the risks posed by BSE might have helped, not only to avoid the dispute, but to provide some empirical check on whether the primary objective of EU policy on BSE should be to maintain a fair open market, or to eradicate the BSE agent from British (and other jurisdictions') beef herds.

Deliberative forms of communication about BSE policy might be considered to be relevant tools for some aspects of policy-making, but there are many other aspects of policy where deliberation could be unnecessary. In so far as the scope and objectives of policy have been explicitly defined and legitimated, much of the subsequent detail of policy could be formulated without necessarily engaging lay citizens in detailed deliberative processes. What may then be sufficient, however, is adequate dissemination of information on how and why particular detailed policies have been selected. That would require transparency, as for example required under the provisions of freedom of information legislation, and pro-

strategies and engaging with public concerns

cedural rules, such as those that oblige expert committees to provide a clear audit trail showing how and why they reached their decisions, where differences of opinion had arisen, and which assumptions and uncertainties were inherent in their conclusions. Risk communication in this sense is not always deliberative but it would sometimes involve dissemination of information about decisions, and the rationale for decisions, in ways that would make it harder, politically and scientifically, for public bodies to claim that the objective of public policy was to ensure adequate food safety whilst in practice acting to promote a different set of objectives.

▾ Methods to bring public opinion into policy-making

The research described in Chapters 4–6 (as well as the theoretical discussion in Chapter 3) provides some useful, if partial, lessons regarding the use of specific methods — focus groups, sample surveys and content analysis of mass media — for understanding and engaging public opinion in policy-making. Each of these methods can be useful at various stages and to meet different rationales in the proposed framework, sometimes alone and sometimes in concert with other methods. It is worth repeating, however, the point made in Chapter 6 that "public opinion is complex and ongoing — it is a process in motion". Although these methods can contribute to understanding public opinion, none can be taken as a "true index" of public opinion.

• Focus group discussions

As discussed in Chapter 4, focus group discussions were effective at accessing people's framing assumptions regarding food safety/risk and how these are formed in social contexts. They illustrated that the "deficit model" of public understanding of risk is not only ineffective but erroneous; the data show that people in all countries had quite sophisticated approaches to risk assessment, including calculations of relative risk.

In terms of risk communication strategies and practices, it is likely that focus groups can provide useful information about how to frame information that needs to be communicated (the upstream stage/instrumental rationale in the co-evolutionary model). In addition, by identifying who is trusted, focus group discussions may also provide useful insights into what parts of society outside official institutions might be effective conduits of risk communication information.

• Surveys of public opinion

As discussed in Chapter 5, public authorities have tended to privilege "one-way" dissemination of information and have not felt particularly compelled to monitor public attitudes. Nonetheless, secondary analysis of sample surveys identified several interesting and potentially useful inputs for risk policy-makers and communications professionals. Although there was no clear consensus regarding the potential content of communication policies (e.g. factors affecting the safety of food products), there were other less equivocal findings pertaining to communication methods, and in particular to sources of information. For example, as regards food safety, consumer organizations were far more trusted than other

Improving communication

sources; teachers, lecturers, and scientists were also deemed to be truthful; meat retailers, too, were considered to be trustworthy sources of information. Moreover, in the realm of government actors, local authorities were perceived by the public as being a more effective guarantor of consumer safety than national or European authorities.

More detailed analysis of survey data at a subsample level could contribute to identifying other important differences, e.g. regarding a specific public's (defined by nationality, social class, media habits, etc.) sensitivity to selected communication contents or means. However, besides their many methodological drawbacks, it should be remembered that the execution of thorough surveys concerning a specific, timely topic requires resources that many policy-makers may not be willing to invest (except in especially critical situations).

• Media analysis

As noted in Chapter 6, content analysis of how the media covered the BSE issue since the early 1980s in the four countries provided useful findings about both the salience and framing of media coverage. Since mass media both mirror public perceptions and contribute to forming them, systematic analysis that monitors these two functions using both quantitative and qualitative methods could aid policy-makers in a number of ways. For example, systematic coding of press materials can provide policy-makers with an index of trust in their activities, or a clearer understanding of how an issue is shaping in the press, in particular by alerting them to

changes in framing and thematic focus. It can also contribute to policy-making if used as a regular input to health intelligence systems, along with information on risks and diseases.

• Potential utility of deliberative and participatory methods

Over recent years there has been much interest in participatory methods and their potential to engage members of the public in dialogue about a range of policy issues, ranging from city planning and health service delivery to food access at the local level. The term "participatory" covers a wide range of tools and techniques. These include visualization and ranking techniques, but are all based on qualitative research methodology. Other new methods are the techniques of deliberative and dialogue methodology, such as deliberative polling. These also are an enhancement of basic qualitative group discussion methods, but are based upon the recognition that lay understanding of complex policy issues is often limited and that it is therefore necessary to provide people with information on these issues before they can deliberate upon them in an informed manner. They also differ in that they are intended not just to extract information from people, but to be interactive and to engage people in dialogue in and about the decision-making processes that affect them.

These participatory and deliberative methods offer much potential, but none has as yet been formally evaluated. Their relevance and efficacy in achieving public involvement, particularly in relation to policy development,

strategies and engaging with public concerns

remain unknown at present (Rifkin et al., 2000). Their ability to access socially hard-to-reach groups, such as ethnic minorities and those on a low income, is also uncertain. Current practice shows that many challenges remain regarding their use in a European context (Draper & Hawdon, 2000).

▾ A research agenda

The importance of having institutional mechanisms where the lessons from this study can be applied cannot be overemphasized. If policy-makers have to think about whether to engage stakeholders and incorporate public perceptions of risk every time an important decision has to be made, the study findings will be a long way from being put into practice. This study suggests that citizens feel health risks and food safety should be looked after by the relevant authorities as a matter of routine, so that their own "rules of thumb" can be applied with some degree of security. They do not wish their opinion sought about every decision that needs to be made. It is for these practical reasons that a research agenda on how to incorporate perceptions of risk into everyday policy-making should give special attention to the testing of innovative arrangements for their institutionalization, and to evaluating their cost and effectiveness.

The co-evolutionary model proposed at the beginning of this chapter could be tested under a number of circumstances. This could include studies evaluating how public perceptions are taken up in policy-making and comparing different methods for achieving this. Factors to be explored as part of the research might include the stage

in policy-making where public perceptions were taken in, the methods used to incorporate perceptions, and the framework assumptions of those commissioning and implementing policies and communication strategies.

Other modifications of existing health information systems could also be tested, particularly new arrangements for gathering intelligence on perceptions of risk and engaging public opinions into policy-making. Such arrangements might include the introduction of awareness/training sessions for staff about the public's and stakeholders' views (and how to access them), the hiring of social science staff into those systems, or the creation of a new type of risk communicator who has skills in gathering intelligence about people's perceptions and engaging them in policy processes. This could conceivably be a function separated from the more usual communication skills, which focus on informing in plain language what science says about risks and interfacing with the media. The inclusion in such systems of indicators of symbolic representation of stakeholder interests (see Chapter 6) could be evaluated, since this study has shown this to be feasible.

Beyond the topics explored in this study, research could also usefully be done on the experience being gained with attempts to institutionalize public participation in decision-making on environmental and health matters. One example is the European Commission directives on Environmental Impact Assessment for projects and Strategic Environmental Assessment for policies, plans and programmes. These formally require the engage-

Improving communication

ment of public opinion in the decisions subject to those assessments (European Commission, undated). Another potential subject for research is the implementation of the international Convention on Access to Information, Public Participation in Decision-making and Access to Justice in Environmental Matters, which entered into force in 2001 (United Nations Economic Commission for Europe, undated).

The assessment of potentially controversial decisions could also form the subject of research aimed at examining and comparing ways of incorporating perceptions of risk into decision-making. Research topics might usefully include issues subject to discretionary decision at the national or subregional level: examples include the implementation of the so-called "second pillar" of the Common Agricultural Policy (CAP)[1] or the assessment of impacts of agricultural science and technology (including genetically modified organisms, or novel foods) on food and nutrition.

▾ Conclusion

Effective risk communication is not about just providing reassurance, as all the jurisdictions in this study have attempted to do. That strategy has been highly problematic. Effective risk communication is not about just reciting regulatory measures either, even if the true basis upon which they have been adopted is made explicit. It is unlikely that it would be achieved solely by better surveillance of public opinion whether through media analyses, surveys or questionnaires, or any other research methodologies. Whilst those tactics would constitute a significant improvement on historical practice, on their own they will not solve the underlying problems of science and governance.

The challenge for effective risk communication is to find other ways in which public concerns can provide input into policy-making, rather than remaining merely an object of policy-making. Public engagement needs to be focused on policy objectives arising from issues such as BSE, on what the strategy to meet those objectives should be, and on how well the ostensible objectives are being met. The new orientation towards dialogue (i.e. effective two-way communication) involves listening to the public, taking ethics seriously, dealing with a range of knowledge, and engaging with democratic citizenship — not just consumerism and choice and information at the point of sale.

The study team hopes that this book makes a contribution to achieving such objectives.

---

[1] Rural development is the so-called "second pillar" of the CAP, with a search for a comprehensive and consistent rural development policy being a priority for Europe. See "Agenda 2000: Reform of the common agricultural policy (CAP)" at http://europa.eu.int/scadplus/leg/en/lvb/l60002.htm.

strategies and engaging with public concerns

References

Agriculture and Environment Biotechnology Commission (2002) *A debate about the issue of possible commercialisation of GM crops in the UK*, draft advice to Government. AEBC/02/06. (http://www.aebc.gov.uk/aebc/about/papers/aebc0206.htm.)

Burgess J et al. (2002) *Some observations and proposals on the 2002–2003 public dialogue on possible commercialization of GM crops in the UK*, for the Public Debate Steering Board meeting, 7 November.

Commission of the European Communities (2000) *Science, society and the citizen in Europe*, SEC, 1973. Brussels, Commission of the European Communities.

Draper A, Hawdon D, eds (2000) *Improving health through community participation: from concepts to commitment*. Proceedings of the Health Education Authority Workshop, 9–10 December 1998. London, The Health Development Agency.

European Commission (undated). *Environmental assessment*. (http://europa.eu.int/comm/environment/eia/home.htm.)

Fiorino DJ (1990) Citizen participation and environmental risk: A survey of institutional mechanisms. *Science, Technology and Human Values*, 15:226–243.

FSA (2002) *Report on the review of scientific committees*, 15 April. (http://www.food.gov.uk/multimedia/pdfs/fsa02_03_04rep.pdf.)

House of Lords (2000) Select Committee on Science and Technology, Third Report, HL Paper 38. *Science and society*. London, Her Majesty's Stationery Office.

Jasanoff S, Wynne B (1998) Science and decision-making. In: Rayner S, Malone EL, eds. *Human choices and climate change: Vol. 1. The societal framework*. Columbus, OH, Battelle Press.

Rifkin SB, Lewando-Hundt G, Draper A (2000) *Participatory approaches in health promotion and health planning: a review*. London, The Health Development Agency.

Stirling A (1998) Risk at a turning point? *Journal of Risk Research*, 1:97.

United Nations Economic Commission for Europe (undated). *Convention on Access to Information, Public Participation in Decision-making and Access to Justice in Environmental Matters*. (http://www.unece.org/env/pp/treatytext.htm.)

Printed in May 2006
by Stabilimenti Tipografici Carlo Colombo S.p.A. - Rome